T0259788

Overcoming AIDS

Lessons Learned from Uganda

a volume in
Research in Global Child Advocacy

Series Editors:
Ilene R. Berson and Michael J. Berson
University of South Florida

Research in Global Child Advocacy

Ilene R. Berson and Michael J. Berson, Series Editors

Childhood in South Asia:
A Critical Look at Issues, Policiesand Programs (2004)
edited by Jyotsna Pattnaik

Advocating for Children and Families in an Emerging Democracy:
The Post Soviet Experience in Lithuania (2003)
edited by Judy W. Kugelmass and Dennis J. Ritchie

Cross Cultural Perspectives in Child Advocacy (2001)
edited by Ilene R. Berson, Michael J. Berson, and Bárbara C. Cruz

Overcoming AIDS

Lessons Learned from Uganda

edited by

Donald E. Morisky
University of California, Los Angeles

W. James Jacob
University of California, Los Angeles

Yusuf K. Nsubuga
Uganda Ministry of Education and Sports

and

Steven J. Hite
Brigham Young University

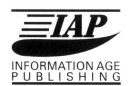

INFORMATION AGE
PUBLISHING

Greenwich, Connecticut • www.infoagepub.com

Library of Congress Cataloging-in-Publication Data

Overcoming AIDS : lessons learned from Uganda / edited by Donald E. Morisky
... [et al.].
   p. cm. -- (Research in global child advocacy)
 Includes bibliographical references and index.
 ISBN 1-59311-471-0 (pbk.) -- ISBN 1-59311-472-9 (hardcover)
 1. AIDS (Disease) in children--Uganda--Prevention. 2. AIDS (Disease) in
adolescence--Uganda--Prevention. 3. AIDS (Disease)--Study and
teaching--Uganda. I. Morisky, Donald E. II. Series: Research in global
child advocacy (Unnumbered)
 [DNLM: 1. HIV Infections--prevention & control--Uganda. 2. Acquired
Immunodeficiency Syndrome--prevention & control--Uganda. 3. Health
Education--methods--Uganda. 4. Child--Uganda. 5. Adolescent--Uganda. WC
503.6 O92 2006]
 RJ387.A25O94 2006
 362.196'97920096761--dc22

                           2006002394

ISBN 13: 978-1-59311-471-8 (pbk.)
        978-1-59311-472-5 (hardcover)
ISBN 10: 1-59311-471-0 (pbk.)
        1-59311-472-9 (hardcover)

Printed in the United States of America

CONTENTS

ACKNOWLEDGMENTS

As the product of several years of collaboration among researchers, practitioners, policy makers, and educators in Uganda, the editors wish to extend thanks to each of the participating organizations and their contributing authors. Appreciation is also extended to Michael and Ilene Berson, who helped encourage us to produce this work.

This book is dedicated to the orphans and street children in Sub-Saharan Africa, who have suffered much from the HIV/AIDS epidemic. It is our hope that this book will help disseminate best practices for overcoming AIDS through a series of case study analyses of organizational and policy lessons learned in Uganda.

PREFACE

The negative impact of HIV/AIDS has been felt world wide, particularly at the family level. Uganda has not been an exception. The AIDS pandemic has in an appalling way affected the lives of youth and children. A number of children have been born with HIV infection over the years. Uganda has an estimated 2 million children orphaned by death of one or both parents, about half of these as a result of HIV and AIDS.

The consequences of HIV/AIDS have been evident in a number of spheres including the disturbing rates of infection among young people. The disease has limited infected and affected individual's ability to enjoy their rights to education, health, enough food, security, and a meaningful life generally within their families and others.

Uganda's multisectoral response is inclusive of young people (children and youth) and prioritizes interventions targeted to children and youth as well as enhancing the capacity of young people generally in the fight against HIV/AIDS. Prevention programs for this category have therefore involved young people themselves in identifying age appropriate messages and engaging in advocacy for behavior change among their peers.

This book highlights a number of lessons drawn over the years in Uganda. The lessons learnt are considered at two critical levels: prevention and mitigation of HIV/AIDS. In the former, lessons related to social and behavioral determinants of HIV among youth, the role of the media in prevention education, capacity enhancement of teachers to provide prevention messages and support in school, the role of religion and family in educating young people, and poverty alleviation are examples of focal areas of discussion.

On the other hand, lessons related to fighting stigma and discrimination, the role played by The AIDS Support Organisation (TASO), equipping youth with prevention and treatment strategies, as well as tackling poverty and the growing problem orphan question are elaborately discussed in this book.

This book will be useful for all actors involved in responding to HIV/AIDS among children, youth, and adults, particularly in addressing the many challenges faced in prevention and mitigation interventions for and by young people globally. The content will also largely benefit policy makers, implementers, and all those directly interfacing with affected and infected youth and children as well as their families.

For the majority of stakeholders, this book should enhance awareness of the needed response for the most vulnerable population group. The lessons learnt should inspire all of us to triple our efforts in the struggle against AIDS, curbing further spread of the disease and mitigating its negative inpact.

Dr. David Kihumuro Apuuli
Director General,
Uganda AIDS Commission

FOREWORD

Overcoming AIDS epitomizes best practices by government, nongovernment, and faith-based organizations in Uganda, in addressing the HIV/AIDS epidemic.

Very few texts offer the breadth of this edited volume. This book is multisectoral in scope in that experts from the Ministry of Education and Sports; Ministry of Health; and Ministry of Gender, Labour and Social Developement have all contributed to this volume. The book also brings together a unique group of contributors who address the Uganda case from both local and international perspectives.

Issues of paramount interest in overcoming the AIDS epidemic are addressed throughtout the text, which include: prevention, HIV/AIDS stigma, integration of HIV/AIDS education into the formal curriculum, and how to reach the masses through formal and informal education efforts. An underlying theme interwoven throughout the book is the continued emphasis on the need for formal and nonformal education in the struggle to fight Africa's worst development crisis. Education is one of the essential ingredients to a successful prevention, treatment, and mitigation strategy in the fight against HIV/AIDS.

Chapters in this volume offer first-hand examples of how to address and overcome the HIV/AIDS epidemic. Although the book focuses on children and youth, the authors also address adult-oriented programs. Papers by Professor Lutalo-Bosa and Rosemary Nabadda of Kyambogo University, Reverand Noll and Jeremy Liebowitz, and ProLiteracy's work address these issues in both formal and nonformal educational settings.

The book builds on the authors' background and vast experiences in implementing HIV/AIDS programs and research. The authors highlight in their papers an understanding of both processes and action in a variety of settings that characterize the diversity of factors responsible for establishing a model HIV/AIDS prevention program. It meets a long standing need. I am confident that it will become a standard text for those involved with HIV/AIDS programs and research for many years to come.

I highly recommend the book to policy makers, educators, researchers, and practitioners in the field of prevention and management of the HIV/AIDS pandemic in society.

Geraldine Namirembe Bitamazire, (MP)
Minister of Education and Sports,
Kampala, Uganda

SERIES EDITORS' INTRODUCTION

As a result of the AIDS epidemic, many nations around the world have faced the demands of caring for a particularly vulnerable population of children, the orphans of parents who have died of AIDS or whose caregivers are terminally ill from the disease. *Overcoming AIDS: Lessons Learned from Uganda* offers an in-depth exploration of this global issue and provides a broad focus on evolving a constructive response to the HIV/AIDS epidemic.

This collaborative resource is the fourth in the *Research in Global Child Advocacy* book series, and it offers readers a glimpse into the experience of children from the perspective of researchers and professionals who diligently work toward crafting a framework for action that is integrated across disciplines. Despite the enormity and intensity of the problem, chapter authors share a commitment to advocate for a better world in which social and economic disparities do not preclude children from experiencing a future that is bright with potential opportunities and hope.

We would like to acknowledge and thank the book editors, Donald E. Morisky, W. James Jacob, Yusuf K. Nsubuga, and Steven J. Hite, for their leadership and dedication in fostering a dialogue about child advocacy and the AIDS epidemic. We also are appreciative of the contributions of Kenneth Carano, a doctoral student at the University of South Florida, who assisted in the editing and revision of the book. George Johnson, our publisher, has provided ongoing support and guidance to this project, and our colleagues from the American Educational Research Association

Special Interest Group on Research in Global Child Advocacy have offered innovative insights to direct the focus of the book series over time. This book provides a beacon to guide child advocates in their struggles to achieve successful outcomes for current generations while honoring the children and families who exhibit courage, resiliency, and an enduring vitality in the face of adversity.

Michael J. Berson
Ilene R. Berson
University of South Florida
Research in Global Child Advocacy Special Interest Group of the
American Educational Research Association

LIST OF ACRONYMS

ABC	Abstinence, Be Faithful, Condoms/Condomize
ACET-AIDS	Care Education and Training
ACP	AIDS Control Programme
ACYC	AIDS Challenge Youth Clubs
ADAA	African Development Aid Association (Ethiopia)
AFSRH	Adolescent-Friendly Sexual and Reproductive Health
AIC-AIDS	AIDS Information Centre
AIDS	Acquired Immunodeficiency Syndrome
ALOZ	Adult Literacy Organization of Zimbabwe (Zimbabwe)
AMREF	African Medical and Research Foundation
ANC	Antenatal Care
ARH	Adolescent Reproductive Health
ART	Antiretroviral Therapy
ARVs	Anti-retrovirals
ASRH	Adolescent Sexual and Reproductive Health
AYA	African Youth Alliance
BCC	Behavior Change Communication
BCI	Behavioral Changes for Interventions
BECCAD	Basic Education, Child Care and Protection, and Adolescent Development
BCP	Behaviour Change Programme
CCATH	Child-Centered Approaches to HIV/AIDS
CEEWA	Council for Economic Empowerment of Women in Africa
CHUSA	Church of Uganda Human Services Agency
COU	Constitution of Uganda
CSC	Consortium for Street Children

EFA	Education for All
FOCA	Friends of Children Association
GIPA	Greater Involvement of People with HIV/AIDS
GOU	Government of Uganda
GYDA	Gulu Youth Development Agency
HEN	Health Education Network
HIV	Human Immunodeficiency Virus
IEC	Information, Education, and Communication
IMAU	Islamic Medical Association of Uganda
ITEK	Institute of Teacher Education Kyambogo (Uganda)
KALA	Kenya Adult Learners Association (Kenya)
LECUSDE	Lesotho Ecumenical Society for Development (Lesotho)
LAI	Literacy and Action International (Ghana)
MAMA	Women's NGO (Ethiopia)
MECUDA	Meta Cultural and Development Association (Cameroon)
MGLSD	Ministry of Gender, Labour, and Social Development (Uganda)
MOES	Ministry of Education and Sports (Uganda)
MOH	Ministry of Health (Uganda)
MRC	Medical Research Council
NACOSA	National AIDS Convention of South Africa
NCDC	National Curriculum Development Centre
NGO	Nongovernmental Organization
OVC	Orphans and Vulnerable Children
PE	Peer Educators
PEARL	Programme for Enhancing Adolescent Reproductive Life
PHC	Primary Health Care
PIASCY	Presidential Initiative on AIDS Strategy for Communication to the Youth
PLI	Philly Lutaya Initiative
PTC	Primary Teachers College
PWA	People living with HIV/AIDS
RCWDA	Rift Valley Children and Women's Development Association (Ethiopia)
RH	Reproductive Health
SHEP	School Health Education Project
SIECUS	Sexuality Information and Education Council of the United States
SPW	Students Partnership Worldwide (United Kingdom)
SRH	Sexual Reproductive Health
SSA	Sub-Saharan Africa
STD	Sexually Transmitted Diseases
STF	Straight Talk Foundation
SYFA	Safeguarding Youth from AIDS
TASO	The AIDS Support Organisation
UAC	Uganda AIDS Commission
UCLA	University of California, Los Angeles
UHS	Uganda Demographic Health Survey
UN	United Nations

UMSC	Uganda Muslim Supreme Council
UNAIDS	Joint United Nations Programme on HIV/AIDS
UNCRC	United Nations Convention on the Rights of the Child
UNDP	United Nations Development Programme
UNESCO	United Nations Educational, Scientific, and Cultural Organization
UNFPA	United Nations Population Fund
UNICEF	United Nations Children's Fund
UPE	Universal Primary Education
UPK	Uganda Polytechnic Kyambogo
USAID	United States Agency for International Development
UYAAS	Uganda Youth Anti-AIDS Association
VCT	Voluntary Counseling and Testing
WFP	World Food Programme
YCS	Uganda Young Christian Students
YWCA	Young Women's Christian Association (Uganda)

CHAPTER 1

INTRODUCTION

**Donald E. Morisky, W. James Jacob,
Yusuf K. Nsubuga, and Steven J. Hite**

Uganda is a country in Sub-Saharan Africa, bounded in the north by Sudan, in the east by Kenya, in the south by Tanzania and Rwanda, and in the west by the Democratic Republic of Congo. Uganda witnessed its first case of AIDS more than 2 decades ago in 1982 at Kasensero, a fishing village along the Lake Victoria shores in Rakai District. The disease of AIDS was then given the local name of *Slim*, reflecting the loss of body weight that characterized the patients. Since this first case in 1982, the country has gone through a tremendous transformation in responding to the AIDS epidemic. There are numerous factors that have contributed to the remarkable success of reducing the prevalence of AIDS from over 30% to its present rate of approximately 7%. The adult HIV prevalence rate is currently 4.1%, representing an eight-fold reduction since the mid-1980s. Over the past decade, HIV infection rates have fallen dramatically, making Uganda one of the very few unequivocal success stories. The most marked decline in HIV prevalence has been among 15-25 year-olds. A strong national government, heavy involvement of nongovernmental organizations, and support from international donors such as the European Union and UNAIDS are some of the reasons for this tremendous success (Okware, Opio, Musinguzi, & Waibale, 2001). In addition, Uganda has become a model for other Sub-Saharan nations currently

Overcoming AIDS: Lesson Learned from Uganda, 1–11
Copyright © 2006 by Information Age Publishing
All rights of reproduction in any form reserved.

addressing the epidemic that has spread across the African continent and now threatens continents throughout the world, particularly Asia (Parkhurst & Lush, 2004). The chapters presented in this book describe and discuss the specifics of the major factors contributing to the successful decline of HIV/AIDS in Uganda.

Overcoming AIDS: Lessons Learned from Uganda consists of 13 well-conceptualized chapters identifying how Ugandan youths have overcome HIV/AIDS in this nation and set a standard for success. The contributors bring to their chapters an understanding of both process and action in a variety of settings that characterize the diversity of factors responsible for establishing a model HIV/AIDS prevention program.

The book is organized into four major sections. Part I provides a historical overview of multisectoral educational initiatives that deal with HIV/AIDS and the destructive influence stigma and discrimination has in facilitating the epidemic. Part II addresses HIV/AIDS educational programs in the formal education sector, including the Ministry of Education and Sports (MOES) and teacher preparation at the Institute of Teacher Education at Kyambogo (ITEK). Part III identifies informal youth and child HIV/AIDS educational programs including nongovernmental agencies such as The AIDS Support Organisation (TASO), ProLiteracy Worldwide, the Ugandan Youth Anti-AIDS Association (UYAAS), the role of faith-based organizations, mass media activities conducted through the Straight Talk Foundation, and psychosocial and behavioral assessments being conducted by the Institute of Social Research at Makerere University and Brigham Young University. Part IV concentrates on how the government is dealing with the growing problem of AIDS orphans and street children.

Chapter 2, "A Multisectoral Strategy for Overcoming AIDS" by Yusuf K. Nsubuga and W. James Jacob, provides a historical overview of HIV/AIDS education programs in Uganda since the mid-1980s. Where HIV and AIDS have traditionally been viewed as primarily a health-related issue, this chapter charts the paradigmatic shift toward a multisectoral response to the epidemic. Much of the multisectoral educational efforts began as extracurricular schemes such as encouraging the formation of school anti-AIDS clubs, school-wide assemblies discussing HIV/AIDS issues, and promotion of the ABC strategy for prevention and mitigation of the epidemic. Only in recent years has the government required that HIV/AIDS be taught in the formal school curriculum. Unlike its East African neighbors, who suffer similar epidemic levels of HIV infection, Uganda received top-level government support once knowledge of the epidemic's severity became known. This support has trickled down to every major governmental sector, including health and education. While the disease continues to pester the Ugandan populous, it is clear that a multisectoral strategy is necessary to overcome the disease.

Yusuf K. Nsubuga and W. James Jacob discuss a major barrier responsible for the lack of progress in Uganda's HIV/AIDS prevention efforts in chapter 3 titled "Fighting Stigma and Discrimination as a Strategy for HIV/AIDS Prevention and Control." The authors begin with an overview of AIDS stigma and how it has permeated societies worldwide and Uganda in particular. Relevant scenarios are presented to provide a glimpse of the difficulties being experiences by different sectors of society and illustrate that inadequate knowledge and information are the culprits responsible for its perpetuity. The authors identify the need for promotion of antidiscrimination laws at community, national, and international levels. They recommend that the HIV/AIDS resolutions passed by the United Nations Human Rights Commission should be disseminated more effectively to heighten awareness and influence behavioral change among the general public.

Chapter 3 also discusses how the government of Uganda is trying to overcome stigma and discrimination through promotion of voluntary counseling, testing, and positive living. The authors describe how stigma and discrimination have forced many HIV positive individuals to go underground and not identify themselves as HIV positive, for fear of blame, shame, and abuse. The government of Uganda has responded proactively to stigma and discrimination by replacing "shame with solidarity and fear with hope." Uganda's unwritten policy of openness has helped to reduce the infection rate to below 5%. It is noted that the government's openness to the epidemic coupled with a high level of political commitment has been a major force in fighting stigma and discrimination.

Evaluating the progress of existing education programs is the focus of chapter 4, written by W. James Jacob, Donald E. Morisky, Steven J. Hite, and Yusuf K. Nsubuga. The chapter identifies key government activities instrumental in reducing both the prevalence and incidence of HIV/AIDS in Uganda. The authors ask the questions, "What is Uganda doing right that so many of its African neighbors are not? What role does education play in reversing the trends of the epidemic? What role will education continue to play in the establishment of a comprehensive program to overcome the epidemic? How can education help with Uganda's orphaned children crisis? The authors identify innovative approaches as to ways the government of Uganda is integrating HIV/AIDS prevention into the secondary school curricula and how these approaches will serve to overcome the dilemma of teacher reluctance to introduce HIV/AIDS prevention curriculum due to the fact that students are not formally examined on this subject matter. The authors further present results of a recently conducted national study to examine the knowledge, attitudes, and practices of secondary students, their teachers and administration officials. Results provide important information on the content areas in HIV/AIDS prevention education which need to be integrated into the secondary school curriculum. Furthermore, insights are provided as to the relative effects of focus group discussions and peer led discussion sessions on HIV/AIDS knowledge, beliefs, and attitudes.

Chapter 5, titled "Preparing a Generation of Teachers for Educating Youth in Uganda" by Rosemary Nabadda and Albert James Lutalo-Bosa, discusses the magnitude of the task required for preparing a generation of teachers in Uganda for educating the youth in overcoming HIV/AIDS. The authors examine the impact of HIV/AIDS on education, responses by the education sector, and challenges in training teachers in the era of HIV/AIDS. The chapter focuses its attention on the effect of HIV/AIDS on staff and students, teacher training curriculum, challenges of training teachers in the era of AIDS and lastly the constraints of training an AIDS competent teacher in Uganda. A key question is the level of responsibility taken by the Ministry of Education and Sports (MOES) in launching the first prevention efforts in 1986, which consisted of media messages and an introduction of HIV/AIDS into the primary school curriculum. In cooperation with the National Curriculum Development Centre, the MOES was able to design, implement, and evaluate the content areas of an HIV/AIDS prevention curriculum at all levels of education. Building competencies and skills of the teachers in Uganda was also a major accomplishment. Kyambogo University in Kampala served as the nexus of innovative teacher training in the country. The authors go on to describe how Kyambogo University responded to the training challenge through several different approaches, including the child-centered approach and AIDS strategies for youth communication.

Several concerns are raised in this chapter with respect to the lack of training and skills for social workers and guidance counselors. It is also noted that teachers need to go beyond the traditional role of instructor and become personal change agents; however it is felt that current teacher training efforts do not adequately prepare teachers for this role.

Chapter 6, "Social and Behavioral Determinants of HIV Education Programs Among Ugandan Youth" by Delius Asimwe and Richard Kibombo from the Institute of Social Research, Makerere University, introduces the third section of this book on nonformal HIV/AIDS education programs in Uganda. The chapter looks at a brief overview of government, faith-based, and local and international programs involved in the prevention effort. Recognizing that HIV's primary transmission is through sexual intercourse, the authors argue for a sexual revolution in societal norms and sexual behaviors. Many of these efforts are only briefly introduced in this chapter; a more comprehensive discussion is found in chapters 7-12, which give several organizational overviews of successful NGOs and FBOs in Uganda.

Perhaps no organization has had a more positive impact on youth and families than The AIDS Support Organisation (TASO) as described in chapter 7. In this chapter, Alex Coutinho, Robert Ochai, Alex Mugume, Lynda Kavuma, and John M. Collins present an organizational overview of TASO and how it has become the preeminent national indigenous not-for-profit nongovernmental organization (NGO) in Uganda. With specific reference to the youth, TASO has been able to initiate a number of very successful interventions targeted to the youth, all centered around the provision of a supportive environment which encourages attendance at school, vocational training, and skills, and the development of the AIDS Challenge Youth Clubs. These youth clubs have been found to have a predominant effect on preventing the further spread of HIV among adolescents. The authors conclude their chapter by providing specific recommendations that address the need for maintaining the high commitment of political leadership for AIDS education and prevention throughout the country.

Lynn R. Curtis is the author of chapter 8, "Equipping Youth With Prevention and Treatment Strategies: Literacy and HIV Initiatives in Uganda and Five Other African Nations." This chapter highlights many of the innovative HIV/AIDS prevention educational initiatives implemented through much of Sub-Saharan Africa generally and Uganda specifically. The ProLiteracy philosophy is based on the premise that individuals learn new concepts through a shared, participatory process, involving focus group discussion, individual assessments, role playing, and interactive session, which in turn raises levels of awareness, knowledge, and skills related to risk reduction. Educational materials are developed and produced which are culturally sensitive and linguistically appropriate to the culture, values, and educational level of the population. ProLiteracy has initiated a program called *Literacy Solutions* that includes a series of English-language, template manuals on learning and action themes that have proven to be extremely popular in the 56 countries that have implemented this program. The training manuals are innovative in the sense that they provide a holistic instructional approach in which the experiences, preferences, and priorities of individuals are tailored to their specific needs. The manuals present a broad perspective of the various social and behavioral determinants of HIV/AIDS, including themes addressing health, economic self-reliance, and human rights. This approach allows the learner to design and implement action plans specific to the developmental needs of their community. The three application areas of this curriculum are the school, community, and church component and all applications have been found to influence significantly the participants' knowledge, awareness, and behavioral intent, leading to reductions in HIV/AIDS risk behaviors. The author presents a well-conceptualized evaluation overview, highlighting specific observable outcomes associated with this program as well as identifying future challenges that remain.

Chapter 9, authored by Sande Ndimwibo and Julie M. Hite is titled "Successful Strategies in HIV/AIDS Prevention: The Case of the Uganda Youth Anti-AIDS Association, 1992-2004." The authors present a comprehensive overview of both formal and informal educational programs utilizing individual cognitive as well as environmental sociostructural approaches. A model program under the direction of the UYAAS highlights many of the significant and innovative approaches the HIV/AIDS prevention effort has been so successful in Uganda. The authors describe the vision, structure, strategies, and successes of UYAAS and provide implications for other HIV/AIDS prevention programs in Uganda as well as other affected nations. UYAAS believes that the most effective approach in HIV/AIDS prevention consists of directly involving the youth in improving their reproductive health status. UYAAS has developed a broad collaborative partnership with national and international agencies that in turn has increased their influence and effectiveness in influencing the reproductive heath status of youth in Uganda. The authors describe how UYAAS has networked with national and international organizations and how their collaborative efforts have significantly influenced the promotion and protection of Uganda youths. The authors describe the utility of the mass media and how this has been a helpful adjunct in communicating the prevention message throughout the country. Additional successful educational strategies consist of training peer educators and local community leaders for various districts, communities, schools, and youth groups. In addition UYASS has provided counselling services to thousands of youth, both in and out of school. The combination of voluntary counselling and HIV testing services, community outreach seminars, and condom procurement and distribution have been predominant factors responsible for the nation's significant decline of HIV/AIDS. UYAAS has established numerous school-based anti-AIDS clubs in Uganda as well as extended microcredit funds to help facilitate income-generating activities and also sets up information and technology programs for these clubs. The clubs engage in extracurricular activities such as sports, drama, games, drawing, and holding regular focus-group discussions on HIV/AIDS and other health-related issues. The authors describe the design, production, and distribution of educational materials as well as address implications of the UYAAS's success with respect to its influence on other HIV/AIDS organizations.

Chapter 10, titled "Maximizing HIV/AIDS Prevention Through the Media: An Analysis of the Straight Talk Foundation" by Catherine Watson, Betty Kagoro, and Beatrice Bainomugisha, provides a comprehensive assessment of the role of the media in influencing the knowledge, attitudes, beliefs, and practices of Ugandan youth with respect to HIV/AIDS high-risk behaviors. The chapter begins with an overview of the determinants and distribution of HIV/AIDS in Uganda. The highly successful ABC (*Abstinence, Be faithful*, if not use a *Condom*) HIV/AIDS prevention recommendations initiated by the Ugandan government are discussed with respect to how this approach has been implemented in the country. The next sections describe the national media-based program in Kampala, Uganda, which has received international attention and revolutionized the national HIV/AIDS programs. The Straight Talk Foundation (STF) originated out of the *Straight Talk* newspaper, which was first published in 1993 (Harding, 2002). The broad objective of the foundation is to improve the mental, social, and physical development of Ugandan adolescents (ages 10 through 19) and young adults (ages 20 through 24). Straight Talk Clubs have also been implemented throughout the country and number over 400. These clubs provide social venues for open discussion about adolescent issues. A recent addition to the Straight Talk mass media approach is the implementation of Straight Talk Radio that literally provides a "wake-up call" to the nation's youth. Each month, the Straight Talk Foundation produces one-half million copies of its *Young Talk* newspapers that are sent to some 13,000 primary schools. Key messages include delaying sex, knowing your rights, avoiding early pregnancy or marriage, staying in school, and preventing HIV/STDs. Another innovative approach includes *Teacher Talk*, which is targeted to primary school teachers with the major goal of fostering a supportive environment at school for adolescent sexual and reproductive health (ASRH) development. A complementary adjunct is *Parent Talk* that helps parents feel comfortable discussing ASRH issues with their children and allowing their adolescent children to express themselves freely. These unique approaches reach both in school as well as the out of school youth and are disseminated throughout the country. The authors discuss an evaluation and monitoring system to assess the impact of the STF on adolescent sexual behaviors.

Jeremy Liebowitz and Reverend Stephen F. Noll's chapter 11 titled "The Role of Religion in Educating Ugandan Youth About HIV/AIDS" provides unique insights into the role of religion and faith-based organizations in reducing the prevalence of HIV/AIDS in the country. First the authors present a historical overview of religious organizations and how they have become involved in primary and secondary education as well as higher education. Having gained trust and acceptance among the popu-

lation, religious organizations have provided a strong foundation for HIV/
AIDS prevention education in the country. The authors discuss how faith-
based organizations have participated in the national HIV/AIDS awareness and prevention program in the nation and the impact they have had
on prevalence. Strengths and weaknesses/challenges are provided as to
how faith-based organizations can become more effective in their outreach efforts. Uganda has a very large Christian population, which is estimated to comprise between 75-90% of the total population. Uganda is a
major center of both HIV/AIDS advocacy as well as ministry group work.
Islam constitutes a smaller community in Uganda, but their work in HIV
prevention activities has been considerable. The work of missionary organizations in Uganda with respect to HIV/AIDS prevention has not been
without controversy. The emphasis on abstinence and faithfulness, perhaps at the expense of condom use, has weakened the overall response to
the epidemic by discouraging one possible source of prevention. Abstinence messages do not always resonate well among the youth, especially
those who are already sexually active. Many religious education programs
have been informal and inconsistent, not relying on integration into the
school curriculum, significantly compromising their sustainability and
outreach efforts. Another controversy raised by the authors includes the
development of curriculum and implementation of teaching strategies.
Most of the AIDS-related knowledge and awareness gained by the youth
has occurred in informal settings such as school organizations, clubs and
social activities. An excellent program discussed in this chapter is that of
"Youth Alive" which identifies a participatory, creative, and involved
youth approach, not just youths as passive recipients of the message but as
developers and deliverers of the message.

   Terry D. Olson and Richard G. Wilkins wrap up the second section of
the book with chapter 12 titled, "The Family, Youth and AIDS: Hope and
Heartbreak for Africa." The authors call for individuals, educators, and
government officials to not only to address but also change existing sexual
beliefs and values in order to overcome the HIV/AIDS epidemic. This
ideological shift unavoidably encounters issues of culture, tradition, religion, and societal norms. Recognizing that psychosocial changes are often
at loggerheads with what is in the best interest of individuals who are
faced with the HIV/AIDS epidemic, Olson and Wilkins persuasively argue
the need to *expose* individuals and families to education issues that can
help them understand and make informed choices in their best interest.
This approach is supported over a traditional development model, where
information is *imposed* on societies, regardless of the intended benefit of
the target population. Olson and Wilkins' have anchored their conceptual
framework by well-established theories, such as the value-expectancy
"Health Belief Model" (Rosenstock, 1974), the theory of reasoned action

(Ajzen, 1985; Ajzen & Fishbein, 1980; Fishbein & Ajzen, 1975; Terry, Gallios, & McCamish, 1993), the theory of planned behavior (Ajzen, 1985, 1991), and social cognitive theory (Bandura, 1986, 1989, 1992). While the AIDS situation portrays a rather bleak picture in much of Sub-Saharan Africa, Olson and Wilkins provide a reason for hope. By building on cultural, familial, and personal values and beliefs that support AIDS prevention, the authors feel that there is a sustainable hope in overcoming the HIV/AIDS epidemic.

Part IV addresses one of the major consequences of the AIDS epidemic in Africa, namely how society will take care of orphans and street children whose parents died of AIDS. Chapter 13 ("Poverty, AIDS, and Street Children in Uganda") by Troy D. Smith and the late Acou Sam Ogojoi present interesting and challenging information as to how street children in Uganda are being affected by poverty and AIDS and how these two factors affect each other. In this chapter, the authors identify reasons for why children choose to live on the streets in urban cities such as Kampala. Amidst the backdrop of over 100 million estimated street children worldwide, the authors discuss how the living habits and behaviors of these children place them at increased risk of HIV/AIDS infection and the initiatives being implemented by governmental and nongovernmental agencies. One of the major reasons why children live on the streets is because of poverty, which leads to abuse, neglect, abandonment, child labor, domestic violence, and crime. Children look for acceptance on the street, employment opportunities, excitement and a sense of autonomy. Because of the marginalized status of children relatively little is known about their HIV/AIDS status, prevalence of the disease, and quantification of high-risk sexual behaviors. Studies have provided evidence that these children are engaged in high-risk behaviors such as unprotected sex and drug use. Due to the low rate of condom use in Uganda condoms are not widely available among the youth.

Chapter 14, "HIV/AIDS and the Growing Problem of Orphanhood: Experiences From Uganda and South Africa" by Christopher B. Meek and W. Joshua Rew, discusses one of the tragic results of the AIDS epidemic—orphanhood. We chose to conclude this book with a chapter that graphically portrays the dismal reality of AIDS orphans in Sub-Saharan Africa, but also offers a glimmer of hope by the success story of Uganda. In this chapter, the authors juxtapose orphanhood trends for both case countries and conclude that while both are considered in crisis, only orphanhood trends in Uganda appear to be improving. Additionally, this chapter acknowledges that while orphanhood in Uganda has and is projected to substantially improve and orphanhood in South Africa appears to be worsening, the outcomes of orphanhood in each country are appalling and deserve discussion. Local and national responses are required to address short-term recovery and long-term prevention.

Considerable interest has been directed to the implementation and evaluation of individual as well as environmental and social-structural interventions directed at HIV/AIDS prevention in high-prevalence countries. In additions, the role of government or political commitment in determining the success or failure of HIV/AIDS policies in Sub-Saharan Africa is of primary interest. This book addresses the many faceted approaches governmental, private, and nongovernmental organizations have undertook these many years to change the direction of HIV/AIDS in Uganda. During the 1990s, Uganda faced a dramatic HIV/AIDS epidemic and at the same time witnessed significant transformations to new political systems. The chapters in this book compare and contrast the ways in which environmental and structural approaches, particularly from nongovernmental organizations can expedite the implementation of effective HIV prevention approaches. We have learned many lessons from Uganda and these provide the impetus and commitment for continued program development and evaluation in support of youth and children overcoming AIDS.

REFERENCES

Ajzen, I. (1985). From intentions to actions: A theory of planned behavior. In J. Kuhl & J. Backman (Eds.), *Action—control: From cognitions to behavior* (pp. 11-39). Berlin, Germany: Springer Verlag.

Ajzen, I. (1991). The theory of planned behavior. *Organizational Behavior and Human Decision Processes, 50*, 179-211.

Ajzen, I., & Fishbein, M. (1980). *Understanding attitudes and predicting social behaviour.* Englewood Cliffs, NJ: Prentice-Hall.

Bandura, A. (1986). *Social foundations of thought and action: A social cognitive theory.* Englewood Cliffs, NJ: Prentice Hall.

Bandura, A. (1989). Perceived self-efficacy in the exercise of control over AIDS infection. In V. M. Mays, G. W. Albee, & F. Schneider (Eds.), *Primary prevention of AIDS: Psychological approaches* (pp. 128-141). Newbury Park, CA: Sage.

Bandura, A. (1992). A social cognitive approach to the exercise of control over AIDS infection. In R. J. DiClemente (Ed.), *Adolescents and AIDS: A generation in jeopardy* (89-116). Newbury Park, CA: Sage.

Harding, G. (2002, March-April). Straight talking about AIDS in Uganda. *The Courier ACP-EU*, pp. 10-11.

Fishbein, M., & Ajzen, I. (1975). *Belief, attitude, intention, and behavior: An introduction to theory and research.* Reading, MA: Addison-Wesley.

Okware, S., Opio, A., Musinguzi, J., & Waibale, P. (2001). Fighting HIV/AIDS: Is success possible? *Bulletin of the World Health Organization, 79*(12), 1113-1120.

Parkhurst J. O., & Lush, L. (2004). The political environment of HIV: Lessons from a comparison of Uganda and South Africa. *Social Science and Medicine, 59*(9), 1913-1924.

Rosenstock, I. M. (1974). Historical origins of the health belief model. *Health Education Monographs, 2,* 328-335.

Terry, D. J., Gallios, C., & McCamish, M. (1993). *The theory of reasoned action: Its application to AIDS-preventive behaviour.* Oxford, England: Pergamon.

PART I

SETTING THE CONTEXTUAL STAGE OF HIV/AIDS IN UGANDA

CHAPTER 2

A MULTISECTORAL STRATEGY FOR OVERCOMING AIDS IN UGANDA

Yusuf K. Nsubuga and W. James Jacob

In response to the escalating HIV/AIDS epidemic in Uganda, the government adopted a multisectoral strategy for the prevention, treatment, and mitigation of the disease. While traditionally viewed as primarily a health problem, Uganda shifted its response towards a collaborated effort in the early 1990s that has included many different government sectors. This cross-sectoral strategy has sometimes been compared to a cocktail strategy, emphasizing that multiple governmental agencies and nongovernmental organizations (NGOs) are united in their efforts for combating the national health crisis.

In this chapter, we provide a historical overview of HIV/AIDS education programs in Uganda since the mid-1980s. While many of the early educational efforts were implemented outside of the official national curriculum, this paper also details the paradigmatic shift toward including it as part of key subjects in the primary and secondary subsectors. We also provide an outline of Uganda's multisectoral education efforts that has and continues to lead to behavioral change communication (BCC) among students. This multisectoral strategy has since been implemented in many

Overcoming AIDS: Lesson Learned from Uganda, 15–42
Copyright © 2006 by Information Age Publishing
15

countries throughout the world and is viewed as a key overarching strategy for curbing the epidemic.

UNIQUE FEATURES OF THE HIV/AIDS EPIDEMIC IN UGANDA

The concern over the HIV/AIDS epidemic in Uganda particularly stems from the high incidence of HIV/AIDS infection among the 15–30 year old age group: the most affected population by the disease. This age group occupies critical positions in families, communities, and society as a whole. Over 80% of the reported AIDS cases are among people aged 15-45, the age group which constitutes the largest part of the potential productive labor force. The illnesses and eventual deaths of people in this age bracket have correspondingly affected the labor force supply and the economy in general through reduction of the family labor force and land under cultivation, income, food security, and children's education opportunities.

Studies have reflected a shift from high to low labor-intensive crops in Sub-Saharan Africa (Gillespie & Kadiyala, 2005; Kapungwe, 2005) and a decline in the production of cash crops and livestock production in some parts of Uganda such as the Rakai District (Food and Agriculture Organization of the United Nations, 2003; Haslwimmer, 1994; MAAIF, 2002; Topouzis, 1994). For a predominantly agriculture-based economy, the consequences of HIV/AIDS are clearly devastating. AIDS has also caused employment insecurity and discrimination in the labor force (Dixon, McDonald, & Roberts, 2002; International Labour Organization [ILO], 2001). The cost of labor at the company level is increasing due to health costs in treatment of opportunistic infections and the recurring training of new employees. Migrant workers, like artisans and those working in large establishments where employees meet regularly for social events, appear to be most at risk. Reasons for this high risk status among migrant workers include being away from their spouse and family for long periods of time increases the likelihood of workers seeking additional partners and engaging in intercourse with sex workers along transportation routes (Decosas & Adrien, 1997; Li et al., 2004; Shaeffer, 1994).

HIV and AIDS have caused a disproportionate loss of trained personnel in all sectors of development. The life expectancy of economically productive Africans is estimated to have dropped from 66 years in the absence of AIDS to approximately 47 years (WHO/UNESCO, 2001). Coupled with the brain drain phenomena where the most skilled health and technology workers opt to leave Uganda and other Sub-Saharan African countries for more affluent opportunities in other countries,

HIV/AIDS has had a huge impact on the human labor force (AED/ USAID, 2003a, 2003b). As a result, HIV/AIDS has touched on every aspect of life and national development in Uganda. In the absence of a cure or vaccine, change in sexual behaviors through education and awareness building remains the most important approach towards preventing HIV/AIDS infection (Malinga, 2000; Mathew, 2004; Tapia-Aguirre, Arillo-Santillán, Allen, Angeles-Llerenas, Cruz-Valdéz, & Lazcano-Ponceet, 2004).

HIV/AIDS in Uganda is one of the current epidemics whose principal route of transmission is heterosexual behavior. Owing to this feature, it mainly affects the sexually active population starting at as early as ages 12–14. This places a heavy responsibility on parents, teachers, schools, communities, and the government to educate youth of the transmission and consequences of HIV/AIDS. Since socioculture values and economic relations underlie sexual interaction between individuals, they have a strong bearing on the spread of the epidemic. Education programs targeted at informing children and youth of the consequences of early unsafe sexual behavior and equipping them with the life skills to prevent them from contracting the virus are key components of combating the continual spread of HIV/AIDS among young people. It is therefore important that the Ministry of Education and Sports (MOES) make effective intervention in AIDS education and awareness building as soon as a child commences primary school. These efforts should be significantly strengthened at puberty and the onset of adolescence.

The Impact of HIV/AIDS on the Community

It is believed that every household in Uganda has in some way been affected by the HIV/AIDS epidemic. At the individual level, there is physical suffering due to sickness and most persons living with HIV/AIDS (PWA) experience stigmatization and discrimination. Savings of PWAs drop as their productivity declines due to absenteeism from work and inability to cultivate. An increase in poverty levels among PWA, as parents are rendered unable to maintain employment and provide for their families (Krueger, Wood, Diehr, & Maxwell, 1990; Whiteside, 2002). Family members also spend most of their productive time caring for the sick and there is increased psychosocial trauma for the affected. Studies also indicate some level of community stigma towards PWAs especially when it comes to care and social support (Kalichman & Simbayi, 2003, 2004; Parker & Aggleton, 2003; Reidpath & Chan, 2005). Extended family structures are becoming apprehensive of extending care to the sick and affected owing to the increasing number of related problems like the increased spending on Medicare.

The demand for palliative care services by PWAs is expected to increase as more people who are infected transition to AIDS. According to the health facility inventory of the Ministry of Health, the annual population per hospital bed was 800, and as of 1997, patients with an HIV/AIDS-related illness occupied more than 55% of hospital beds. Health workers also experience psychosocial stress due to fear of being infected. Others exhibit stigma, which might result in a proportion of PWAs being turned away. Use of traditional medicine as a form of therapy for AIDS is steadily growing and there is a notable positive change in the attitude towards the role of traditional medicine (Gbodossou, 2001). Antiretroviral (ARV) therapy has been proven to prolong productive lives of PWAs, but has only been privately available in authorized health facilities in the country by a few PWAs.

According to the Uganda AIDS Commission (2004), "The impact of HIV/AIDS on young people is multidimensional" (p. 11). Several of the ways children and youth are affected by the epidemic include the need to drop out of school, take care of sick family members, early marriages, stigmatization and discrimination, and the loss of family inheritance through orphanhood.

Women are the largest group affected by the HIV/AIDS virus. Women have typically been disadvantaged biologically, socially, and economically in terms of HIV/AIDS (Erben, 1990; Rivers & Aggleton, 1998; UNAIDS/UNFPA/UNIFEM, 2004). The large vaginal mucosal surface area of women increases chances of infection during sex; men transmit HIV more effectively to women than vice versa. In addition, they are at a greater risk of receiving contaminated blood and blood products during pregnancy and delivery. Further, women are more exposed to risky situations due to their dependence on men for socioeconomic survival, and they generally have limited access to formal education and information regarding HIV/AIDS (Bulman, Coben, & Van Anh, 2004; Gillis, 1999). Women have traditionally played the role of caregiver, bearing the burden of caring for the sick and the affected, often foregoing economically productive activities to fulfill such duties. The lack of knowledge of how HIV/AIDS is spread, coupled with the lack of control over sexual behavior of the male, has increased the risk to women. Culturally, men have viewed sex as a rite of passage, a way to establish masculinity and virility and as such have engaged in multiple sexual relationships, including polygamy and sex with commercial sex workers. Some men have engaged in homosexuality and many others in unprotected penetrative sex, which has increased their vulnerability to HIV infection, thereby increasing the risk of infection to his female spouse or partners.

Educational Obstacles: Domestic Violence and Ethnic Conflicts

Even with all of Uganda's success in battling the HIV/AIDS epidemic, ethnic conflicts, domestic violence, and rebel warfare continue to limit opportunities for Ugandan youth and are predictors for spreading HIV among adolescents. Annette Richardson (2001) identifies how African youth educational opportunities have continuously suffered primarily due to ethnic conflicts and domestic violence (see also AED/USAID, 2003b). Unchecked rebel advances on schools and small villages, has led to thousands of displaced persons and refugees. Like Uganda's civil war-riddled past, adjacent countries are stricken with histories of war and genocide that have resulted in human rights violations and sexual violence toward women and children (Amnesty International, 2004; Human Rights Watch, 2002).

In the Great Lakes Region and Uganda, people migrate primarily due to civil conflict and in search for better job and trading opportunities. In 2001, there were 700,000 internally displaced persons and 224,000 refugees residing in Uganda (Basara & Kaija, 2002). The infamous Lord's Resistance Army (LRA), headed by Joseph Kony, has engaged in an armed rebellion in the Northern Region of Uganda for nearly 2 decades. Often the LRA will target youth in schools. Girls are targeted to become sex slaves; young men are compelled to join ranks with the LRA in a form of forced recruitment (De Temmerman, 2001).[1] Those who resist LRA terrorist-like activities are either killed or left to fend for themselves after their village has been rampaged. While the government of Uganda has fought the LRA with the national military, several districts in the Northern Region are vulnerable to lawless rebel advances.

THE CURRENT STATE OF HIV/AIDS IN UGANDA

By the end of 2003, UNAIDS estimated a total of 530,000 PWA in Uganda. Of these, 450,000 were adults and approximately 84,000 were children 14 years or younger. Of the total estimated adults living with HIV/AIDS, approximately 270,000 were females and 260,000 were males (UNAIDS/WHO, 2004b). Heterosexual contact constitutes 75–80% of new HIV infections in Uganda. Mother-to-child transmission, including breast feeding constitutes 15–20% of new HIV infections. The use of blood, blood products, and aseptic conditions in health facilities only constitutes 2–4% of new HIV infections, while sharing nonsterile sharp-piercing instruments with an HIV-infected person constituted less than 1% (Ministry of Health, MOH, 2000). The MOH's *STD/HIV/AIDS Surveillance Report* (2003b) indicated a total of 60,974 AIDS cases (children and adults) reported to the AIDS Control Programme (ACP) Surveillances Unit during the year 2002. Urbanicity plays a role in the overall antenatal prevalence rates. In 2001, the cumulative prevalence rate was 6.5%, closely comparing with 6.1% in 2000. The rates for urban and rural sites varied, however, where urban sites were at 8.8% and rural locations 4.2% respectively compared with 8.7% and 4.2% in 2000 (Uganda AIDS Commission, 2003).

Cumulative AIDS deaths since the beginning of the epidemic were estimated at 947,552 as of December 2001; of these, 852,797 were adults and 94,755 children. Adult female deaths were estimated at 425,644 and males at 427,153. Where Uganda's adult HIV-prevalence rate peaked much earlier than most other countries, Uganda maintains the highest proportion of AIDS orphans in the world (Uganda AIDS Commission, 2003).

Estimates of new infection rates are rare in Uganda. Longitudinal community studies are therefore required in this area. Estimating incidence requires following-up with cohorts of initially healthy people tracking the rate at which they become infected. Studies in Rakai and Masaka Districts show rates of less than 2% (i.e., less than 20/1000) HIV-uninfected adults become infected in the course of 1 year in a rural general population (Kayita & Kyakulaga, 1997). These studies also show that the incidence rate in Masaka and Rakai is lower than it was in the 1980s. A study of 2,300 secondary school students in Gulu found HIV incidence of 2.8% of every 1,000 persons (Accorsi, Fabiani, Lukwiya, Corrado, Awil Onek, & Declich, 1998). The decline in HIV prevalence in younger individuals (15 and under) may indicate increased prevention efforts. If this were to be true, it would mean that increased efforts are required to reduce the HIV-infection rate to zero among the 12–19 year olds. By implication, this would demand more aggressive but harmonized efforts by the MOES.

It was also noted that since almost 50% of the new HIV/AIDS infection rates fall in the age group of 15–25 (MOH, 2001), the education sector becomes a key tool for HIV/AIDS intervention efforts. The education sector is also the second largest governmental sector in terms of working population, with up to 130,000 primary school teachers and over 36,000 secondary teachers. This is a very large work force, which, if well equipped with HIV/AIDS education, can constitute a great force of agents of change in the school system and in the community at large.

Declining Trends in HIV/AIDS Prevalence

Generally recognized as an HIV/AIDS success story, Uganda has documented a decline in adult prevalence rates from 1993 onward. In

1985, prevalence among antenatal clinic attendees was at 11% of the total population. This figure rose to nearly 30% in 1992 and then began its decline in the mid-1990s (MOH, 2001). Adult prevalence in Uganda at the end of 2003 was estimated at 4.1% in rural areas by UNAIDS/WHO (2004b).[2] In the rural areas where trends in the past exhibited a mixed pattern of stabilization and decline, prevalence rates appear to be clearly declining. For example in Gulu District's Lacor Hospital in Northern Uganda, trends among antenatal attendees have fallen from 27.1% in 1993 to 16.3% in 1997 and 11.9% in 2002. The decline is more significant in the young age group of 15–25 years (MOH, 2003b).

There is reported increased knowledge on HIV/AIDS with two out of three persons able to cite at least two acceptable ways of protection against HIV. There is an increase in the proportion of sexually active persons who ever used condoms, reported reduction in the number of sexual partners, and an increase in the average age of first sexual experience. Voluntary counseling and testing (VCT) services have been expanded to different parts of the country as one of the major prevention and support interventions. VCT services are being integrated into health services at the district level. Blood safety from HIV has increased to more than 98%. The heath sector has developed guidelines on syndromic management of STDs, increased training for service providers, and integrated STD service within primary health care (PHC) and maternal/child health and family planning services. A mother-baby package containing essential safe motherhood requirements has been introduced. A project involving a comprehensive package of care before, during, and after delivery involving administration of antiretroviral drugs has also been piloted to target mother-to-child transmission, and the country has participated in HIV vaccine development and trials for a number of years.

HIV/AIDS, CHILDREN, AND YOUNG PEOPLE

AIDS is the fourth leading cause of death among the under-five population and may significantly increase infant mortality by 75% and under-five mortality by more than 100% if mother-to-child transmission of HIV is not contained. Compounding the situation, AIDS has accounted for approximately 1,700,000 orphans since the epidemic began. With a population of 26.7 million, this is a daunting figure (Hyde, Ekatan, Kiage, & Barasa, 2002b; UNAIDS/WHO, 2004b). These children and young people experience orphanhood at an age when parental guidance and support are needed. Traditional support systems are failing to cope with the

Table 2.1. Situational Analysis at Global, Regional, and National Levels

	Global Estimates	Sub-Saharan Africa	Uganda Estimates
Total Number of PWA	39.4 million[a]	25.4 million[a]	530,000[b]
Adults	37.2 million[a]	23.4 million[b]	450,000[b]
Women	17.6 million[a]	13.3 million[a]	270,000[b]
Children < 15 yrs.	2.2 million[a]	1.9 million[b]	84,000[b]
People Newly Infected With HIV/AIDS	4.9 million[a]	3.1 million[a]	60,974
Adults	4.3 million[a]		56,451
Women	2.3 million[a]		30,347
Children < 15 yrs.	640,000[a]		4,523 < 12 yrs.
Total AIDS Deaths Since Beginning of Epidemic	21.9 million[a]		947,552[c]
Adults	17.6 million[a]		852,797[c]
Women	8.9 million[a]		427,153[c]
Children < 15 yrs.	4.3 million[a]		94,755[c]
AIDS Deaths	3.1 million[a]	2.3 million[a]	78,000[b]
Adults	2.6 million[a]		
Women	11.2 million[a]		
Children	500,000[a]		
AIDS Orphans < 15 yrs.	15.0 million[b]	12.3 million[b]	940,000[b]

Sources: MOH (2003a), Uganda AIDS Commission (2003), UNAIDS (2004), UNAIDS/ UNICEF/USAID (2004), UNAIDS/WHO (2001, 2004a, 2004b), UNICEF (2002).
a2004 Estimate
b2003 Estimate
c2001 Estimate

increasing number of orphans, which has resulted in an increase in the number of street children and child-headed families as school dropout rates increase.

Young people's vulnerability is mainly attributed to initiation of sex in their lives at an early age where most of the sexual encounters are without the benefit of consistent and correct condom use and in some cases a result of rape or defilement. There has also been an increase in sexual abuse by adults who think young people are free of HIV, which has resulted in girls being more infected and affected than boys (UNAIDS/ UNFPA/UNIFEM, 2004). Infected children and young people frequently experience stigmatization and discrimination that is often carried with them throughout the duration of their lives.

YOUTH SEXUAL BEHAVIOR AND
MODES OF HIV/AIDS TRANSMISSION

A number of studies carried out by the National Curriculum Development Centre (NCDC) and other organizations dealing with adolescents' sexuality reveal that a substantial percentage of adolescents in Uganda become sexually active early in life. The average age for sexual intercourse debut for both males and females is 15 and 16 years. Findings also reveal that some male children ages 15–19 begin having sexual intercourse between ages 10 and 14. There is high risk and incidence of STDs including HIV/AIDS among the youth resulting from early sexual involvement and unsafe sex practices (Uganda HIV/AIDS Partnership, MOH, Uganda AIDS Commission, & MEASURE Evaluation Project, 2004; UNFPA, 2003).

The *Demographic and Health Survey 2000/2001*, shows that children in Uganda become sexually active at a very early age. According to the survey, by age 15, 23% of girls were already sexually active. The cumulative percentage of sexually active women increases steadily to reach 92% by age 25. The percentage of sexually active men, who are sexually active by the same age, is 81%. The average age at first sexual intercourse, for women 20–49 years is 16.7 and the corresponding figure is 18.8 years for males (Uganda Bureau of Statistics & ORC Macro, 2001). This confirms that women start having sex earlier than men, with a difference of about 2 years. By implication, the girl child is more at risk of HIV infection than the boy child of the same age group. Young women aged 15–24 are at a higher risk of HIV infection than men owing to an earlier age of their first sexual experience, and overall, about 54% of the reported AIDS cases are females (MOH, 2001).

Designing interventions and education programs for youth must first identify the underlying root causes and reasons of youth transmission of STDs and HIV/AIDS. The major concerns regarding early sexuality are the misconceptions held by youths about the consequences of participating in sexual behavior at early ages, which has been identified as a key contributing factor to the continued transmission of HIV/AIDS. Several studies have been conducted to better understand youth perceptions regarding sexual behavior in Uganda (Asiimwe, Kibombo, &

Neema, 2003; Hulton, Cullen, & Khalokho, 2000; Stoneburner & Low-Beer, 2004). Some of the responses from our research findings reveal that youth base their decision to engage in sex primarily from the information and misconceptions perpetuated by other youth. Both males and females noted that if they do not engage in sex, their fertility may be affected, resulting in barrenness for females and sterility in males. Males expressed a concern for proving manhood and ensuring their ability to produce children as well as preventing the release of fluids from private parts, such as nocturnal emissions. Youth also reported peer pressure as another reason to engage in early sexual behavior. Respondents noted that one should be sexually active once one knows enough to protect oneself and that waiting for marriage was too long to wait. While some female respondents noted that they engaged in early sexual behavior to ensure marriage at a later time. There was also a fear that if one took too long to have sex, respondents would not find love in a relationship.

In response to existing knowledge gaps among youth, it is essential for them to receive more information on reproductive health from parents, teachers, and other members of the civil society. During a focus group discussion among secondary students in Mbarara, some of the areas in which youths requested to have more information were:

- consequences of early sexual behavior;
- mother-to-child vertical transmission of HIV/AIDS;
- how to avoid risky situations such as drugs and alcohol;
- various stages of the maturation process in human beings;
- information on protective devices like condoms and how to use them;
- dangers of self medication;
- knowledge on legal procedures to be taken in case of rape and defilement;
- symptoms, mode of transmission, and sources of treatment and counseling for STDs and HIV/AIDS;
- process of human conception and how the variables of gender, age, and frequency and timing of intercourse relate to this process; and
- safe sex practices and how to avoid pregnancy. (Nsubuga, 2004)

As portrayed in the responses above, youth are not only interested in sex but also in how to avoid obtaining STDs and HIV/AIDS, pregnancy, and other consequences of sex.

HIV/AIDS AND THE EDUCATION SECTOR IN UGANDA

Programs to Mitigate the HIV/AIDS Epidemic in the Education Sector

The declining trends in prevalence and new infections demonstrate positive signs that HIV/AIDS programs are reaching target audiences. Many of these target audiences exist at the school level and the formal national education curriculum has and will continue to play a pivotal role in informing children, young adults, and the community of how to protect themselves against the spread of HIV/AIDS. Available literature and data indicate that the MOES and its partners have designed and implemented several projects directed towards mitigation of the impact of HIV/AIDS since 1986. In the remaining portion of this chapter, we will provide salient examples of these projects. The advent of the HIV/AIDS pandemic gave impetus for the development of several multisectoral government and nongovernmental initiatives to prevent the spread of the virus in addition to alleviating its adverse effects. These multisectoral, education-based projects include the School Health Education Project (SHEP), Population and Family Life Education, Life Skills Initiative, and the Presidential Initiative on AIDS Strategy for Communication to Youth (PIASCY).

School Health Education Project (SHEP)

The SHEP initiative was one of the very first initiatives by the MOES designed to focus on sexual reproductive health (SRH) including HIV/AIDS prevention in schools. It was started in 1986 in recognition of the potential contribution schools could make in the mitigation of the epidemic. Therefore this was a school-based program and consisted of two major components: the primary health education syllabus and the family life and education syllabus. The primary health education syllabus focused on HIV/AIDS and STD prevention while the family life and education syllabus focused on human reproduction, parenting skills, and moral and ethical values. The SHEP curriculum covered a wide range of topics ranging from sociocultural beliefs to STDs and HIV/AIDS. Table 2.2 lists the full range of topics covered in the SHEP curriculum. SHEP's comprehensive and versatile curriculum provided basic knowledge on general health, and sexual and reproductive health. However, the vast nature of the curriculum may have clouded the quantity and quality of information taught to the target groups in terms of HIV/AIDS prevention and control. In the same way, an evaluation of the SHEP project in 1994

Table 2.2.   SHEP Curriculum

Growth and Development	STD/HIV/AIDS	Bacterial, Viral, and Fungal Diseases
Family Planning and Contraceptives	Immunization	Food and Nutrition
Sociocultural Attitudes and Beliefs	Hygiene	Exercise, Sex, and Recreation
Sexual Harassment and Abuse	Pollution	Family and Relationships
Marriage and Parenthood	Reproduction	Common Childhood Illness
Water Sources and Protection	First Aid	Responsible Sexual Behavior
Environmental Sanitiation	Abortion	Antisocial Behavior

identified that while the curriculum was quite successful in promoting knowledge, it was not having any measurable influence on student behavior. An NCDC official concurred with this assessment and added, "Curriculum components impart knowledge but do not transform attitudes and behaviour. Schools teach knowledge for passing examinations not skills for behaviour change" (Balinda, 2002).

A second major problem raised in the evaluation of SHEP was teachers' embarrassment and inability to address certain topics regarding sexual and reproductive health. The sociocultural and religious backgrounds of teachers made some uncomfortable while articulating issues of sexual and reproductive health to pupils and students. Culturally, teachers are socialized not to talk openly about sensitive sexual issues especially with children. Often it is difficult to unlearn the attitudes of teachers in a short amount of time; it takes time to deal with the many psycho-social and cultural barriers that exist in an educational context. There were very limited efforts to orient teachers into the delivery of packages. Issues like attitude clarification, language use, religious perspectives, and strategies to overcome cultural barriers to communication about sex hindered the preparation of teachers to develop the SRH packages in the curriculum developed under the SHEP project.

Relating to this challenging context, a female teacher in one of the core primary teacher training colleges was quoted saying: "Sex education is good but because of our upbringing we feel that it is immoral." Therefore although the curriculum was rich, delivering it appropriately was affected by attitudinal, language, and sociocultural barriers that had to be unlearned before it could be effectively implemented to foster both knowledge and behavior change. Similarly the evaluation brought forth the issue of inappropriate methodology as a barrier to effective teaching of attitudes that would lead to behavior change. Under this, the primary data sources did not only emphasize the nonapplication of methodological triangulation but also highlighted issues relating to approaches to sex education in different cultural settings (Sengendo & Sekatawa, 1999). They argued that SHEP did not provide answers to the heterogeneous cultural and religious backgrounds of schools, the heterogeneous environments surrounding schools, and the multiplicity of school types. These heterogeneous aspects led evaluators to question how to approach sexual and reproductive health education in religious settings, in different school types (i.e., single-sex schools, day and boarding schools), or the surrounding environment of bars and cinemas near many school premises.

Evaluations of SHEP suggest not only the need for methodological flexibility and triangulation but also the need for contextualization of the curriculum to the different school and community settings. After realization of these weaknesses, SHEP was abandoned in 1994 prior to achieving its primary objective—to integrate health education into the primary, secondary, and higher education subsectors' curricula (Kiirya, 1998). However, many lessons were learned from the project. To make an effective program the SRH education needs to be a nonexaminable subject and utilization of a life skills approach by putting emphasis on developing teachers' abilities to use participatory methodologies and making the language of instruction flexible and adaptable to the heterogeneity of the students, school, and community. These lessons led to the development of other education programs.

Population and Family Life Education Program in the Uganda Formal Education System

The Population and Family Life Education Program in the formal education system began in 1990. Jointly implemented by the MOES, NCDC, and UNFPA, the program can be divided into two major historical phases:

1. Population and Family Life Education Curriculum Development Approach (1990–1996).
2. Adolescent Reproductive Health Guidance and Counseling in School (1997–2000).

Curriculum Development Approach

The initial curriculum development phase had the overall goal of creating awareness of the relationship between population and development among in-school youths, teachers, parents of students, and other community members. One of the most effective ways to achieve this objective was through an information, education, and communication (IEC) strategy in which population messages were integrated into various school subjects of social studies and science at the primary school level and in biology, geography, religious education, agriculture, and home economics at the secondary school level.

The major topics of this curriculum integration program included: Family Life Education, Population Information & Data, Population Distribution, Structure and Dynamics, Population & Environment, Population and Resource Balance, Gender Roles and Development, and Sociocultural Beliefs and Practices. The issues of STDs and HIV/AIDS were highlighted and tackled effectively in the Family Life Education topic which had the overall objective of making youth aware of dangers associated with premarital sex, including early pregnancy, STDs, HIV/AIDS, and dropping out of school.

The immense task of reviewing all school syllabi for primary, secondary, and tertiary institutions has been an ongoing effort at the NCDC since 1996. To date there is a primary school syllabus, which was launched in 1999. The secondary education curriculum review has been planned to take into account HIV/AIDS issues since 1995. As of 2006, all primary, secondary, and higher education subsectors will have integrated population and family life issues into their respective curricula.

Adolescent Reproductive Health and Counselling

The MOES, NCDC, and UNFPA have jointly implemented an Adolescent Reproductive Health and Counseling project nationwide since 1998. The Ministry of Health, through its IEC unit of the Reproductive Health Program, provided overall coordination including the provision of training manuals and medical personnel who worked as resource persons and trainers. The overall goal of this project has been to use IEC as a key strategy in the development of beliefs, attitudes, values, knowledge, and skills acquisition that leads to safer reproductive health practices by youth.

At the onset of the project in 1998, a baseline survey titled "Reproductive Health in School Curriculum" was carried out in a number of primary, secondary, and tertiary institutions. The survey was conducted at participating schools and through focus group discussions. Teachers, administrators, parents, and youth were included in the survey and focus group discussions. Through the survey a number of reproductive health-related problems were identified, including:

- lack of proper and adequate information on human sexuality;
- students are exposed to uncensored mass media and sex related films;

- information, schools, and student hostels prematurely expose adolescents to environments that encourage adolescents to start sex;
- peer influence;
- economic factors that force girls into prostitution or accepting to engage in sex in return for money and other material things; and
- lack of parental care in reproductive health guidance and counseling.

Early sexual involvement among adolescents—due largely to the lack of guidance and counseling on human sexuality by parents, teachers, religious and other civic leaders—has led to continuing prevalence of teenage pregnancy, unwanted pregnancies and related complications, and STDs including HIV/AIDS among young people. The main strategy of the project was to establish an effective communication support system through reproductive health guidance and counseling services in both the primary and secondary pilot schools. The project implemented a holistic approach to introduce students and communities to the reproductive health curriculum. In addition to training of school teachers in the area of reproductive health, the reproductive health strategy also provided training on how to effectively communicate and teach the curriculum. Peer educators were selected in secondary schools and trained in the reproductive health curriculum. They also had to reorient the music and drama curriculum to incorporate the aspects of the reproductive health curriculum through the composition of music and drama productions. These changes required the instruction of district and school administrators to realize and impress the importance of the curricular changes and the need for establishing reproductive health counseling services within the schools. This led to community outreach and the involvement as well as the instruction of parents on reproductive health and the need for their support and instruction of their children as they develop emotionally, physically, and intellectually through the various stages of adolescence. In order to better incorporate teachers, parents, and school administrators in this process and present a clear and understandable message regarding reproductive health, development and distribution of the reproductive health IEC materials were provided to teachers and students. In an attempt to measure the effectiveness of the program a system was developed to monitor and evaluate the performance of the trained personnel in schools and assess the impact of the counseling service on the students.

Guidance and Counseling

The guidance and counseling component has been ongoing for some time in the education system. Its major focus has been the creation of structures for the appointment of senior female and male teachers in both primary and secondary schools.[3] Currently, many primary and secondary schools have these structures in place but they are operating without clear-cut policy guidelines. However, as Karen A. Hyde, Andrew Ekatan, Paul Kiage, and Catherine Barasa (2002a) note, most of the opportunities for counseling and guidance were directed towards the girl child. The key issues discussed included prevention of pregnancy among school girls, sexual harassment, and personal hygiene, especially during menstruation. The major strength of this initiative is that girls have had more opportunities to receive some information and advice about sexual and reproductive matters. It is, however, important to note that boys are still in the addendum and not in the preface of this initiative.

The short fall of the guidance and counseling program lies in the approach/strategy of giving guidance and counselling in large group settings. This affects purposeful expression of feeling and critical psycho-socio issues by the pupils and students. At the secondary school level, focus group discussion responses often indicated moderate levels of mistrust of teachers by students on grounds of confidentiality. There was also no confidential space available in many schools for counseling and guidance of students, making opportunities for personal counseling extremely limited. The other issue raised involved the selection of senior women and men teachers. In some schools there was a mismatch between the teachers students felt comfortable talking to and those teachers who were actually selected. This situation sometimes caused conflicts and discordance between teachers. Although this program does appear to be reaching female youth and providing information regarding sexual and personal health, there remains a gap between informing students and integrating this knowledge into behavior.

Since the establishment of the Reproductive Health Guidance and Counseling in some of the country's schools, there have been indicators of closer interaction between teachers and the adolescents under their care, especially regarding the discussion of SRH matters. School headteachers have endeavored to create private rooms where counseling can be done in private as well as allocating sufficient time for counselors to meet with different groups of children. Teachers who have gone through training, have acquired basic communication and counseling skills and reports show that a number of issues on relationships, hygiene, and career are being effectively handled in a friendly atmosphere. The trained teachers report that the training has sharpened their knowledge of human reproduction process and consequently their teaching of science and social studies subjects, which have population issues in their content. Other teachers in schools have been well sensitized by their colleagues who went through the guidance and counseling training and there is evidence of collective efforts to improve the health of adolescents. Group guidance sessions on various reproductive health topics, especially STDs and HIV/ AIDS, have been implemented and children are obtaining knowledge about the dangers of early sexual involvement. The guidance and counseling of adolescents is contributing to a campaign for the retention of the enrolled Universal Primary Education (UPE) pupils, especially girl children, in upper primary classes.

A number of parents are being helped by counselors to have meaningful and open communication with their children regarding SRH issues. Some parents are reporting improvement in their children's behavior. While some students in the formal school system have the benefit of being exposed to SRH knowledge and information, many others are missing this opportunity because of the financial limitations cited earlier.

Life Skills Initiative

Through experience for the last years, it has become increasingly clear that knowledge alone does not change behavior. The dangers of such a gap have become even more apparent with the onset of HIV/AIDS. As a result, the government of Uganda, in conjunction with UNICEF, saw the need to teach children life skills required for coping with the world in which they live. The Life Skills Initiative was established after an impact evaluation of SHEP found that while children's knowledge on health issues had increased significantly, there was no corresponding behavior change. The missing link was identified as life skills to assist the children to translate knowledge into positive health behaviors.

The objectives of the Life Skills Initiative are to develop skills among youth in the areas of interpersonal relationships, self awareness and self esteem, problem solving, effective communication, decision making, negotiating safe sex, maintaining chastity, resisting peer pressure, critical thinking, and formation of friendships. The major strategy adopted was to infuse life activities into the existing syllabi in schools and higher education institutions rather than developing and implementing a separate life skills curriculum in each subsector. Life skills in the context of the Life Skills Initiative were defined as personal and social skills required by young people to function confidently and competently with themselves, with colleagues, and with the wider community.

HIV/AIDS Education Through Drama

HIV/AIDS messages were also carried out through drama performances in large school assemblies. The plays were written and played in both primary and secondary subsectors, the Riddle for primary and Hydra for secondary. However, lessons learned included adopting a life skills approach. Drama performances have a potentially powerful affect on both performers and the audience, by addressing sensitive topics that are often difficult or culturally unacceptable to discuss or portray by another means.

PIASCY

In early 2002, President Yoweri Kaguta Museveni proposed a way to improve communication on HIV and AIDS to young people. The President's concerns were that in spite of the great success Uganda had attained in containing the situation, this might reverse if children did not continue to receive enough appropriate and correct information. This initiative became known as the Presidential Initiative on AIDS Strategy for Communication to Youth (PIASCY).

PIASCY calls for a strategy to help school-going youth become AIDS competent. In a country where over half the population is 16 years or younger, the strategy takes advantage of UPE. Under UPE almost all children of primary age are in school. The President's vision included a component where head teachers addressed school assemblies on HIV/AIDS every 2 weeks. All teachers are then expected to take the discussion into classrooms and clubs.

The PIASCY program has allowed school administrators and researchers to open a dialogue with students and to increase awareness of the problems, challenges, and questions facing youth in regards to HIV/AIDS. It became apparent that there is a high incidence of STDs, including HIV/AIDS, resulting from early sexual involvement and unsafe practices, thus emphasizing the need to provide sex education at the earliest level possible. The dialogue allowed investigators to see that pupils and students have misconceptions about the consequences of early sexuality and that there continues to be an inadequate amount of counseling and guidance from schools and families. This lack of counseling and guidance appeared from two sources—parents and teachers. Some parents and teachers expressed that they had made wrong choices and had messed up their own lives, and the resulting guilt prevented them from counseling children about sexual matters.

To compound this situation, many teachers do not feel adequately prepared to provide instruction on reproductive health to their students. Although teachers provide reproductive health knowledge in subjects like science, biology, and religious education, this education has generally been superfluous. The majority of teachers do not have adequate knowledge of SRH issues and therefore they place little emphasis on crucial issues like HIV/AIDS, STDs, and family planning as they are not well informed on these issues. Furthermore, the increasing hostility directed towards children and youth by guardians and step parents have forced many young people to look for people outside the home who are friendly to them and willing to provide wanted and needed material things.

This provides students with few options as to where they obtain their knowledge regarding SRH. Although information provided by peers may not be reliable, students often seek advice from peers because they are highly accessible and are often viewed as nonthreatening. In addition, contemporary mass media often carry sex-related materials and literature that motivate students to experiment.

These issues have led researchers to identify a mismatch between the demands and supply for the project's services; additionally, children respond more positively to IEC messages and materials when they are involved in the development process. This increases the relevance of the curriculum to the students' perceived needs. Through student participation in the PIASCY program, students identified four areas of limited knowledge: (1) information and knowledge regarding legal procedures in case of sexual abuse; (2) the process of human conception and how variables like age, gender, frequency, and timing of sexual intercourse relate to this process; (3) information regarding the possible earliest time by age that students should know about STDs, their modes of transmission, and sources of treatment; and (4) accurate information regarding reproductive health to clear misconceptions about abstinence from sex.

PIASCY is such a large government initiative that its full implementation will take time to reach the entire education sector. The first stage of the implementation process has focused on ensuring the following three programs nationwide: (1) that each school holds HIV/AIDS-related assemblies once every 2 weeks, (2) that the standard prevention messages are shared to and understood by students, and (3) establishing AIDS clubs which serve as conduits for open discussion and delivering messages to all students. Another focus of the initiative relates to the production of materials that are age appropriate for students at primary and secondary schools. Although the initiative was first introduced at the primary subsector in 2003, in-service training of secondary teachers did not begin until 2004 and 2005. A series of handbooks were prepared by the MOES (2004a, 2004b, & 2004c) for teachers and students in 2004. To ensure that these messages are reaching the student masses, the production of HIV/AIDS materials, and the in-service training of new and existing teachers is a multiyear and ongoing process.

Extracurricular Activities

In addition to national education programs, the MOES has partnered with the governmental, private, and volunteer sectors of society to promote multisectoral knowledge and understanding programs regarding SRH and sexual behavior in terms of HIV/AIDS. As part of the PIASCY program, NGOs, private organizations, and foundations have been invited into schools to provide additional instruction, training, and exposure to the topics of reproductive health and HIV/AIDS awareness. In addition, most schools invite special visitors to give talks at least once a term. Visitors come form various NGOs and faith-based organizations (FBOs). Some of the more common NGOs that partner with Ugandan schools include the AIDS Information Centre (AIC), The AIDS Support Organisation (TASO), Uganda Youth Anti Aids Association (UYAAS), Student Partnership Worldwide, Kiteetika Rural Women's Association (KIRWA),[4] and ProLiteracy Worldwide.

The major activities included giving testimonies about PWA to raise awareness. Organizations provided counseling regarding means of protecting oneself against infection of HIV/AIDS and other STDs. The organizations distributed leaflets and other IEC materials, especially *Straight Talk*, *Young Talk*, and *Teacher Talk* newspaper inserts. In the urban schools, films like *More Time* were shown and discussed with the students.

Although these activities were reported to be useful, educating, and interesting, pupils and students were more impressed and touched by testimonies of PWA. Teachers also acknowledged that PWA testimonies were generally viewed as more persuasive, effective, and had significantly impacted the students and teachers.

One such PWA organization is the Philly Lutaya Initiative (PLI) that tests individuals for HIV/AIDS. Similar to the PLI, an organization known as Networks of People Living with AIDS meets with student groups. This network is intended to give AIDS a human face and awaken the students and pupils to its realities. In an attempt to inform students of services available for individuals impacted by HIV/AIDS, the Uganda Network on Law Ethics and HIV/AIDS was established to provide an appropriate legal and ethical response to HIV/AIDS. It currently assists in mitigating discrimination, stigmatization, and abuse of human rights. In an attempt to increase rural knowledge in regards to reproductive health and HIV/

AIDS, the African Medical and Research Foundation (AMREF) delivers a school health and AIDS prevention program to rural schools.

The Straight Talk Foundation (STF) publishes newspapers directly related to reproductive health and HIV/AIDS. The foundation has influenced the sexual behaviors of many people through the publications of *Straight Talk*, *Young Talk*, and *Teacher Talk*, which currently reaches over 1 million young people in primary and secondary schools. STF has a two-fold mission to help keep adolescents be safe and be able to communicate for better health by: (1) increasing understanding of adolescence regarding sexuality and reproductive health, and (2) promoting safe sex and child and adolescent rights. TASO contributes to promoting openness about HIV/AIDS through its concept of "Living positively with AIDS." It adopted this approach in response to fear, denial, and stigma that were paralyzing community responses to the HIV/AIDS epidemic in Uganda.

MULTISECTORAL STRATEGIES FOR THE WAY FORWARD

Given the knowledge gained by previous experience and the devastating impact of the epidemic on all governmental sectors, it is envisaged that NGOs, governmental sectors, and schools will intensify their response to the HIV/AIDS epidemic. This united effort is accomplished primarily through developing and enforcing policies and legal and regulatory provisions relevant to the epidemic. In the education sector, this will be accomplished through reviewing the curriculum, aiming at incorporating issues related to HIV/AIDS in syllabus and reading materials, and developing an advocacy, mobilization, and welfare strategy relevant to the epidemic for students and staff. The MOES will strengthen the human and institutional capacity for all target audiences to access AIDS services (information, education, counseling, and health care). This will be made possible through adequate planning and managing an entire range of HIV/AIDS interventions under its purview, including the establishment of an HIV/AIDS collection, documentation, and management system of all data relevant to the epidemic in education and sports institutions. The MOES has also developed a sector-specific policy for addressing HIV/AIDS and a workplace policy and program.

There are several factors that contribute to the behavioral change communication (BCC) students receive through a multisectoral strategy for overcoming AIDS. Figure 2.1 portrays a model of the various elements that exist in Uganda to reach the mass student body in the formal primary and secondary education system. Government commitment, multisectoral collaboration between government sectors, political stability, and a democratic society are all precursors for an effective HIV/AIDS educa-

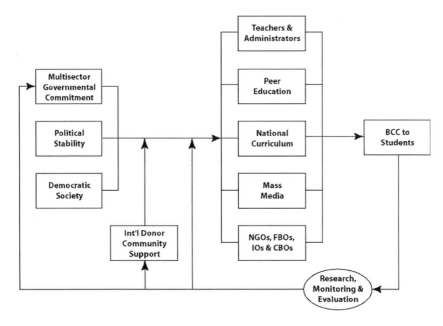

Figure 2.1.   Multisectoral Model for Behavioral Change Communication in the Ugandan Education System.

tion campaign. Although geographic pockets of Uganda continue to suffer from political strife—such as the war-torn Northern districts—since Museveni overthrew the Obote regime in the mid-1980s, Uganda has maintained a relatively stable political environment. Governmental leadership in Uganda recognized the magnitude of the HIV problem early and resolved to confront it openly. Leadership also realized the scarcity of knowledge that existed among the general population and determined to address this knowledge gap through multiple avenues, including the education system.

Due in large part to political support and a stable environment, the international donor community has widely recognized Uganda as a model Sub-Saharan African country in the fight against AIDS. Ugandan government officials are regularly asked to contribute to regional and global HIV/AIDS strategy initiatives in order to share what they have learned with other countries. School administrators and senior male and female teachers serve as counselors to students about HIV/AIDS issues. This is an important counselor-patient relationship, especially when students learn for the first time that they are HIV-positive through school-supported voluntary counseling and testing programs. Teacher training institutes are actively preparing the next generation of teachers with adequate information and life skills to help integrate HIV/AIDS information into their classes. In-service training seminars are an important part of the MOES's ongoing strategy for teaching the existing primary and secondary level teaching force about prevention, counseling, and treatment of the disease.

Because of the sensitive nature of discussing sexual matters in schools, peer education forums are often an effective avenue for the dissemination of information. Anti-AIDS student clubs provide students with the opportunity to discuss sex education issues among friends and peers. Although HIV/AIDS has not always been part of the national curriculum, the PIASCY program emphasizes the integration of HIV/AIDS information as a fundamental part of primary and secondary education level curricula in Uganda. At the secondary education level, HIV/AIDS is being integrated into five key subjects already being offered to students. School-wide assemblies are hosted on a bimonthly basis where key issues are discussed about the nature and prevention of the disease. Handbooks and other ICE materials are made available to teachers and students that provide age-appropriate information to students.

Mass media has perhaps a greater impact on the dissemination of health-related information to the masses than any other medium. Newspapers, radio programs, television shows and infomercials, and pamphlets all serve as effective education mediums in reaching students and youth in Uganda. NGOs, FBOs, international organizations (IOs), and community based organizations (CBOs) play a crucial IEC role in the nonformal and formal education sectors. The Straight Talk Foundation, for instance, offers multimedia outlets, including national newspaper inserts and radio programs in English and several local languages. The AIDS Support Organisation (TASO) provides counseling and IEC to schools through training programs, peer education programs, and the establishment of student clubs. Another organization that trains schools on how to establish and keep clubs running is the Uganda Youth Anti-AIDS Association (UYAAS). FBOs are particularly influential in the education sector as a large and increasing number of private schools are church owned and operated. In their ability to bring in qualified researchers, practitioners, and program operating funds, IOs also play an important role in educating students about HIV/AIDS. Often IOs will partner with Ugandan-based NGOs, FBOs, and CBOs to help sustain already existing education networks.

Each of the items identified in Figure 2.1 is an essential element in the student BCC process. Underlying each of these elements is an atmosphere of openness about the AIDS epidemic. Only when a disease of this magnitude is dealt with openly at the national, community, school, and personal levels can sustainable results be realized. Research is an essential component that provides the necessary feedback on the monitoring and evaluation of program effectiveness. Are students really learning through school-wide assemblies? Does inclusion of HIV/AIDS-related material in the national curriculum actually change student behavior? Which organizations that work with schools are most effective in helping students change behavior? These questions and many more will need to be answered through sound empirical research on the multisectoral model for BCC.

CONCLUSION

It is now clear that apart from being a major health problem, HIV/AIDS is an enormous development issue and a potential security crisis. In Sub-Saharan Africa and in Uganda in particular, the epidemic poses a serious threat to achievements so far gained in reducing poverty, provision of basic education, and is thus an obstacle to the realization of national development goals and the education for all goals. In an effort to revitalize and expand any country's societal response against HIV/AIDS, countries and ministries must build and strengthen a multisectoral capacity for coordination, planning, and implementation at all levels. While national multisectoral responses are important they are not sufficient in dealing with HIV and AIDS. As the influence of HIV spans across geographical boundaries so must prevention and care programs. Stepping up advocacy for HIV/AIDS with particular emphasis on political leadership at all levels and addressing the AIDS orphans crisis are essential to an effective strategy in addressing the problems presented by the HIV/AIDS pandemic.

NOTES

1. During a national HIV/AIDS education study, conducted jointly by the MOES and the editors (W. James Jacob, Donald E. Morisky, Steven J. Hite, and Yusuf K. Nsubuga), the LRA attacked an all-girls secondary school that was randomly selected to participate in the study of 76 Ugandan secondary schools. Over 30 girls were taken by the army. After some time, most girls were released, but only after suffering through continuous group rape and physical abuse.
2. Although the national antenatal clinics reported these findings, some urban clinics reported much higher figures. For instance, at Old Mulago Hospital's STD Sentinel Clinic reports show a much higher percent over the same time period. In 1989, HIV prevalence among patients was at 44.2%. This figure peaked in 1990 at 44.6% and then started a decline reaching 35.9% in 1995, 20.5% in 2000, and reach 19.0% at the end of

2002 (over a 50% decline in HIV prevalence since 1989 and 1990). For more information on Uganda's HIV prevalence rates by location, see the Ministry of Health's *STD/HIV/AIDS Surveillance Report* (2003).

3.   Senior male and female teachers are generally assigned at each secondary school in Uganda. They serve as counselors with boarding and day students regarding issues of school management, hygiene, sexual and reproductive health, and discipline. Often senior teachers are not the most qualified or informed teachers on SRH issues. In other cases, senior teachers may not have personality characteristics so necessary for students to confide sensitive issues such as SRH topics, relationships with a boyfriend or girlfriend, and other personal issues.

4.   KIRWA was established by a group of female teachers in Wakiso District who target predominantly rural schools and communities. KIRWA activities include offering sex education in rural schools, instructing parents and teachers about prevention strategies and how to treat someone with AIDS, and offering microcredit opportunities and training to parents and guardians who adopt AIDS orphans. The MOES has identified KIRWA as an effective NGO that has made a substantial impact in the rural areas of Wakiso District.

REFERENCES

Accorsi, S., Fabiani, M., Lukwiya, M., Corrado, B., Awil Onek, P., & Declich, H. (1998). HIV sero-survey in medical ward. In *Coping with the impact of the AIDS epidemic in Northern Uganda: Analysis of six years of activities of Lacor Hospital, Gulu (1992–97)* (pp. 57–61). Rome: Instituto Superiore di Sanità.

AED/USAID. (2003a). *The health sector human resource crisis in Africa: An issues paper.* Washington, DC: Author.

AED/USAID. (2003b). *Multisectoral responses to HIV/AIDS: A compendium of promising practices from Africa.* Washington, DC: Author.

Amnesty International. (2004). *Rwanda, "marked for death,": Rape survivors living with HIV/AIDS in Rwanda.* New York: Author.

Asiimwe, D., Kibombo, R., & Neema, S. (2003). *Focus group discussions on social cultural factors impacting on HIV/AIDS in Uganda.* Kampala, Uganda: Makerere Institute of Social Research.

Balinda, M. (2002). *Integration of HIV/AIDS into the national curriculum.* Paper presented at the Collin Hotel, Mukono, Uganda.

Basara, R., & Kaija, D. (2002). The impact of HIV/AIDS on children: Lights and shadows in the "successful case" of Uganda. In G. A. Cornia (Ed.), *AIDS, public policy and child well-being* (pp. 1–73). Florence, Italy: UNICEF.

Bulman, D., Coben, D., & Van Anh, N. (2004). Educating women about HIV/AIDS: Some international comparisons. *Compare, 34*(2), 141–159.

Decosas, J., & Adrien, A. (1997). Migration and HIV. *AIDS, 11*(Suppl. A), S77–S84.

De Temmerman, E. (2001). *Aboke girls: Children abducted in Northern Uganda.* Kampala, Uganda: Fountain.

Dixon, S., McDonald, S., & Roberts, J. (2002). The impact of HIV and AIDS on Africa's economic development. *British Medical Journal, 324*(7331), 232–234.

Erben, R. (1990). The special threat to women. *World Health*, 7–9.

Food and Agriculture Organization of the United Nations. (2003). *HIV/AIDS and agriculture: Impacts and responses. Case studies from Namibia, Uganda and Zambia.* Rome: Author.

Gbodossou, E. V. A. (2001). *Involvement of traditional healers as IEC (information, education, communication) in the prevention of HIV/AIDS.* Dakar, Senegal: PROMETRA.

Gillespie, S., & Kadiyala, S. (2005). *International conference on HIV/AIDS and food and nutrition security: From evidence to action.* Washington, DC: International Food Policy Research Institute.

Gillis, L. (1999). *Women and HIV prevention: Review of the research and literature.* Toronto: Community Research Initiative of Toronto.

Haslwimmer, M. (1994). Is HIV/AIDS a threat to livestock production? The example of Rakai, Uganda. *World Animal Review, 80*(81), 92–97.

Hulton, L. A., Cullen, R., & Khalokho, S. W. (2000). Perceptions of the risks of sexual activity and their consequences among Ugandan adolescents. *Studies in Family Planning, 31*(1), 35–46.

Human Rights Watch. (2002). *The war within the war: Sexual violence against women and girls in Eastern Congo.* New York: Human Rights Watch.

Hyde, K. A. L., Ekatan, A., Kiage, P., & Barasa, C. (2002a). *HIV/AIDS and education in Uganda: Window of opportunity?* Kampala, Uganda: Rockfeller Foundation.

Hyde, K. A. L., Ekatan, A., Kiage, P., & Barasa, C. (2002b). *The impact of HIV/AIDS on formal schooling in Uganda—Summary report.* Nairobi, Kenya: Centre for International Education, University of Sussex Institute of Education; Downtown Printing Works.

International Labour Organization (ILO). (2001). *An ILO Code of Practice on HIV/AIDS and the world of work.* Geneva, Switzerland: Author.

Kalichman, S. C., & Simbayi, L. C. (2003). HIV testing attitudes, AIDS stigma, and voluntary HIV counselling and testing in a Black township in Cape Town, South Africa. *Sexually Transmitted Infections, 79*(6), 442–447.

Kalichman, S. C., & Simbayi, L. C. (2004). Traditional beliefs about the cause of AIDS and AIDS-related stigma in South Africa. *AIDS Care, 16*(5), 572–580.

Kapungwe, A. (2005). Household food security and nutritional status in Zambia: Policy challenges. *African Insight, 35*(1), 36–43.

Kayita, J., & Kyakulaga, J. B. (1997). *HIV/AIDS status report, Uganda.* Kampala: Uganda AIDS Commission.

Kiirya, S. (1998). *HIV/AIDS in Uganda: A comprehensive analysis of the epidemic and the response.* Kampala, Uganda: Makerere Institute for Social Research.

Krueger, L. E., Wood, R. W., Diehr, P. H., & Maxwell, C. L. (1990). Poverty and HIV seropositivity: The poor are more likely to be infected. *AIDS, 4*(8), 811–814.

Li, X., Fang, X., Lin, D., Mao, R., Wang, J., Cottrell, L., et al. (2004). HIV/STD risk behaviors and perceptions among rural-to-urban migrants in China. *AIDS Education and Prevention, 16*(6), 538–556.

Malinga, F. (2000). *Actions taken by Ministry Of Education and Sports to cope with the impact of HIV/AIDS*. Paris: International Institute for Educational Planning (IIEP).

Mathew, T.-J. (2004). Senegal renews its campaign against AIDS. *Contemporary Review, 285*(1664), 167–169.

MAAIF. (2002). *The impact of HIV/AIDS on agricultural production and mainstreaming HIV/AIDS messages into agricultural extension in Uganda*. Rome: Food and Agriculture Organization of the United Nations.

Ministry of Education and Sports (MOES). (2004a). *Presidential initiative on AIDS strategy for communication to youth (PIASCY), helping pupils stay safe: A handbook for teachers, P3–P4*. Kampala, Uganda: Author.

MOES. (2004b). *Presidential initiative on AIDS strategy for communication to youth (PIASCY), helping pupils stay safe: A handbook for teachers, P5–P7*. Kampala, Uganda: Author.

MOES. (2004c). *PIASCY handbook for students of secondary schools*. Kampala, Uganda: Artec Consult and Author.

Ministry of Health (MOH). (2000). *HIV/AIDS surveillance report*. Kampala, Uganda: Author.

MOH. (2001). *HIV/AIDS Surveillance Report*. Kampala, Uganda: STD/AIDS Control Programme, Ministry of Health.

MOH. (2003a). *Policy for reduction of the mother-to-child HIV transmission in Uganda*. Kampala, Uganda: Author.

MOH. (2003b). *STD/HIV/AIDS surveillance report*. Kampala, Uganda: Author.

Nsubuga, Y. K. (2004, November). *Addressing HIV/AIDS concerns among young people in schools*. Focus group discussion, Mbarara, Uganda.

Parker, R., & Aggleton, P. (2003). HIV and AIDS-Related stigma and discrimination: A conceptual framework and implications for action. *Social Science & Medicine, 57*(1), 13–24.

Reidpath, D. D., & Chan, K. Y. (2005). A method for the quantitative analysis of the layering of HIV-related stigma. *AIDS Care, 17*(4), 425–432.

Richardson, A. (2001). Social injustice: The irony of African schooling disruption. In M. J. Berson & I. R. Berson (Eds.), *Cross cultural perspectives in child advocacy* (pp. 1–25). Greenwich, CT: Information Age.

Rivers, K., & Aggleton, P. (1998). *Adolescent sexuality, gender and the HIV epidemic*. New York: United Nations Development Programme.

Sengendo, J., & Sekatawa, E. K. (1999). *A cultural approach to HIV/AIDS prevention and care* (No. 1). Paris: UNESCO.

Shaeffer, S. (1994). *The impact of HIV/AIDS on education: A review of literature and experience*. Paris: UNESCO.

Stoneburner, R. L., & Low-Beer, D. (2004). Population-level HIV declines and behavioral risk avoidance in Uganda. *Science, 304*(5671), 714–718.

Tapia-Aguirre, V., Arillo-Santillán, E., Allen, B., Angeles-Llerenas, A., Cruz-Valdéz, A., & Lazcano-Ponce, E. (2004). Associations among condom use, sexual behavior, and knowledge about HIV/AIDS: A study of 13,293 public school students. *Archives of Medical Research, 35*(4), 334–343.

Topouzis, D. (1994). *Uganda: The socio-economic impact of HIV/AIDS on rural families with an emphasis on youth*. Rome: Food and Agriculture Organization of the United Nations.

Uganda AIDS Commission. (2003). *The HIV/AIDS epidemic: Prevalence and impact*. Kampala: Uganda AIDS Commission.

Uganda AIDS Commission. (2004). *The revised national strategic framework for HIV/AIDS activities in Uganda, 2003/04–2005/06: A guide for all HIV/AIDS stakeholders*. Kampala: Author.

Uganda Bureau of Statistics, & ORC Macro. (2001). *Uganda demographic and health survey 2000/2001*. Calverton, MD: Authors.

Uganda HIV/AIDS Partnership, MOH, Uganda AIDS Commission, & MEASURE Evaluation Project. (2004). *AIDS in Africa during the nineties: Uganda. Young people, sex, and AIDS in Uganda*. Chapel Hill, NC: MEASURE Evaluation, Carolina Population Center, University of North Carolina at Chapel Hill.

UNAIDS. (2004). *2004 report on the global AIDS epidemic*. Geneva, Switzerland: Author.

UNAIDS/UNICEF/USAID. (2004). *Children on the brink 2004: A joint report of new orphan estimates and a framework for action*. Washington, DC: USAID.

UNAIDS/UNFPA/UNIFEM. (2004). *Women and HIV/AIDS: Confronting the crisis*. Geneva, Switzerland: Authors.

UNAIDS/WHO. (2001). *AIDS epidemic update*. Geneva, Switzerland: Authors.

UNAIDS/WHO. (2004a). *AIDS epidemic update*. Geneva, Switzerland: Authors.

UNAIDS/WHO. (2004b). *Uganda epidemiological fact sheets on HIV/AIDS and sexually transmitted infections*. Geneva, Switzerland: Authors.

UNICEF. (2002). *Orphans and other children affected by HIV/AIDS*. New York: Author.

UNFPA. (2003). *State of world population 2003*. New York: Author.

Whiteside, A. (2002). Poverty and HIV/AIDS in Africa. *Third World Quarterly, 23*(2), 313–332.

CHAPTER 3

FIGHTING STIGMA AND DISCRIMINATION AS A STRATEGY FOR HIV/AIDS PREVENTION AND CONTROL

Yusuf K. Nsubuga and W. James Jacob

BACKGROUND OF AIDS STIGMA

HIV and AIDS are currently regarded as the leading challenges to global development and world health. The pandemic has not only claimed millions of lives but continues to cause direct and indirect suffering among people everywhere. The management of its dynamics and magnitude has been further complicated by the stigma associated with HIV/AIDS and discrimination that disrupts most of the interventions aimed at mitigating the effects not only on individual health but also on socioeconomic life. Uganda's recently registered successes in reducing the prevalence of HIV can be attributed partly to the efforts to address this issue and ability in enabling Ugandans to overcome stigma and discrimination through promotion of voluntary counseling, testing, and positive living (UNAIDS/WHO, 2004). It is, however, important to recognize that stigma and discrimination associated with disease are not new; both have existed

Overcoming AIDS: Lessons Learned from Uganda, 43–59
Copyright © 2006 by Information Age Publishing

throughout recorded history but have been exacerbated with the rise of the AIDS epidemic. Throughout this chapter, we use the term *AIDS stigma* to represent all types of HIV/AIDS-related stigma, discrimination, and prejudice.

This chapter begins with an overview of AIDS stigma and how it has permeated societies worldwide and Uganda in particular. It then defines several types of AIDS stigma and concludes by providing a list of strategies that have helped Ugandans deal with this issue. This chapter is intended to help eliminate AIDS stigma, since it is a leading impediment in many nations, and it only exacerbates the situation people living with HIV or AIDS (PWA) face.

Understanding the dynamics associated with AIDS stigma requires looking at the disease from the internal perspective of those who are living through the cruel realities associated with the AIDS epidemic. The following three scenarios highlight different elements associated with AIDS stigma.

> One afternoon my daughter, who was in Primary 6, came back home crying and she came straight to my room and asked, "Dad, is it true that I have AIDS?" I wondered what had happened at school and later found out that since my daughter had been sick for some days a teacher had rebuked her for not finishing her homework and in the process expressed concerns aloud about the persistent illness of my daughter and asked if she had AIDS. (Parent of a student in Kampala, Uganda, 2004)

In the second case, a European-based fishing company had planned to subject all its employees to mandatory HIV testing. They argued that their clients in Europe and elsewhere wanted to be assured that workers were free from the virus and considered healthy enough to handle the fish. Upon hearing about this organizational policy, the government of Uganda immediately intervened, and the testing did not take place.

The third AIDS stigma case happened when 15 participants in the 11th International Conference for People Living with HIV/AIDS, which was held in Kampala, Uganda, were returning to their homes in India. They had reached Mumbai airport at 2:00 p.m. and were in line for immigration clearance when six of them were taken out of the line and asked to present a yellow fever certificate. According to Indian AIDS activists, six of the participants told the medical officers of the immigration department they were HIV positive. The six individuals were then detained, taken by rickshaw to a nearby hospital, and locked up without access to proper sanitation, medication, food, or water. In reaction to this third incident, Stuart Flavell, international coordinator for the Global Network of People Living with HIV/AIDS, one of the international organizations mobilized to seek help for the detainees, commented:

What has happened is abhorrent. These people were singled out for mistreatment because they are HIV positive. How else can you explain that the other travelers coming from Uganda were not put in quarantine? This incident is yet more evidence of the discriminatory and inhuman attitude of some government officials against people living with HIV/AIDS. (Bushee & Hale, 2003)

These three examples illustrate the reality of stigma and discrimination and indicate that these tend to be perpetuated by a lack of adequate information regarding HIV and AIDS. Discrimination causes isolation and marginalization of people living with HIV/AIDS.

Over the past decade, the international community has emphasized fighting AIDS stigma because it is widely recognized as one of the most imperative obstacles to overcome in conquering the AIDS epidemic (Cameron, 1993; Chesney & Smith, 1999; Goldin, 1994; Herek, Capitanio, & Widaman, 2002). Stigma has been noted by human rights activists as one of the major barriers which continues to undermine efforts to stop the spread of the AIDS virus. Public health leaders criticized public health care for PWA, saying many often receive poor or no treatment because of the stigma surrounding the disease (Herek, Capitanio, & Widaman, 2003). In many countries, discrimination prevents people who are known to have HIV from accessing education or employment opportunities or from caring for their families. Regarding AIDS stigma, Peter Piot (2001) commented at the World Conference Against Racism, Racial Discrimination, Xenophobia, and Related Intolerance, "People living with HIV are part of the solution, not part of the problem—they are the world's greatest untapped resource in responding to the epidemic" (p. 1). HIV/AIDS-related stigma comes from the powerful combination of shame and fear; shame because the sex or drug injections that transmit HIV are surrounded by taboo and moral judgment, and fear because AIDS is a relatively new epidemic and considered deadly. Responding to AIDS with blame or abuse of people living with AIDS simply forces the epidemic underground, creating the ideal conditions for HIV to spread. The only way to make progress against the epidemic is to replace shame with solidarity and fear with hope.

In most countries, there are well-documented cases of PWA being discriminated against and sometimes even denied access to services on the grounds of their serostatus. At workplaces in education, healthcare, and the community, people may not understand that HIV cannot be transmitted through everyday contact with people who have the virus or AIDS, and they may not know that infection can be avoided by the adoption of relatively simple precautions. This lack of knowledge can lead people to discriminate against those who are either infected or presumed to be infected with HIV.

The Declaration of Commitment adopted by the United Nations General Assembly Special Session on HIV/AIDS in June 2001 highlights global consensus on the importance of fighting AIDS stigma to prevent and control the spread of HIV/AIDS.[1] Participants identified stigma, silence, discrimination, and denial, as well as a lack of confidentiality, as factors that undermine prevention, care, and treatment efforts. AIDS stigma further increases the negative impact of the epidemic on individuals, families, organizations, communities, and nations (see also King, 1989; Malcolm, Aggleton, Bronfman, Galvao, Mane, & Verrall, 1998; Muyinda, Selley, Pickering, & Barton, 1997). The Special Session concluded that nations should develop and implement multisectoral national strategies and financing plans to combat HIV/AIDS, plans that address the epidemic in forthright AIDS-stigma goals: conform stigma, silence, and denial; address gender- and age-based dimensions of the epidemic; and eliminate discrimination and marginalization. Also, by 2003, nations should create or strengthen laws, regulations, and other measures to eliminate all forms of discrimination against PWA and to ensure the full enjoyment of all human rights and fundamental freedoms by PWA. Nations attending the Special Session also agreed to extend aid to members of vulnerable groups—in particular, access to education, inheritance, employment, health care and other social services, prevention, support and treatment, information, and legal protection—while respecting their privacy and confidentiality (United Nations, 2001).

A *Progress Report* (UNAIDS, 2003) on the UN General Assembly Special Session shows that progress has been made in some Member States, but much work remains.[2] In the *Progress Report*, Peter Piot mentioned that

> a majority of countries worldwide have no legal protection in place to prohibit discrimination against vulnerable populations, and more than one-half of countries in Sub-Saharan Africa do not have laws to prevent discrimination on the basis of a person's HIV-positive status. (p. 7)

This figure is discouraging in the battle to curb AIDS stigma. While the Uganda constitution prohibits any form of discrimination, which can be broadly interpreted to include HIV-discrimination, there is no specific legislation to prevent discrimination against PWA. Only 38% of countries worldwide have adopted HIV-antidiscrimination laws (p. 10). The Uganda Ministry of Justice is spearheading a general HIV law that will include a section on HIV/AIDS-antidiscrimination. While establishing antidiscrimination legislation is helpful it is often not sufficient to prevent AIDS stigma. There is a need for the sensitization and education of the masses that stigma and discrimination will only drive the disease underground and eventually create a greater negative impact than would be realized in an open and accepting society. There is also a need to educate PWA about positive living, basic hygiene, food preparation, and helping secure children's inheritances after a parent dies of AIDS. Throughout the world, the shame and stigma associated with the HIV/AIDS epidemic have silenced open discussions in respect to both its causes and appropriate responses. This has caused those infected and affected by HIV/AIDS to feel guilty, ashamed, and unable to express their views or fight for their innate human rights.

DEFINING AIDS STIGMA AND DISCRIMINATION

Stigma can be defined in many ways and has existed for thousands of years in recorded society. Examples of disease-related stigma include treatment of those with leprosy, cholera, and syphilis (Valdiserri, 1987, 2002). Stigma is a social phenomenon which includes the holding of derogatory social attitudes or cognitive beliefs, the expression of negative effects, or the display of hostile or derogatory behaviors toward individuals or members of a group because of their association with or link to that group. Stigma is also a discrediting attribute that reduces the overall status of an individual in society, often leaving the victim without adequate familial or social support (Goffman, 1963). Discrimination, on the other hand, is a negative action based on a preexisting stigma that creates isolation. In the case of HIV and AIDS, stigma and discrimination are results of one's positive serostatus or association with the effects of the deadly human immunodeficiency virus.

AIDS stigma is a social construct that can take on many different forms, causing victims to be rejected, isolated, blamed, or ashamed (Alonzo & Reynolds, 2002). Individuals, groups, and societies are involved in stigmatizing others, which frequently occurs in the absence of conscious awareness or thought (see Figure 3.1). Often systematic and part of reinforcing existing societal norms and divisions, AIDS stigma hurts PWA, AIDS orphans, and those suspected of being infected with HIV. In some cases, association with PWA, illness, or the death of a relative or friend can also subject individuals to stigma. AIDS stigma is harmful to those facing the realities of the problem around which it exists, and sufferers often experience socioeconomic inequalities as well.

Many social factors influence how people might react to situations that potentially trigger AIDS stigma. These include individual levels of HIV/AIDS knowledge, positive and negative experiences with PWA, time of exposure with PWA, personal values, ethics, religious and traditional beliefs. Organizational culture is also a factor that influences how managers, employees, and potential employees view and deal with AIDS

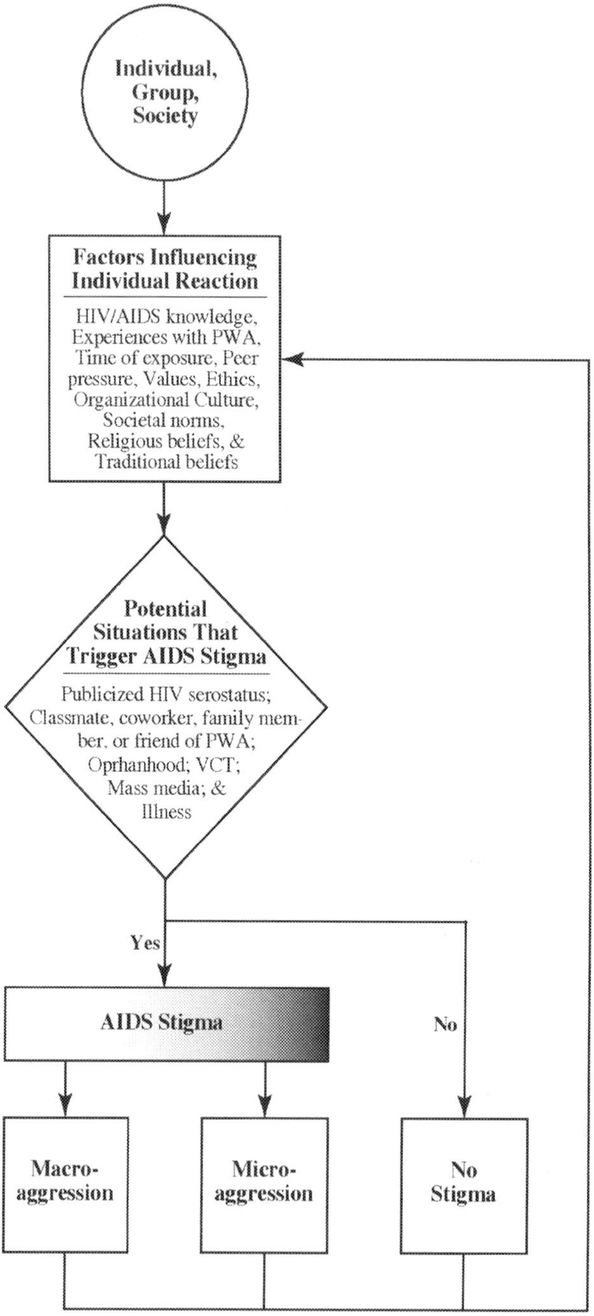

Figure 3.1.   AIDS Stigma Reaction Model

stigma.[3] While many private and government organizations have adopted anti-AIDS stigma policies, this has unfortunately not permeated all organizations throughout Uganda.[4] Peer pressure is another powerful factor that can impact people's reactions toward PWA, AIDS orphans, and friends/family members of PWA.

Although not the only scenarios where individuals might encounter one form of AIDS-related stigma, Figure 3.1 does provide several common potential situations that trigger AIDS stigma. These situations include publicizing one's HIV serostatus; during an individual's voluntary counseling and testing (VCT) experience; association with a classmate, coworker, family member, or friend of a PWA; association with AIDS orphans; stigma due to one of several mass media mediums including radio, television, Internet, or newspaper;[5] and illness that might be perceived as one who is suffering from AIDS symptoms.

AIDS stigma can be portrayed and experienced in many ways that mirror a spectrum, ranging from *nonaggressions* to *macroaggressions*. Keeping a child out of school, quarantining a person in an airport because he or she is HIV positive, or forcing an employee to take a blood-screening test to determine his or her serostatus are examples of AIDS macroaggression stigmas. There are also many other less obvious or even subconscious types of AIDS stigma that are based on a concept first introduced in the critical race theory literature called *microaggressions* (see for instance, Gordon & Johnson, 2003; Solorzano & Yosso, 2003; Villalpando, 2003). These can be more subtle, and they include verbal innuendos or negative body language expressed toward PWA. Comments like "they" or "them" versus "us" place PWA in a stigmatized state by forcing them into an "other" category. Continuously staring at or not wanting to sit by a student who is known to have HIV, or not being willing to play sports with PWA or their family members are forms of AIDS microaggression stigma. Microaggressions are day-to-day incidences that add up and eventually take a toll on a person's self-esteem, reputation, and interactions with others. If people encounter one of the situations portrayed in Figure 3.1 and react in a nonaggressive manner then they are considered to have no stigma attached to their reactions. Increased HIV/AIDS knowledge or associations with PWA are general predictors to reacting with no stigma when encountering one of the potential situations that triggers AIDS stigma in this model (Crawford, 1996; Kalichman & Simbayi, 2003).

There are different stages and levels of aggression an individual might have with AIDS stigma. For instance the first encounter an individual has with PWA is usually different than the second, tenth, or centennial encounter. The more time of exposure an individual has with PWA may decrease the amount of stigma reaction from an individual. Thus the feedback loop portrayed in Figure 3.1 shows a return from an AIDS stigma experience—be it a macroaggression, microaggression, or no stigma/nonaggression experience—adds to an individual's cumulative experience, portrayed in the box containing various factors influencing individual reactions to HIV/AIDS.

AIDS stigma is an obstacle to the prevention, treatment, and mitigation of HIV and AIDS. In many of the hardest hit countries, government officials, practitioners, and citizens—including those most affected by the epidemic—often continue to look the other way when HIV/AIDS victims are stigmatized because of the rejection, discrimination, and shame attached to AIDS (UNAIDS, 1998). AIDS stigma can be categorized into three main subgroups: *self-stigma*, *felt stigma*, and *enacted stigma* (Brown, Macintyre, & Trujillo, 2003; Jacoby, 1994; Malcolm et al., 1998; Scrambler, 1998; Scrambler & Hopkins, 1986).[6]

Self-Stigma

Self-stigma is the process whereby PWA impose feelings of difference, inferiority, and unworthiness on themselves. In many cases, self-stigma breeds hatred, shame, and blame and perpetuates self-pity and "unexplained" stress. One person with AIDS once expressed the following about her situation upon discovering that she had been infected with HIV:

> The way I saw myself fundamentally changed in a matter of minutes. I thought that I was marked, different from everyone else. I felt dirty, ashamed, and guilty. I wasn't sure why I felt guilty; it just felt like an appropriate response. (High School Teacher in Mbarara, Uganda, 2004)

Perhaps no one feels self-stigma more than at the time of his or her initial diagnosis of HIV. This situation is significantly amplified if the individual lacks a strong support mechanism, such as family, friends, classmates, and coworkers. Self-stigma only increases when a person is already highly vulnerable to low self-esteem. In some instances, individuals have dual or multiple stigmas, which are perpetuated through a negative synergistic or vicious-cycle effect. Sometimes individuals have preconceived misunderstandings or mythical beliefs about HIV and AIDS (Brown et al., 2003; Herek, 2002).

Self-stigma manifests itself in feelings of shame, dejection, self-doubt, guilt, self-blame, and inferiority. It perpetuates loss of self-esteem, confidence, and refusal of help from others, causing high levels of stress, anxiety, and denial. This jeopardizes the possibility for affected individuals to seek much-needed care, support, and treatment. The very nature of HIV transmission denotes for many a manner of self-induced infection (Sontag, 1989) or a violation of societal morals (Brandt, 1991).

Despite its destructive impact on the psyche of an individual, there are various ways to overcome self-stigma. Individuals faced with this situation can effectively benefit from peer support as well as from quality health care and counseling services. Self-stigma can be further overcome by disclosing HIV status to loved ones, by remaining productive in the family or community, and by learning more about HIV and AIDS. Access to antiretroviral treatment (ART) for those in need of medication and a genuine respect of the rights of all PWA help overcome self-stigma. In workplaces, supervisors can train and employ people who are HIV positive. In schools, teachers and administrators should be sensitive to the individual needs of their students; they should extend support to students who are HIV positive or who have parents who are suffering from the disease.

Felt Stigma

Felt stigma is when PWA or those affected by HIV/AIDS (such as family members, friends, or coworkers) experience fear associated with negative societal perspectives of HIV, AIDS, or other characteristics that are commonly associated with the disease (promiscuity, homosexuality, infection, parents with AIDS, etc.). For children, the stigma associated with being labeled an "AIDS orphan," or having a parent with HIV or AIDS, can cause psychological distress, isolation, and depression. A person may hide his or her HIV serostatus to avoid being discriminated against or ostracized by friends, family, and society (Brown et al., 2003). Felt stigma can also affect those who potentially could or would associate with PWA (Green & Platt, 1997; Simmoff, Erlen, & Lidz, 1991; Snyder, Omoto, & Crain, 1999).

Enacted Stigma

Enacted stigma are feelings that come from intentional acts of discrimination (Jacoby, 1994). Equally destructive to one's ability to effectively cope with infection or the effects of AIDS, enacted stigma is manifested in physical and social isolation by family, friends, and community. It is usually caused by gossiping or name-calling and can take the form of insults, judgment, blame, and condemnation. Individuals encounter a loss of rights and decision-making power, and sometimes stigma-by-association affects the whole family. HIV/AIDS-affected individuals suffer from enacted stigma when they receive cruel looks from others or unequal job opportunities and when they at times fail to maintain much-needed healthy social relationships.

The nature and intensity of AIDS stigma is shaped by the social construction of the epidemic in different locales. Stigma therefore needs to be discussed in its cultural context. Thomas et al. (2005) report on the results of a clinic-based study aimed at understanding stigma among 203 HIV-positive individuals in Chennai, South India. This study identifies the impact of stigma on the quality of life among these individuals as well as the gender implications of stigma. It was noted that the actual stigma experienced among individuals infected with HIV was much less (26%) as compared to the fear of being stigmatized or perceived stigma (97%). Internalizing of stigma was found to have a highly significant negative correlation with quality of life in the psychological domain and a significant negative correlation in the environmental domain. However individuals who did experience actual stigma seemed more determined to live and experience an above moderate quality of life. The implication of this study encourages HIV-infected individuals to rise above stigma, avoid internalizing their stigmatized feelings and work toward a better quality of life. Health providers need to address these issues in their care for HIV infected individuals.

FEATURES AND CAUSES OF AIDS STIGMA

Stigma is value laden, and it can be blatant or subtle (i.e., microaggressions), but it always results in a loss of status. It compromises human rights and is characterized by denial, ignorance, and fear (Panos Institute, 1990). All of these come from stereotyping, labeling, or pointing out differences between "us" and "them." The separation of "them" and "us" often leads to a victim being shunned, isolated, or rejected. Stigma is debilitating and gives PWA an inferior status.

Because AIDS stigma is described by its attributes, it is important to analyze some of its fundamental underlying causes. AIDS stigma primarily results from unawareness, misconceptions, or fears about the disease. AIDS stigma has perpetuated moral judgments and assumptions about the sexual behavior of PWA, as well as questions about their associations with illicit sex, alcohol, and drugs (Valdiserri, 2002; Walker & Booker, 2002). In some cases, stigma and discrimination have links with religion and the belief that HIV/AIDS is a punishment from God. In other words, AIDS stigma is the result of many factors: ignorance, intolerance, prejudice, absence of a widespread treatment or cure, irresponsible portrayal of the epidemic in the media, fears about death, and deep-rooted taboos about sexuality, illness, and drug use.

AIDS STIGMA BREEDS SILENCE

AIDS stigma has disastrous effects, ranging from mild microaggressions to serious violence, even death. It perpetuates isolation, dropping out of school, depression, suicide, alcoholism, violence, loss of employment, and diminished self-esteem. In relation to HIV/AIDS, stigma limits an individual's ability to get tested for HIV and thus affects that individual's access to treatment and care (Mill, 2003; Raveis, Siegel, & Gorey, 1998; Sowell Lowenstein, Moneyham, Demi, Mizuno, & Seals, 1997). In cases where quality counseling has not been provided, stigma can lead to the break-up of families and relationships. It therefore jeopardizes the potential of infected and affected people to live positively with HIV and AIDS. Stigma and discrimination breed silence about the deadly virus, and yet the first weapon needed is openness. Individuals become reluctant to open up for fear of the consequences and cannot, therefore, seek needed help and support. Unsafe behavior and practices could be perpetuated and, as a result, further promote the risk of infection.

Instigating and supporting AIDS stigma against PWA is a violation of human rights (Aggleton, 2000; Goldin, 1994; Herek, 2002; Mann, Tarantola, & Netter, 1992). Stigmatization places the oppressed in a different category from the rest of society, and in most cases, this categorization is subordinated to the societal norm. Armen H. Merjian (2002) described this phenomenon as akin to the creation of a "new class of individuals subject to widespread and often virulent prejudice and discrimination" (p. 117). PWA have experienced the negative aspects of AIDS stigma in virtually every area of their lives—education, employment, civil rights, and security (physical and emotional)—areas that are generally recognized as fundamental human rights for all.

Uganda's unwritten culture toward HIV and AIDS, often referred to as its *policy of openness*, has infiltrated the country's multiple cultures and ultimately has helped curb the overall HIV infection rates. Openness and widespread public support, coupled with a high level of political commitment, can help fight stigma and discrimination. When AIDS came to Africa, some countries—for tourism and other reasons—refused to admit that they faced a health epidemic. A majority of them have remained in that state of denial for a long time. This attitude provides fertile ground for the spread of the disease. In Uganda, because of the policy of openness, a number of people went public and announced their serostatus, which gave HIV/AIDS a human face and helped fight stigma and discrimination. The ability to be forthright about one's serostatus is essential in the fight against AIDS. Both local and national entities—governments, nongovernmental organizations (NGO), and ethnic groups—must be committed to this atmosphere of openness.

One such person known for his openness toward the disease was the renowned Ugandan artist Philly Bongolay Lutaya. Philly was a Ugandan musician based in Sweden who, in 1989, declared publicly that he was living with the virus that causes AIDS. He was the first Ugandan to give AIDS a human face. Philly turned suffering into an opportunity to help the rest of the world understand the reality of HIV/AIDS. For several months following his open declaration, Philly toured the country, performing his music and giving testimonies in schools, colleges, and other places. He hoped young people would listen to his warnings and live morally so as to avoid the pain and suffering associated with AIDS.

The crusade that Philly launched contains the essence of Uganda's current perspective on the fight against stigma and HIV/AIDS. His efforts were not in vain. Today the Philly Lutaya Initiative (PLI) has been founded on his philosophy of openness. Members of the PLI continue to conduct AIDS education campaigns in schools and provide other information to show how one can combat HIV-related stigma, discrimination, and denial.

The government of Uganda has won acclaim for its approach to the epidemic. It has also developed the concept of living positively with HIV/AIDS. Many people who went public and overcame the stigma and discrimination associated with HIV/AIDS are now able to live productive lives. It was on these principles of openness that The AIDS Support Organisation (TASO) was established in 1987. TASO was created by 16 original members, 12 of whom had HIV, to be primarily a counseling and support organization for PWA throughout the country. TASO has since grown to become the largest AIDS-oriented NGO in Africa and is recognized around the world as a leader and innovator in HIV/AIDS care and support.

STRATEGIES TO COUNTER AIDS STIGMA

We need to promote antidiscrimination laws at community, national, and international levels. The various international human rights treaties, conventions, and covenants that many countries have signed, as well as HIV/AIDS resolutions passed by the United Nations Human Rights Commission, should be more effectively disseminated in order to create awareness, influence change, and inform the general public about the law reform process.

Health care provision practices also need to be reviewed. The general health sector and its service organizations should be encouraged to review their policies, professional codes of conduct, and practices to prevent and redress stigma and discrimination (Mill, 2003; Woodhead, 2003). Training of health care providers is necessary to deal with AIDS stigma; policies and procedures also need to be established for action against those who breach agreed upon policies.

In the workplace, employees and employers should be sensitive to issues regarding stigma, discrimination, and people's rights with respect to HIV and AIDS. This will help reduce stigma and promote the positive attitudes necessary for an effective work environment and, above all, a healthier life.

We need to let people know the basic facts about HIV transmission, prevention, and management. Ignorance distorts the facts and breeds only fear, which in turn perpetuates AIDS stigma. A joint UNICEF, UNAIDS, and WHO (2002) study of 40 countries indicated that 50% of youth worldwide do not know how to protect themselves against HIV infection. There is a continuous need to provide accurate information to decrease misconceptions and fight unnecessary discrimination.

PWA and those affected by the epidemic bear the consequences and face the negative effects of AIDS stigma continually in their lives. Sharing such experiences humanizes the disease, allows communities to under-stand how HIV/AIDS impinges upon lives, and allows others to reflect on how they and their society are responding to the pandemic. These actions affect lives especially at the immediate family level. It is common for sib-lings, who in many instances are also parents, to die from the disease. Many children are orphaned because of AIDS, since most people who die from the epidemic are between ages 25–40. Thus immediate family mem-bers are called on to raise orphaned nieces and nephews. For children, this may mean living in a new home with an aunt, uncle, or other close relative. Because finances are generally limited among immediate family members, they are even scarcer for newly acquired AIDS-orphaned chil-dren. Those whose spouses have died recently will often remarry. In this scenario, it is likely that the remaining spouse of a partner who died from AIDS is also HIV positive. Thus the new spouse is likely to acquire the dis-ease, further perpetuating this vicious cycle.

Faith-based organizations and churches are also powerful sources of external influence in reducing the stigma of AIDS. Until recently, the Catholic church in South Africa remained silent or, worse still, adopted a theology that contributed to the stigma and discrimination faced by those who are HIV-positive. However, church leaders have taken a more positive public stance on education, prevention, care, support, and lobbying for treatment (Haddad, 2005).

AIDS stigma issues should constitute a central part of HIV/AIDS pre-vention and care programs at the individual, family, community, and national levels. All outreach work on this issue should discuss stigma, dis-crimination, and any human rights violations that result from them. Peer and outreach educators should be taught to address the issue of stigma and discrimination in their daily work.

The role of access to ART in the normalization of HIV/AIDS, as it moves from being categorized as a fatal disease to a chronic, manageable one, needs to be highlighted. Fear, one of the building blocks of stigma, can be reduced when people come to understand that having HIV or AIDS is not an automatic death sentence.

In conclusion, with a focus on stigma and discrimination, the world AIDS Campaign hopes to encourage people to break the silence and to break through barriers to effective HIV/AIDS prevention and care. Only by confronting stigma and discrimination will the fight against HIV/AIDS be won. We need to have communities and workplaces where people do not react negatively to news that a neighbor is HIV positive or that a family is dealing with the effects of AIDS. This will lead to an increased desire for sufferers to establish their status as HIV positive and will encourage victims to be open about the pandemic so that they can become a more solid force in fighting the spread of HIV/AIDS.

NOTES

1. The 189 UN member states adopted the Declaration of Commitment on HIV/AIDS and outlined a Millennium Development Goal to halt and begin to reverse the HIV/AIDS epidemic by 2015.

2. This is the first of several reports by UNAIDS on the state of the Declaration of Commitment. It is recognized as the most comprehensive assessment of national, regional, and global responses to HIV/AIDS.

3. We define organizational culture as a set of unwritten laws that exist within all organizations, that reflect on how an organization is both formally and informally operated. Examples of organizational culture include employee attire; socialization processes; established organizational norms; and treatment of minorities, disadvantaged groups, women, the elderly, and children at organizational facilities. D'Amelio, Raffaele D'Amelio, Perito, Biselli, Natalicchio, and Kingma (2001) note that only 17% of 121 sample countries had established laws that protect PWA in the workplace, at school, and at public facilities and events.

4. In some instances teachers, employees, and workers have been released from their jobs because their respective HIV-seropositive status was publicized. Unfortunately this type of AIDS stigma phenomenon is not limited to the workplace and occasionally spouses are divorced and family members ostracized when they are known to be HIV positive.

5. The media has had an immense impact on shaping the way the public views HIV and AIDS. For more information on how the media has affected the public image of AIDS, see Sander L. Gilman (1988) and Genevieve Paicheler (1992).

6. We recognize that other HIV/AIDS-related stigma categorizations have been used in the literature. The three subgroups we use in this chapter—self-stigma, felt stigma, and enacted stigma—are overarching and encompass other categorizations we have found in the literature. Theodore de Bruyn (2002) identifies three different subgroup categories worth noting—*institutional*, *noninstitutional*, and *structural stigma and discrimination*. Institutional stigma is similar to our definition of organizational culture or situations of stigma that occurs at the workplace, at school, or at a public venue or government operated facility. Noninstitutional stigma involves interpersonal relations with friends, family members, and the community in which one resides or interacts. De Bruyn's final subgroup, structural stigma and discrimination, incorporates both the institutional and noninstitutional subgroups but relates directly to issues of gender, ethnic identity, and socioeconomic status.

REFERENCES

Aggleton, P. (2000). *HIV and AIDS-related stigmatization, discrimination and denial: Research studies from Uganda and India*. Geneva, Switzerland: UNAIDS.

Alonzo, A. A., & Reynolds, N. R. (2002). Stigma, HIV and AIDS: An exploration and elaboration of a stigma trajectory. *Social Science & Medicine, 41*(3), 303–315.

Brandt, A. M. (1991). AIDS and metaphor: Toward the social meaning of epidemic disease. In A. Mack (Ed.), *In time of plague: The history and social consequences of lethal epidemic disease* (pp. 91–110). New York: University Press.

Brown, L., Macintyre, K., & Trujillo, L. (2003). Interventions to reduce HIV/AIDS stigma: What have we learned? *AIDS Education and Prevention, 15*(1), 49–69.

Bushee, J. M., & Hale, F. (2003). *HIV positive travelers singled out for quarantine in mumbai scheduled for release*. Amsterdam: Global Network of People Living with HIV/AIDS.

Cameron, E. (1993). Legal rights, human rights and AIDS: The first decade. *AIDS Analysis Africa, 3*, 3–4.

Chesney, M. A., & Smith, A. W. (1999). Critical delays in HIV testing and care: The potential role of stigma. *American Behavior Science, 42*, 1162–1174.

Crawford, A. M. (1996). Stigma associated with AIDS: A meta-analysis. *Journal of Applied Social Psychology, 26*(5), 398–416.

D'Amelio, R., Raffaele D'Amelio, E., Perito, O., Biselli, R., Natalicchio, S., & Kingma, S. (2001). A global review of legislation on HIV/AIDS: The issue of HIV testing. *Journal of Acquired Immune Deficiency Syndromes, 28*(2), 173–179.

de Bruyn, T. (2002). HIV-related stigma and discrimination: The epidemic continues. *HIV/AIDS Policy & Law Review, 7*(1), 8–14.

Gilman, S. L. (1988). *Disease and representation: Images of illness from madness to AIDS*. Ithica, NY: Cornell University Press.

Goffman, E. (1963). *Stigma: Notes on the management of spoiled identity*. New York: Simon & Shuster.

Goldin, C. S. (1994). Stigmatization and AIDS: Critical issues in public health. *Social Science and Medicine, 39*, 1359–1366.

Gordon, J., & Johnson, M. (2003). Race, speech, and a hostile educational environment: What color is free speech? *Journal of Social Philosophy, 34*(3), 414–436.

Green, G., & Platt, S. (1997). Fear and loathing in health care settings reported by people with HIV. *Sociology of Health & Illness, 19*(1) 70–92.

Haddad, B. (2005). Reflections on the church and HIV/AIDS: South Africa. *Theology Today, 62*(1), 29–37.

Herek, G. M. (2002). Thinking about AIDS and stigma: A psychologist's perspective. *Journal of Law, Medicine & Ethics, 30*, 594–607.

Herek, G. M., Capitanio, J. P., & Widaman, K. F. (2002). HIV-related stigma and knowledge in the United States: Prevalence and trends, 1991–1999. *American Journal of Public Health, 92*(3), 371–377.

Herek, G. M., Capitanio, J. P., & Widaman, K. F. (2003). Stigma, social risk, and health policy: Public attitudes toward HIV surveillance policies and the social construction of illness. *Health Psychology, 22*(5), 533–540.

Jacoby, A. (1994). Felt versus enacted stigma: A concept revisited. *Social Science and Medicine, 38*(2), 269–274.

Kalichman, S. C., & Simbayi, L. C. (2003). HIV testing attitudes, AIDS stigma, and voluntary HIV counselling and testing in a Black township in Cape Town, South Africa. *Sexually Transmitted Infections, 79*(6), 442–447.

King, M. B. (1989). Prejudice and AIDS: The views and experience of people with HIV infection. *AIDS Care, 1*(2), 137–143.

Malcolm, A., Aggleton, P., Bronfman, M., Galvao, J., Mane, P., & Verrall, J. (1998). HIV-related stigmatization and discrimination: Its forms and contexts. *Critical Public Health, 8*(4), 347–370.

Mann, J. M., Tarantola, D. J. M., & Netter, T. W. (1992). *AIDS in the world.* Cambridge, NY: Harvard University Press.

Merjian, A. H. (2002). The court at the epicenter of a new civil rights struggle: HIV/AIDS in the New York Court of Appeals. *St. John's Law Review, 75*(1), 115–124.

Mill, J. E. (2003). Shrouded in secrecy: Breaking the news of HIV infection to Ghanaian women. *Journal of Transcultural Nursing, 14*(1), 6–16.

Muyinda, H., Selley, J., Pickering, H., & Barton, T. (1997). Social aspects of AIDS-related stigma in rural Uganda. *Health and Place, 3*(3), 143–147.

Paicheler, G. (1992). A problem for sociological research: Society facing AIDS. *Current Sociology, 40*(3), 11–23.

Panos Institute. (1990). *The 3rd epidemic: Repercussions of the fear of AIDS.* Budapest, Hungary: Author.

Piot, P. (2001, September). *Press Release.* Paper presented at the World Conference against Racism, Racial Discrimination, Xenophobia and Related Intolerance, Durban, South Africa.

Raveis, V. H., Siegel, K., & Gorey, E. (1998). Factors associated with HIV-infected women's delay in seeking medical care. *AIDS Care, 10*(5), 549–562.

Scrambler, G. (1998). Stigma and disease: Changing paradigms. *The Lancet, 352*(9133), 1054–1055.

Scrambler, G., & Hopkins, A. (1986). Being epileptic, coming to terms with stigma. *Sociology of Health and Illness, 8*, 26–43.

Simmoff, L. A., Erlen, J. A., & Lidz, C. W. (1991). Stigma, AIDS and quality of nursing care: State of the science. *Journal of Advanced Nursing, 16*, 262–269.

Snyder, M., Omoto, A. M., & Crain, A. L. (1999). Punished for their good deeds: stigmatization of AIDS volunteers. *American Behavior Science, 42*, 1175–1192.

Solorzano, D., & Yosso, T. J. (2003). Critical race and LatCrit theory and method: Counter-storytelling. *International Journal of Qualitative Studies in Education, 14*(4), 471–495.

Sontag, S. (1989). *AIDS and its metaphors*. New York: Farrar, Straus and Giroux.

Sowell, R. L., Lowenstein, A., Moneyham, L., Demi, A., Mizuno, Y., & Seals, B. F. (1997). Resources, stigma, and patterns of disclosure in rural women with HIV infection. *Public Health Nursing, 14*(5), 302–312.

Thomas, B. E., Rehman, F., Suryanarayanan, D., Josephine, K., Dilip, M., Dorairaj, V. S., & Swaminathan, S. (2005). How stigmatizing is stigma in the life of people living with HIV: A study on HIV positive individuals from Chennai, South India. *AIDS Care, 17*(7), 802–817.

UNAIDS. (2003). *Progress report on the global response to the HIV/AIDS epidemic, 2003*. Geneva, Switzerland: Author.

UNAIDS/WHO. (2004). *Uganda epidemiological fact sheets on HIV/AIDS and sexually transmitted infection*. Geneva, Switzerland: Author.

UNICEF, UNAIDS, and WHO. (2002). *Young people and HIV/AIDS: Opportunities in crisis*. New York: UNICEF.

United Nations. (2001). *Declaration of commitment on HIV/AIDS*. New York: United Nations General Assembly Special Session on HIV/AIDS.

Valdiserri, R. O. (1987). Epidemics in perspective. *Journal of Medical Humanities Bioethics, 8*, 95–100.

Valdiserri, R. O. (2002). HIV/AIDS stigma: An impediment to public health. *American Journal of Public Health, 92*(3), 341–342.

Villalpando, O. (2003). Self-segregation or self-preservation? A critical race theory and Latina/o critical theory analysis of a study of Chicana/o college students. *International Journal of Qualitative Studies in Education, 16*(5), 619–646.

Walker, W. T., & Booker, S. (2002, November 28–December 4, 2002). AIDS: Discrimination is deadly. *The New York Amsterdam News*, p. 13.

Woodhead, K. (2003). Fighting AIDS stigma: Caring for all. *British Journal of Perioperative Nursing, 13*(6), 255–261.

PART II

HIV/AIDS EDUCATION PROGRAMS IN THE FORMAL EDUCATION SECTOR

CHAPTER 4

EVALUATION OF HIV/AIDS EDUCATION PROGRAMS IN UGANDA

**W. James Jacob, Donald E. Morisky,
Steven J. Hite, and Yusuf K. Nsubuga**

This chapter begins with a review of research that has been published on HIV/AIDS education programs in Uganda. It discusses governmental support for educational initiatives from the mid-1980s to the present. Within this context of descriptive literature and policy, we introduce a national study conducted among students ($N = 883$), teachers ($N = 443$), and administrators ($N = 217$) at 76 secondary schools in 2002–2004. Findings indicated a significant knowledge difference between groups: students having a significantly lower understanding compared with teachers and administrators on how to prevent becoming infected with HIV and how to treat HIV/AIDS. Intervention programs were implemented, and students who participated significantly increased their overall HIV/AIDS knowledge, supporting the effectiveness of in-class discussions on the topic. Results also indicated a moderate increase in knowledge levels of teachers and administrators who participated in the intervention group.

Overcoming AIDS: Lessons Learned from Uganda, 63–83
Copyright © 2006 by Information Age Publishing

INTRODUCTION AND OVERVIEW

Impacting over half of Uganda's approximately 26 million people under the age of 16, the education sector plays a prominent role in the HIV/AIDS epidemic. Believed to be the epicenter of AIDS in the 1970s and 1980s (Mbulaiteyea, Mahe, Ruberantwari, & Whitworth, 2002; Mugyeni, 2002), Uganda has had a long history of AIDS involvement. Fortunately, Uganda has experienced much success in recent years in curbing the epidemic. Yet many questions remain on how to best keep the disease from escalating: What are some of the sociostructural and environmental forces in Uganda which are driving down the prevalence of HIV/AIDS that can benefit neighboring countries? What role does education play in reversing the trends of the epidemic? What role will education continue to have towards overcoming the epidemic? How can education help with Uganda's orphaned children crisis?

The Ministry of Education and Sports (MOES) first introduced HIV/AIDS prevention campaigns on a national level in 1986. Activities introduced included various media messages targeting youth, HIV/AIDS education in the primary curriculum, and school theatrical performances that depicted real-life scenarios facing youth. School plays were held in over 8,500 primary schools nationwide, while additional performances were translated and presented in 12 local languages (Malinga, 2000). While a syllabus was written for instruction at the secondary level, this did not enter the formal curriculum until later (Jacob, Mosman, Hite, Morisky, & Nsubuga, 2006). The advent of universal primary education (UPE) in 1997 created an ideal pedagogical moment to reach the majority of children in the country. Thus Uganda policy makers embraced education as an essential medium for disseminating HIV/AIDS prevention information. In 1995, the government instigated a life skills program in the curriculum focusing on adolescent needs and behavior consequences.

At the primary level[1] students are introduced to instruction on sexually transmitted diseases and HIV/AIDS prevention (Ministry of Health, 2001). This most regularly occurs in the upper primary level grades, where students are entering adolescence. Two additional handbooks were introduced at the primary level in 2003—a resource handbook for teachers and a student handbook with 24 key messages. President and Mrs. Yoweri Museveni proposed a new education program that would disseminate HIV/AIDS prevention, treatment, and mitigation information to students on a more sustained basis. The culmination of this initiative was a multisectoral project called *PIASCY*—Presidential Initiative on AIDS Strategy for Communication to Youth. PIASCY has several components including head-teachers holding schoolwide assemblies biweekly. Using the *PIASCY Handbook for Teachers* as a guide, teachers were asked to incorporate these messages into their respective classrooms throughout the school year. Where PIASCY originally targeted UPE students, it also is an adaptable model for introducing HIV/AIDS instruction at the secondary subsector level. In addition to the teacher's handbook, student handbooks have also been produced, one for the lower secondary students (Senior 1 to 4 grade levels) and one for the upper secondary students (Senior 5 to 6 grade levels).

MOES and teacher training institutions have developed a curriculum strategy to integrate HIV/AIDS instruction initially into five subjects and eventually into every subject offered in secondary schools. Our findings show that one of the most common criticisms teachers and students have had toward HIV/AIDS instruction as part of the formal classroom instruction is that it has never been included as an examination topic for the secondary leaving examinations.[2] Thus many teachers could not justify holding class discussions regarding HIV issues, as they had only a certain amount of time to prepare students with the subject matter for exam preparation. Similarly many students felt that wavering from the class subject matter was not a good use of class time. Discussions about HIV and AIDS were thus entrusted to nonformal education mediums, even among students in the formal education system.[3] Making HIV/AIDS part of the official curriculum will help obviate this criticism shared by teachers and students.

The five secondary school subjects that have HIV/AIDS instruction integrated into their curriculum since the beginning of the 2004 school year include biology; health science and life skills; English; literature; and music, dance, and drama.[4] While the MOES is striving to implement HIV/AIDS instruction in all subjects, this has not yet been realized. HIV/AIDS prevention, treatment, and control issues woven into the curriculum seem like a good fit to help link the subject matter with students' actual lives.

Relatively few research studies have been published on education and the HIV/AIDS epidemic (Hyde, Ekatan, Kiage, & Barasa, 2002). Among the studies conducted, most are limited to a case within a single district (De Walque, 2004; Kinsman, Harrison, Kengeya-Kayondo, Kanyesigye, Musoke, & Whitworth, 1999; Kinsman et al., 2001; Kirby et al., 1994; Shuey, Babishangire, Omiat, & Bagarukayo, 1999) or a case study of two Central Region Districts (Hyde et al., 2002). All of these studies have relatively limited sample sizes. The limited generalizability of the findings of these studies amplifies the need for a broader examination of the epidemic through an educational lens. The study discussed in this chapter helps fill this need by examining secondary education programs in twelve districts, three from each of Uganda's main geographic regions.[5]

METHODS

School Selection Process

From the official MOES list of secondary schools consisting of a total of 1,948 schools, 76 secondary schools were randomly selected and stratified by geographic region, urbanicity,[6] and type of school (government or private).[7] Schools selected were evenly distributed among the four main geographic regions, with a slightly larger number of schools in the Central Region because it contains the largest portion of the population. Selection was also evenly distributed between rural and urban schools, except for districts that were almost entirely urban (i.e., Kampala District). Private and government schools were evenly stratified at 38 schools each.

Study Participants

Participating administrators ($N = 217$), teachers ($N = 433$), and students ($N = 883$) were randomly selected from the master enrollment and teacher roster lists at the sample schools to receive questionnaires (see

Table 4.1.   Characteristics of Sample Secondary Students

	Frequency	Percentage
Gender		
Female	443	50.2
Male	440	49.8
Age		
12–14	112	12.7
15–17	409	46.3
18–20	332	37.6
21–26	30	3.4
Urbanicity		
Urban	488	55.3
Rural	395	44.7
Geographic Region		
Central	299	33.8
Eastern	212	24.0
Northern	156	17.7
Western	216	24.5
Governance		
Government	466	52.8
Private	417	47.2

Table 4.2.   Characteristics of Sample Administrators and Teachers

	Administrators		Teachers	
	Frequency	Percentage	Frequency	Percentage
Gender				
Female	46	21.2	119	27.5
Male	171	78.8	314	72.5
Experience (in years)				
1–3	64	29.5	146	33.7
4–6	63	29.0	105	24.2
7–9	34	15.7	63	14.6
10–12	16	7.4	54	12.5
13–15	10	4.6	28	6.5
16 or more	30	13.8	37	8.5
AIDS Training				
Yes	165	76.0	339	78.3
No	52	24.0	94	21.7
Urbanicity				
Urban	119	54.8	239	55.2
Rural	98	45.2	194	44.8
Geographic Region				
Central	70	32.2	141	32.6
Eastern	54	24.9	107	24.7
Northern	39	18.0	77	17.8
Western	54	24.9	108	24.9
Governance				
Government	116	53.5	231	53.3
Private	101	46.5	202	46.7

Tables 4.1 and 4.2). Response rates for the pre and posttreatment surveys were 95.2 and 89.9% for administrators, 95.0 and 79.2% for teachers, and 96.5 and 91.1% for students. The student sample was further stratified by gender and grade level. Quantitative information was complemented by qualitative, in-depth interviews, allowing triangulation of data with randomly selected administrators ($N = 10$), teachers ($N = 38$), and students ($N = 50$) from the sample participants. While this chapter primarily focuses on the intervention program and overview of this study, two additional articles written by the editors discuss qualitative findings associated with administrator, teacher, and student perspectives on effective educational strategies for overcoming HIV/AIDS in schools (Jacob, Mosman, Hite, Morisky, & Nsubuga, 2006; Jacob, Mosman, Morisky, Hite, & Nsubuga, 2006). A follow-up focus group was held the following year with participants from each of the 76 schools, to determine the level of

integration of HIV/AIDS instruction into their formal or extracurricular activities.

IRB Approval

This study conformed to three institutional review boards (IRBs) during the planning, implementation, and evaluation stages: the University of California, Los Angeles; Uganda's MOES; and Brigham Young University. All members of the research team assured responsibility for continuing review of ongoing research to ensure that the rights and welfare of human subjects were protected. The research team gave participating schools two tuition and fees scholarships to help educate students who have been orphaned by having one or both parents die from HIV/AIDS. Prior to participating in this study, selected students, teachers, and administrators all signed consent forms endorsed by the UCLA Office for Protection of Research Subjects.

Advisory Committee

The research team met regularly with members of an advisory committee from the onset of this study and kept the committee informed as the study progressed. National and regional government, religious, and community leaders, and representatives from the study populations joined our advisory committee and offered helpful advice, including a wider perspective on the Ugandan educational context. The committee was responsible for revising wording and selecting questions included in the study relevant to the Uganda context. Absence of an advisory board in developmental stages was a crucial drawback of the Kinsman et al. (2001) study on rural secondary schools in Masaka District, Uganda.

Instruments

The baseline and follow-up questionnaires were based on WHO/UNESCO's *School Health Education to Prevent AIDS and STD—A Resource Package for Curriculum Planners* (WHO/UNESCO, 1999). Questionnaires were administered in a group setting to approximately 21 participants randomly selected from each school, consisting of students ($N = 12$, two from each *form* or "grade level"), teachers ($N = 6$), and administrators ($N = 3$). Because of the relatively small sample size from each school, we did not experience difficulty in maintaining confidentiality and integrity of responses. The questionnaires were administered and monitored both by members of our research team and by school administrators. Instruments used unique identification numbers linking subjects between pre and postquestionnaires and identifying individuals participating in the study's intervention. The names of subjects participating in this study were never used in the coding or data collection process and would not be distributed in any way to government or other organizations. The interval between baseline and follow-up interviews was between 6 weeks and 2 months; and intervals between baseline questionnaire and interventions were between 2 weeks and a month.

Theoretical foundations of the study questionnaires and in-depth interviews included the theory of reasoned action (Ajzen, 1985; Ajzen & Fishbein, 1980; Fishbein & Ajzen, 1975; Fishbein, Middlestadt, & Hitchcock, 1991; Terry, Gallios, & McCamish, 1993) and the information-motivation-behavioral skills model (Fisher & Fisher, 1992). Both frameworks have been combined to form what is known as the behavioral changes for interventions (BCI) model (King & Wright, 1993), used in the development and planning stages of intervention programs. Knowledge acquisition, attitude development, motivational support, and skills development are the primary antecedents of this model.

Pilot Test of Questionnaire and Intervention

Our research team pilot tested the questionnaires at a local secondary school in Mukono. The pilot study consisted of an initial visit during which we administered the questionnaire to randomly selected students, teachers, and administrators. We went through the questionnaire with participants and received feedback on each of the consent, questionnaire, and intervention processes. The questionnaire was fine-tuned to improve alignment of the wording and phrasing of questions with Ugandan cultures and contexts. A second visit to this school was arranged to conduct focus groups related to our intervention program with two groups of participants: one with students and a second with teachers and administrators. We separated the two groups so that students could feel comfortable discussing HIV/AIDS issues openly without having their teachers and administrators in the same room. Group members who participated in this pilot intervention agreed that this was the best type of format to get students, teachers, and administrators to participate openly and candidly.

Intervention

An intervention program was then facilitated in 26 of the schools selected from our sample. This intervention was developed jointly by W. James Jacob, Donald E. Morisky, and Lynn R. Curtis, Vice President of ProLiteracy Worldwide International Programs.[8] The research team facilitated a learner-guided discussion around the topics needed to clarify and increase awareness of HIV/AIDS issues among the various participant groups. This intervention approach included a focus group strategy based on participatory methods which ultimately culminated in action decisions by the participants.

The problems connected with HIV/AIDS extended into every facet of life. Systematically addressing these problems requires an approach that accounts for intersection and overlap. Traditionally, international development initiatives have focused in one of six areas—education, health, economic self-reliance, environment, peace, or human rights. While each of these areas is crucial to promoting individual and community development, permanent solutions are found not in advancing one single area, but in empowering people to effectively integrate them all within a given local or national context. Increasingly, local contexts are being impacted by globalization of trade, technology, and economies. A combined, democratic approach provides the foundation for needed empowerment.

We used Jacob and Curtis' *Overcoming AIDS Manual* (2002), published by ProLiteracy Worldwide, which guided our research in facilitating the focus groups in discussions associated with multiple HIV/AIDS topics. Participants were divided into two groups—one consisting of students and another of teachers and administrators. Unlike Robina Mirembe's (2002) focus groups that separated male and female students, we included voices of both genders in both groups, due to the sexual nature of matters being discussed. Our interventions add to the findings of an earlier study using focus groups conducted by Kinsman et al. (2001) in rural schools in Masaka District, Uganda. Yet unlike the findings in the Kinsman et al. study, our focus groups were well attended, interactive using small-group dynamics, and intellectually invigorating, in which they ultimately led to action agreed upon by group consensus.

ProLiteracy Worldwide has developed a unique approach that combines education with cutting-edge strategies for human development (see Figure 4.1). Known as *Literacy for Social Change*, this approach integrates fundamental skills, critical thinking, cultural expression, and action to help individuals and communities to assess their material and social needs and to implement solutions to pressing local problems. *Literacy for Social Change* is a holistic instructional approach that accounts for the experiences, needs, preferences and priorities of individual learners and

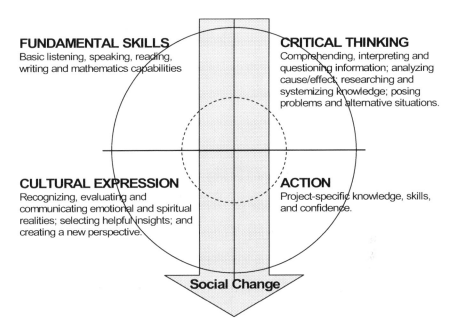

FUNDAMENTAL SKILLS
Basic listening, speaking, reading, writing and mathematics capabilities

CRITICAL THINKING
Comprehending, interpreting and questioning information; analyzing cause/effect; researching and systemizing knowledge; posing problems and alternative situations.

CULTURAL EXPRESSION
Recognizing, evaluating and communicating emotional and spiritual realities; selecting helpful insights; and creating a new perspective.

ACTION
Project-specific knowledge, skills, and confidence.

Social Change

Figure 4.1.   Literacy for Social Change Approach. Reprinted from Jacob and Curtis (2002, p. iii), with permission from Proliteracy Worldwide.

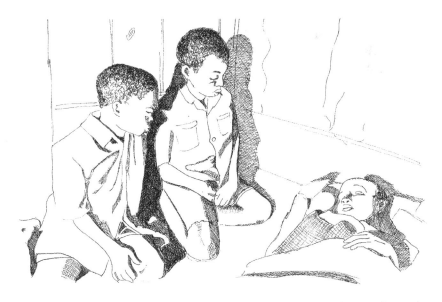

Figure 4.2.   Organizing for the Care of Orphans Code. Drawn by Natalie Jacob and reprinted from Jacob and Curtis (2002, p. 57), with permission from Proliteracy Worldwide.

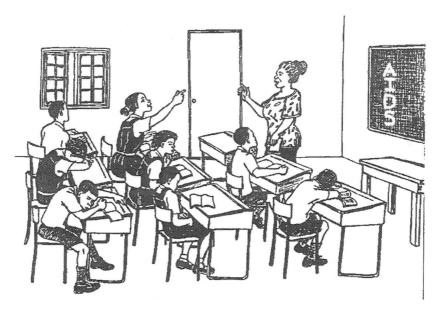

Figure 4.3.   What Role Should Schools Have in Helping to Overcome AIDS
Code. Drawn by Operation Upgrade, Durban, South Africa in Jacob and Curtis
(2002, p. 9), with permission from Proliteracy Worldwide.

their communities. Our education intervention process begins in a group
setting where local facilitators use *codes* (pictures or learning activities)
that reflect realities from the learners' lives. These locally produced codes
address relevant issues pertaining to a particular area of community
development (see Figure 4.2).

Based on theories established by Paulo Freire (1971) and Frank
Charles Laubach (Curtis, 1990, 1996; Laubach, 1967), codes educate
and empower people in a variety of international and development contexts. Codes are a powerful tool for facilitating group discussions. Figure 4.2, one of several codes we used during interventions, portrays two
secondary-aged school children caring for a parent dying from AIDS.
The code drew out strong emotions and feelings from a majority of the
intervention participants. Discussion topics ranged from how to help
family members and others with AIDS to what to do if one or both parents die.

Linking the discussion to schools and to the formal education sector,
we used a code that asked what role schools should take in helping to
overcome the epidemic (see Figure 4.3). This code helped participants
discuss what is being taught in their respective schools and what should

be taught. Often discussions led to participants agreeing that schools could be more active in their teaching and classroom discussions regarding the topic. Helping integrate HIV/AIDS education topics into previously set curriculum was a common action commitment of participant groups that used Figure 4.3 during their intervention focus group discussion. This commitment affirms that administrators, teachers, and students are willing to support the MOES's plan to integrate HIV/AIDS instruction into the existing formal curriculum.

Within the use of these codes, learners generate a dialogue based on questions that guide them from observation to reflection to action. These layers of questions provide a structure that generates key ideas as the substance of the discussion is built on participants' own experiences. As a result, learners exercise ownership of the ideas and internalize and apply important information readily.

Using this information, learners then design and implement action plans that address their individual and community needs. These plans include strategies for preventing HIV/AIDS, improving education, promoting human rights, starting health clinics, digging clean-water wells, forming microcredit and cooperative business ventures, overseeing reforestation projects, and carrying out a host of other participant-generated efforts. More significant than these observable action projects, however, is a base of new skills, information, values, and confidence that enables learners to continue development plans and efforts long after the outside agents are gone.

As part of the discussion and implementation of community action plans, participants also take part in learning activities. Based on codes using the *Literacy for Social Change Approach*, facilitators help learners produce action plans relating to development themes, which are then used in a range of reading and writing practice exercises. These learning activities are meaningful not only because they are based on the learners' own experience, but also because they address individual and schoolwide critical daily challenges, often going beyond the classroom to form a crucial aspect of solutions to shared concerns.

Facilitators guide the focus groups by following a sequence designed to generate discussion and critical thinking on various levels. This pattern of questioning is called *FAMA* (Facts, Association, Meaning, and Action):

1. **Facts:**   Questions that draw on the physical or sensory aspects of the code and allow participants to sharpen their observation and enter the discussion easily.

2. **Associations:**   Questions that refer to personal experiences of individual participants and the shared experience of the group.

3. **Meaning:**   Questions that help participants flesh out principles, ideas, and values represented in the code.

4. **Action:**   Questions that encourage participants to apply the discussion in their daily lives and allow them to plan to accomplish specific objectives.

The research team facilitating the discussions took special care to guide participants into the leading issues addressed in the first questionnaire. They were careful not to linger on issues that they were convinced participants already knew. Facilitators were also careful to insure that the participants were clear about the main issues addressed in the intervention, which were predominantly established by group interests and relevancy, and were largely generated by discussion.

FINDINGS

Although our data include findings on the curriculum, knowledge, attitudes, skills, and intentions of participants, the remainder of this chapter examines the impact of our intervention program on participant knowledge. The knowledge index consists of 46 questions, broken into five primary constructs: general knowledge, modes of HIV transmission, prevention strategy beliefs, self-efficacy beliefs, and treatment (see Table 4.3).

Prequestionnaire findings highlight a significant variability between groups, with 68.8% of teachers and 67.7% of administrators scoring *high* on the knowledge index, compared with only 28.1% of student participants ($X^2 = 269.20$ $p < .001$). Older students tended to perform better than younger students, especially comparing the oldest students with the youngest. Where Uganda secondary schools enroll students ranging from ages 12 to 26, many students are sexually active, unmarried young adults (Hogle, Green, Nantulya, Stoneburner, & Stover, 2002). It is generally better to compare knowledge between ages rather than grade levels, as students may range 5 to 10 years within a grade level. Where grade level comparison is somewhat misleading, age tends to provide a more accurate picture among secondary school students.

Urbanicity was a clear indicator for participant knowledge. Where 33.0% of urban students had a high knowledge index score, only 22.0% of rural students scored high ($X^2 = 17.69$ $p < .001$). Participants from the Central Region tended to score higher than those from the other regions, except among administrators. Among Eastern Region Administrators, 77.8% scored high, compared with only 51.9% and 59.0% of Western and

Table 4.3. Prequestionnaire Knowledge Index Scores by Stratification

	Administrators (%)			Teachers (%)			Students (%)		
	N	High	X^2	N	High	X^2	N	High	X^2
Aggregate Scores	217	67.7		433	68.8		883	28.1	
Gender									
Female	46	67.4	.08	119	77.3	8.44*	443	24.6	9.07*
Male	171	67.8		314	65.6		440	31.6	
Age									
12–14							112	16.1	68.97***
15–17							409	20.0	
18–20							332	39.4	
21–26							30	56.7	
Urbanicity									
Urban	119	74.0	4.98	239	71.1	8.58*	488	33.0	17.69***
Rural	98	60.2		194	66.0		395	22.0	
Geographic Region									
Central	70	77.1	13.55*	141	77.3	8.72	299	32.4	16.60*
Eastern	54	77.8		107	67.3		212	20.3	
Northern	39	59.0		77	63.6		156	27.6	
Western	54	51.9		108	63.0		216	30.1	
Governance									
Government	116	69.8	.20	231	74.5	10.58**	466	31.3	5.68**
Private	101	65.4		417	62.4		417	24.4	

*p < .05; **p < .01; ***p < .001

Northern Regional Administrators respectively ($X^2 = 13.55 \ p < .05$). Participants from government schools were distinctly higher in all categories than were participants from private schools.

Control and intervention groups were established; comparisons between these two groups are provided in Tables 3.4 and 3.5. All groups performed better on the postquestionnaire than they did in their first attempt. This is probably due to knowledge gained by repetitive testing bias, as the participants had been exposed to and thence were somewhat familiar with the material as it was readministered.

The increase of knowledge among students in the intervention group (up 19.4% from the pretest) was striking compared the performance of the control group, which only rose 4.8%. Male students improved their knowledge indexes the most from the intervention, gaining 24.2% compared to 14.0% by female intervention students. This trend did not hold true for students in the control group, as both genders had moderate increases: 4.6% and 5.6% among female and male students respectively.

Administrators in the intervention group, which showed a combined 3.9% increase, actually improved their scores moderately less overall than did administrators in the control group, which realized a 6.9% increase. Teachers in the intervention group (up 8.8% from the pretest) had a marginally higher increase than teachers in the control group (up 7.5%).

Tables 4.4 and 4.5 highlight subgroup differences between male and female participants in knowledge index scores. Males tended to have

Table 4.4.   Knowledge Index Scores: Control Groups

	Administrators (%)			Teachers (%)			Students (%)		
	N	High	X^2	N	High	X^2	N	High	X^2
Prequestionnaire									
Female	25	60.0	.56	61	75.4	5.73	282	20.9	10.05**
Male	122	63.9		231	61.9		302	30.5	
Combined Total	147	63.3		292	64.7		584	25.9	
Postquestionnaire									
Female	23	73.9	.20	50	80.0	3.55	271	25.5	7.65*
Male	108	69.4		184	70.1		269	36.1	
Combined Total	131	70.2		234	72.2		540	30.7	

*$p < .05$; **$p < .01$

Table 4.5.   Knowledge Index Scores: Intervention Groups

	Administrators (%)			Teachers (%)			Students (%)		
	N	High	X^2	N	High	X^2	N	High	X^2
Prequestionnaire									
Female	21	76.2	.40*	58	79.3	.61	161	31.1	.968
Male	49	77.6		83	75.9		138	34.1	
Combined Total	70	77.1		141	77.3		299	32.4	
Postquestionnaire									
Female	21	85.7	6.54*	48	85.4	2.07	144	45.1	4.56
Male	42	78.6		60	86.7		120	58.3	
Combined Total	63	81.0		108	86.1		264	51.8	

*$p < .05$

higher prequestionnaire scores than females among administrators in both the control and intervention groups, but lower than females among teachers in both groups. Yet when administrators and teachers took the post test questionnaire, females outperformed males in both control and intervention groups. Female administrators improved by 13.9% and 9.5% respectively in control and intervention groups. Male students maintained a larger percentage of high knowledge index scores on both tests in both control and intervention groups. Why the gender knowledge gap exists in the student control and intervention groups is somewhat puzzling. Female students in our sample tended to be slightly younger, with an average age of 16.6 compared with the average male student at 17.3 years. Since older students generally scored higher on the pretest than did younger students, this age difference may be one reason why male students generally scored higher than female students.

DISCUSSION

It is difficult to infer why students in the intervention group gained more knowledge than the administrators and teachers between pre and postquestionnaires, as the same intervention protocol was followed for all three groups. Although the same codes and settings were used among all intervention groups, discussions and group action items did often vary between administrator and teacher intervention groups and student intervention groups.

Establishing and maintaining a learner-friendly atmosphere was a key element to intervention success. Learning was found to be most effective as participants freely expressed their ideas, feelings, and experiences. Such open participation can stimulate genuine learner ownership of the concepts discussed and inspire action and change. Goals agreed upon by all groups included the following three themes: (1) to abstain from sexual intercourse during school years and until marriage; (2) once married, to be faithful to one's spouse; and (3) to hold regular peer education seminars and club meetings to discuss various HIV/AIDS topics. Although these were common action items that the group as a whole voted to adopt, there was often a vigorous discussion—and in some cases debate— prior to the group adopting something as a creed. Teachers and administrators were also interested in discussing ways to include HIV/AIDS instruction in their classes; their group action goals generally targeted a pedagogical perspective. Students tended to focus mostly on behavioral commitments to prevention and treatment.

Teachers, administrators, and students of all intervention schools expressed a deeply felt need and desire to participate in open, safe dialogue about HIV/AIDS. Although HIV/AIDS was not part of the official secondary education curriculum or syllabus at the time of this intervention, head teachers generally welcomed open dialogue associated with the AIDS epidemic. The only negative responses, which were few, were over limited time of already over-burdened administrators and teachers. Students for the most part showed great interest in attending and participating in HIV/AIDS discussions, and the topic often rekindled varied emotions, memories, and first-hand experiences from all participants. All participants had friends, kin, or both who had suffered in one way or another from the disease. For example, the picture shown in Figure 4.2 portrays two children caring for their dying parent which often sparked poignant and meaningful discussions amongst focus group participants.

The first session for persons living with HIV or AIDS (PWA) generally provoked intense emotional responses (debate, tears, laughter, surprise, etc.), accompanied by expressions of relief and enthusiasm for at last having a safe forum for learning and discussion about HIV/AIDS. Many schools committed to maintain this dialogue as part of regular extracurricular activities among students, teachers, and administrators.

Participants expressed new awareness, knowledge, and skills related to avoiding high-risk behavior. Many questions were asked regarding modes of transmission, myths, and sexually appropriate behavior. As sessions continued, participants frequently expressed intent to engage in new, more supportive behavior toward PWA. Participants often proposed individual or group action to provide support or encouragement to PWA or to help AIDS orphans. Participants also shared recent discussions they had been having with peers, neighbors, and family members regarding HIV/AIDS.

Participants often described improved communications and relationships emerging with parents, siblings, children, extended family, neighbors, fellow-students, teachers, and coworkers as a result of new HIV/AIDS conversations they were having in direct response to assignments coming from these sessions. The intervention accelerated organizational action and mobilized additional local resources to provide initial exposure to PWA's materials and training. Incentive grants generated an enthusiastic, active organizational response and stimulated participating schools to launch expanded and improved HIV/AIDS programs. In the process they mobilized additional programmatic resources for prevention and treatment than had originally existed or been planned at the schools.

Most participants felt that the MOES should make HIV/AIDS instruction a formal part of the national curriculum and thus included on secondary national examinations at the Ordinary and Advanced levels. This somewhat controversial approach has been debated for nearly two decades, especially after the School Health Education Program (SHEP) recommended that HIV/AIDS should be a nonexaminable topic and thus excluded from the formal education leaving examinations. Many teacher and administrator participants provided qualitative feedback in focus groups, and in response to the questionnaires they stated that they would like to spend more time on HIV and AIDS in the classroom but were already constrained to teach the subject matter required by the MOES and examinable on their Ordinary- and Advanced-level examinations.

STUDY LIMITATIONS

All groups improved their knowledge index scores between pre and postintervention questionnaires. This may have been due to a repetitive testing bias to exposure to the same test material (Nelson, Gordon, Simmons, Goldberg, Howland, & Hoffman, 2000). The study could have been strengthened by attempting to limit this bias by not informing participants beforehand of the posttest date. Yet the authors and advisory board decided it was necessary to risk the influence of repetitive testing bias in order to schedule all study activities in advance to accommodate the busy schedules of school administrators, teachers, and students. Administrators and teachers were particularly pressed for time and many had to miss an entire class or two to participate in each phase of the study.

CONCLUSION AND IMPLICATIONS FOR THE FUTURE

Uganda has a rich history for addressing HIV/AIDS issues in the education sector. Although this educational heritage has been primarily at the extracurricular level, some HIV/AIDS curricular initiatives have been produced in the primary subsector. At the beginning of the 2004 school year, integration of HIV/AIDS issues in five subjects and a teacher handbook for instruction has been developed and implemented at the secondary level. Beginning in 1986, the government instigated a national program facilitating epidemic discussions through extracurricular activities, including mass media, drama, and peer education. Where these extracurricular programs have helped over the years in curbing the overall infection rate among sexually active adults, additional gains can still be achieved through the education sector. Other recent educational initiatives, like President Museveni's PIASCY, will undoubtedly yield long-term knowledge increases among students at the primary and postprimary levels. Still more needs to be done at the secondary level, where students are faced with adolescent decisions about sexual activity and health.

This chapter has looked at a national secondary school study on administrator, teacher, and student knowledge about HIV and AIDS. Students scored significantly lower overall than their teachers and administrators in both pre and postquestionnaires; yet students attending the intervention realized a higher knowledge increase on the postquestionnaire than both administrator and teacher intervention groups. Focus group discussions using a learner-guided approach yielded strong knowledge gains. This FAMA approach focused on understanding HIV/AIDS issues through group discussion and critical thinking activities that ultimately lead to application and action. Students in the control group, along with teachers and administrators, also realized moderate knowledge gains between pre and postintervention questionnaires.

Participants continuously shared with the authors that they were too pressed on time to include HIV/AIDS instruction on a regular basis in their classrooms. School structural constraints—such as lack of sufficient time and the fact that HIV/AIDS instruction is not currently examinable subject matter—was the most common response. Teachers and administrators had difficulty justifying necessary chunks of time on the subject because they were already stretched to their limit to teach examinable subject matter. Based on these qualitative findings, we support the movement to integrate HIV/AIDS instruction into the formal, examinable curriculum. What could be more relevant to the needs of students than a topic that so deeply impacts their families, friendships, and relationships with their future spouse and children? Many students board at their schools and are not able to receive instruction on HIV/AIDS from their parents. Day students can also benefit from in-school HIV/AIDS instruction, as they can take information home to help educate siblings, parents, and community members about how to deal with the epidemic. We are not suggesting an entire subject devoted to HIV/AIDS and other diseases, but feel the subject should be better integrated into key courses that students are taking anyway.

NOTES

1. The primary level in Ugandan schools is comparable to the elementary level in the United States, with grades ranging from Primary 1 (P1) to Primary 7 (P7), comparable to kindergarten through sixth grade in U.S. schools.

2. Secondary level examinations include the Uganda Certification of Education (UCE) Examination at the *Ordinary* or *O* level (i.e., consisting of Senior 1 to 4 grade levels) and the Uganda Advanced Certificate (UAC) at the *Advanced* or *A* level (i.e., Senior 5 to 6 grade levels).

3. Students generally obtained information from peers, the radio, newspapers such as *Straight Talk* or *Young Talk*, or from senior women and men teachers. Karen A. L. Hyde, Andrew Ekatan, Paul Kiage, and Catherine Barasa (2002) found that male students generally obtained HIV/AIDS information from the radio, while female students tended to obtain information from discussions with senior women teachers.

4. There are efforts in place to integrate PIASCY into the formal curriculum but it has not yet been accomplished or documented. Currently the training of teachers is being accomplished mainly through MOES-led workshops where teachers are instructed to integrate aspects of HIV/AIDS in these five subjects while teaching. A forthcoming secondary-level curriculum review will examine this integration process in detail.

5. Uganda is separated into four key geographic regions: the semiarid dry Northern Region; the semiarid Eastern Region; the Central Region, consisting of the moist lake, crescent zone bordering Lake Victoria; and the semiarid Western Region.

6. The term *urbanicity* was coined in 1974 by W. Allen Martin (1976). Unlike other terms that deal with urban issues (i.e., urbanism and urbanization), urbanicity includes the ecological context of a geographical location, considering the social and economic dominance in the spatial area.

7. As of September 2004, there were 784 government aided and 2,055 private secondary schools in Uganda.

8. ProLiteracy Worldwide is the world's oldest and largest nongovernmental literacy organization. Its international programs are based upon a Freirean conscientization process of democratic education where empowerment among participants and relevance in subject matter taught are the dual goals in the education process.

REFERENCES

Ajzen, I. (1985). From intentions to actions: A theory of planned behavior. In J. Kuhl & J. Backman (Eds.), *Action—control: From cognitions to behavior* (pp. 11–39). Berlin, Germany: Springer Verlag.

Ajzen, I., & Fishbein, M. (1980). *Understanding attitudes and predicting social behaviour*. Englewood Cliffs, NJ: Prentice-Hall.

Curtis, L. R. (1990). *Literacy for social change*. Syracuse, NY: New Readers Press.

Curtis, L. R. (1996). *Picturing change*. Syracuse, NY: New Readers Press.

De Walque, D. (2004). *How does the impact of an HIV/AIDS information campaign vary with educational attainment? Evidence from rural Uganda*. Washington, DC: World Bank.

Fishbein, M., & Ajzen, I. (1975). *Belief, attitude, intention, and behavior: An introduction to theory and research*. Reading, MA: Addison-Wesley.

Fishbein, M., Middlestadt, S. E., & Hitchcock, P. J. (1991). Using information to change sexually transmitted disease-related behaviors: An analysis based on the theory of reasoned action. In J. N. Wasserheit, S. O. Aral, & K. K. Holmes (Eds.), *Research issues in human behavior and sexually transmitted diseases in the*

AIDS era (pp. 243–257). Washington, DC: American Society for Microbiology.

Fisher, J. D., & Fisher, W. A. (1992). Changing AIDS-risk behavior. *Psychological Bulletin, 111*, 455–474.

Freire, P. (1971). *Pedagogy of the oppressed*. New York: Continuum.

Hogle, J., Green, E. C., Nantulya, V., Stoneburner, R., & Stover, J. (2002). *What happened in Uganda? Declining HIV prevalence, behavior change, and the national response*. Washington, DC: USAID.

Hyde, K. A. L., Ekatan, A., Kiage, P., & Barasa, C. (2002). *The impact of HIV/AIDS on formal schooling in Uganda—summary report*. Nairobi, Kenya: Centre for International Education, University of Sussex Institute of Education; Downtown Printing Works.

Jacob, W. J., Mosman, S. S., Hite, S. J., Morisky, D. E., & Nsubuga, Y. K. (2006). Reforming the national curriculum: Evaluating HIV/AIDS education programmes in Ugandan secondary schools. *Development in Practice*.

Jacob, W. J., Mosman, S. S., Morisky, D. E., Hite, S. J., & Nsubuga, Y. K. (2006). HIV/AIDS education: What African students say is effective. *Families in Society*.

King, A. J. C., & Wright, N. P. (1993). *AIDS and youth: An analysis of factors inhibiting and facilitating the design of interventions*. Review commissioned by GPA/WHO.

Kinsman, J., Harrison, B., Kengeya-Kayondo, J., Kanyesigye, E., Musoke, S., & Whitworth, J. (1999). Implementation of a comprehensive AIDS education programme for schools in Masaka District, Uganda. *AIDS Care, 11*, 591–601.

Kinsman, J., Nakiyingi, J., Kamali, A., Carpenter, L., Quigley, M., Pool, R., et al. (2001). Evaluation of a comprehensive school-based AIDS education programme in rural Masaka, Uganda. *Health Education Research, 16*(1), 85–100.

Kirby, D., Short, L., Collins, J., Rugg, D., Kolbe, L., Howard, M., et al. (1994). School-based programmes to reduce sexual risk behaviours: A review of effectiveness. *Public Health Reports, 109*(3), 339–360.

Laubach, F. C. (1967). *Thirty years with the silent billion*. Westwood, NJ: Revell.

Malinga, F. (2000). Uganda: Designing communication and education programs to combat HIV/AIDS. *ADEA Newsletter, 12*(4), 13–14.

Martin, W. A. (1976). *The conceputalization and measurement of urbanization*. Unpublished doctoral dissertation. Austin, University of Texas at Austin.

Mbulaiteyea, S. M., Mahe, C., Ruberantwari, A., & Whitworth, J. A. G. (2002). Generalizability of population-based studies on AIDS: A comparison of newly and continuously surveyed villages in rural southwest Uganda. *International Journal of Epidemiology, 31*(5), 961–967.

Ministry of Health. (2001). *Primary School teacher's guide on STDs/HIV/AIDS prevention education*. Kampala, Uganda: STD/AIDS Control Programme, Ministry of Health.

Mirembe, R. (2002). AIDS and democratic education in Uganda. *Comparative Education, 38*(3), 291–302.

Mugyeni, P. N. (2002). HIV vaccine: The Uganda experience. *Vaccine, 20*(15), 1905–1908.

Nelson, L. S., Gordon, P. E., Simmons, M. D., Goldberg, W. L., Howland, M. A., & Hoffman, R. S. (2000). The benefit of houseofficer education on proper medication dose calculation and ordering. *Academic Emergency Medicine, 7*(11), 1311–1316.

Shuey, D. A., Babishangire, B. B., Omiat, S., & Bagarukayo, H. (1999). Increased sexual abstinence among in-school adolescents as a result of school health education in Soroti District, Uganda. *Health Education Research, 14*(3), 411–419.

Terry, D. J., Gallios, C., & McCamish, M. (1993). *The theory of reasoned action: Its application to AIDS-preventive behaviour.* Oxford, England: Pergamon.

WHO/UNESCO. (1999). *School health education to prevent AIDS and STD a resource package for curriculum planners.* Rio de Janeiro, Brazil: CECIP.

CHAPTER 5

PREPARING A GENERATION OF TEACHERS FOR EDUCATING YOUTH IN UGANDA

Rosemary Nabadda and Albert James Lutalo-Bosa

The international community has acknowledged Uganda's contribution to the world in response to the HIV/AIDS pandemic across the continent of Africa. This chapter presents several national interventions toward saving the youth from this killer disease. Kyambogo University, as an institution at the forefront of teacher training in Uganda, has had a strong influence on the preparation of teachers for educating the youth. Teacher training has never been more challenging than in the last two decades when trainers have had to cope with the impact and demands of the AIDS pandemic.

Formal education is acquisition of knowledge, skills, and attitudes for the survival and well-being of the recipients. To promote goals stated in this definition, governments of countries set up timely reviews or ongoing commissions to examine the arrangement of their education systems and curricula, with the intention of making these systems relevant to the needs of their societies. According to the late Fredrick Harbirson, as quoted by Todaro (2000),

Overcoming AIDS: Lessons Learned from Uganda, 85–102
Copyright © 2006 by Information Age Publishing

Human resources constitute the ultimate basis for the wealth of a nation's capital and natural resources are passive factors in production. Clearly, a country which is unable to develop the skills and knowledge for the well-being of its people and for utilization of this knowledge in the national economy will not be able to develop in anything. (p. 326)

To develop sound human resources requires a good educational system. As a teacher training institution, Kyambogo had to adjust its curriculum to prepare the teachers for the task of meeting the HIV/AIDS-related needs of the people.

This chapter examines teacher preparation in Uganda in the context of needs created by the spread of HIV/AIDS. It considers the effects of HIV/AIDS on staff and students, adaptations in the teacher-training curriculum, challenges of training teachers in the area of AIDS, and constraints encountered in training an AIDS-competent teacher in Uganda at this time. Finally it looks forward to the hopes for future progression and competence.

IMPACT OF HIV/AIDS ON THE EDUCATION SECTOR

It is relevant to reflect on the impact the AIDS epidemic has had on the education sector in Uganda before examining the preparation of teachers. The spread of HIV/AIDS has affected both the numbers of teachers and capacity to train and manage them, as well as the demand for education created by numbers and characteristics of the school-age population.

Research has shown that prolonged illness and deaths due to illness account for 9% of the teacher losses in Uganda. However, data are inadequate to discern the proportion of prolonged illness and death that can be directly attributed to AIDS (Amone, Bukuluki, Bongomin, & Oyabba, 2003). In 1998, the Ministry of Education and Sports (MOES) reported 16.5% of primary school teachers, trained and untrained, left the schools through transfers, promotions, and the pursuit of further studies or career advancement. The highest teacher attrition from all causes was in 1997, when it reached 25% among primary school teachers and 31% among secondary school teachers (Hyde, Ekatan, Kiage, & Barasa, 2002).

Absenteeism due to AIDS-related illness is also a common problem attributed to the AIDS epidemic. Many absences are necessitated by school responsibilities, as well as personal sickness, family sickness, and funeral attendance. According to the Uganda Demographic Health Survey (UHS) (2001), 14% of Ugandan children under 18 years of age are orphans. In 2002 it was estimated that 1,078,000 children of primary school age (6–14 years) had lost one or both parents to AIDS, which is 17% of all children in the age group (Kamal, 2002).

Children have often been stopped from attending school so they could nurse and care for the sick. The resulting frequent absenteeism can lead not only to poor performance but to dropping out from school altogether (Kaweesa, 2002). Quality of education is being affected by frequent absenteeism of teachers and heavy responsibilities of children orphaned by AIDS who must care for young siblings. Further, the cost of education, especially in secondary schools, has become an obstacle for those children orphaned by AIDS or whose parents are incapacitated by AIDS (Kaweesa, 2002).

RESPONSE TO HIV/AIDS BY THE MINISTRY OF EDUCATION AND SPORTS

A number of initiatives have been undertaken to expand AIDS prevention education, mainly through curricula at different levels of formal education in Uganda. The MOES launched its first HIV/AIDS prevention efforts in 1986 by mainly targeting primary schools with media messages and specific curriculum (Malinga, 2000). In 1987 the School Health Education Project (SHEP) was launched by UNICEF, aimed at reducing STD and HIV among the youth in primary school classes. A total of 8,000 primary school teachers were trained in AIDS prevention. However, at the end of the project in 1994, the overall objective of integrating health education in primary, secondary, and tertiary curricula had not been achieved because the program had been poorly designed (UNICEF, 1998).

The government undertook a review of the primary school curriculum in the late 1980s. Although the curriculum incorporated topics on sexual reproductive health, according to Hyde et al. (2002), it included very little reference to HIV/AIDS. With support from UNICEF, different teaching and learning materials—such as health kits for primary schools, primary teachers colleges, and secondary schools—were developed and produced (Kaweesa, 2002). In 1995, the MOES designed another program known as Basic Education, Child Care and Adolescent Development (BECCAD) to focus mainly on life skills. This program trained teachers from secondary schools, national teachers colleges, and 40 Grade 2 teachers colleges (UNICEF, 1998). Equipping teachers and fully involving them to fight AIDS among the youth remains a daunting challenge for a country like Uganda. Gaps still exists in communicating accurate information on the subject of AIDS. According to Cogan (2003),

The HIV/AIDS crisis has highlighted the inadequacy of preventive education in the developing world. . . . If preventive education is to alter young
people's attitudes and behaviour, the school must engage in practical terms
with the resource factors which determine the health of the community to
which its pupils belong and at the same time communicate in the classroom
essential information about these issues. (pp. 3, 7)

Contributions and Achievements
of the National Curriculum Development Centre

The National Curriculum Development Centre (NCDC) is a corporate
body of the MOES of the government of Uganda. The Center is responsible for inter alia development of curriculum for various levels of education in Uganda. Among its functions are designing and evaluating the
curricula at all levels of education and recommending and implementing
necessary change. The NCDC intervened in the HIV/AIDS prevention
education by implementing the Adolescent Reproductive Health Project
(UGA/97/P11, 1997–2000) in schools. The project, funded by the government of Uganda in collaboration with the UN Population Fund (UNFPA),
involved training teachers to integrate population and family life education in career subjects.

The project made reproductive health (RH) activities available in
schools by training 63 primary school teachers and 59 secondary school
teachers, in addition to school guidance counselors, 24 school club
patrons, and 40 RH peer mobilizers. These activities, along with other
RH services, enabled teachers to reach many vulnerable young people
with information about preventing STDs, HIV, and AIDS. Learners in the
project schools expressed their appreciation for the RH services. They
found the services satisfactory and were willing to comply with the
requirement that they change their behavior. The larger community
expressed satisfaction and support as well. The success of the NCDC program has demonstrated that pupils can be made aware of RH problems
and how to handle them through RH sessions in schools. In addition to
the teacher-student involvement, the program has been enhanced by the
participation of guidance and counseling staff.

TEACHER TRAINING IN UGANDA

Teacher training in Uganda began in 1877 when Christian missionaries
introduced formal education in the country. Ugandan teachers needed
training in order to teach in the new schools. In 1889 formal teacher edu-

cation classes were established at particular schools then called *central schools*. Eventually, separate teacher training schools were set up. By 1920, teacher training colleges had been established in many parts of Uganda (Ssekamwa, 1997). At present, primary school teachers are trained at Grade 3 primary teachers colleges. For lower primary school, candidates who have completed 4 years of secondary education follow a 2-year course leading to the Grade 3 teacher's certificate. Upper primary school teachers who hold the Uganda certificate of education follow a 1-year course leading to the Grade 4 teacher's certificate. Secondary school teachers are trained at the national teachers colleges, universities and the Institute of Teacher Education Kyambogo (ITEK) in a program lasting 2 years. There is also a 3-year upgrading course for Grade 4 teachers leading to the Grade 4 teacher's certificate (International Association of Universities, 2004).

Since 1987, ITEK had been running bachelor of education courses. Kyambogo University is a new university established in July 2003 by the *Universities and Other Tertiary Institutions Act*. The university was created by a merger with two other tertiary institutions, the former Uganda Polytechnic Kyambogo (UPK) and ITEK. Affiliated with 10 national teachers colleges and 47 primary teachers colleges, Kyambogo University coordinates programs and accredits students. The faculty of education is responsible for enhancing the professionalism of in-service and preservice teachers by enriching their training experience and their managerial skills in the education arena. Today Uganda is undergoing substantial educational reform, and the faculty of education of Kyambogo University is at the center of these reforms in respect to curriculum innovation.

RESPONSE OF THE KYAMBOGO UNIVERSITY COMMUNITY TO HIV/AIDS

Since 2002, Kyambogo University has stepped up services in addressing the issue of HIV/AIDS in the community. These services are predominantly student and health centered. They address mostly information, prevention, treatment, and counseling. Voluntary counseling and testing (VCT) for HIV has been fully integrated into the existing health services and the community has fully embraced and utilized the services. HIV/AIDS prevention education is given to incoming students during orientation week by the university's medical staff. In addition to these health services, the university has trained over 80 student peer educators in communicating information concerning skills in RH and development. Kyambogo University students of the Languages and Literature Department wrote poems on the theme of HIV/AIDS "Stigma and Discrimination" for World AIDS Day 2003. The Student Performing Arts Group has been instrumental in educating the community about AIDS through poems, dramatic monologues, songs, fashion shows, and drama. University administration has recognized the need to develop a university wide HIV/AIDS policy, and the process has already begun.

TRAINING OF AIDS-COMPETENT TEACHERS

Various Kyambogo University departments have already taken steps to integrate relevant aspects of HIV/AIDS in their academic programs. The bachelor of guidance and counseling degree program in the Department of Psychology offers an HIV/AIDS care and counseling course. The program targets primary and secondary school teachers, primary teachers college tutors, and lecturers in tertiary institutions (Kyambogo University, 2002). The Department of Biological Sciences has just produced a syllabus considering the demands of society that HIV/AIDS be given special attention under the areas of health and disease (Kyambogo University, 2003).

The Department of Adult and Community Education (CACE) has included under the section of community health education an area on HIV/AIDS. This program targets teachers from primary and secondary institutions. The same information has been integrated into the bachelor's degree program for the academic year 2004–2005. Similarly, the faculty of special needs has included HIV/AIDS information in its curriculum (Kyambogo University, 2004b).

Another intervention to raise HIV/AIDS awareness is the CCATH (Child-Centred Approaches to HIV/AIDS), coordinated by Child-to-Child Uganda under Kyambogo University. The major objective of CCATH is to support children affected by HIV/AIDS by using child-centered approaches, in their schools. The project has been implemented at 13 primary schools in Uganda, using a series of HIV/AIDS awareness activities, including training teachers in child-centered approaches. Below are the achievements of CCATH Uganda and lessons learned during implementation.

Achievements

- An increased number of children now have open dialogue at home with parents and peers about HIV/AIDS.
- Children are more confident and motivated, and they aspire for opportunities in life.

- Children are able to share more openly the HIV/AIDS of their parents without fear in HIV/AIDS clubs and groups. About 2,000 children are involved in clubs in the 13 participating schools.
- Children in some of the beneficiary schools have set up an emergency fund whereby they contribute money for food and clothing to their needy friends.
- Child-to-Child has been involved in formulating the education sector HIV/AIDS policy.
- Child-to-Child Uganda's approaches and methods have been included in the Presidential Initiative in AIDS Strategy for Communication to Youth (PIASCY).

Lessons Learned

- Children's voices are louder and clearer when they work in groups like peer clubs.
- Teachers participate in the fight against HIV/AIDS if provided with the right information and support.
- There are great gains when the children are given a chance to participate actively in activities designed for them. (Ngobi, 2004)

When teachers graduate and are posted to different schools across the country, they are expected to guide and offer psychosocial support to the youth under their care, in addition to their teaching. The majority of teachers who find themselves with increased workloads, however, may not be able to meet these objectives. Yet teaching and learning about HIV/AIDS prevention needs to be highly interactive, with broad participation of young people, teachers, and surrounding communities.

Formal Curriculum for Teacher Preparation in the Context of AIDS.

Dissemination of information and skills connected to RH and HIV/AIDS by teachers is vital. With more than 50% of all new HIV/AIDS infections among children and youth in their formative years, institutions of learning are a logical place to reach young people who are at risk. The struggle everywhere is to provide them access to information and training that will reduce their vulnerability to AIDS. Educators are key in presenting valuable information about reproductive health and HIV/AIDS to the adolescent group. But to do so successfully, they need to comprehend what they teach, attain good teaching practices, and identify with what is developmentally and culturally correct.

Teachers are often the most important people, apart from family members, with whom young people interact on a daily basis. In an era of HIV/AIDS, teachers play an even more significant role as they provide accurate information and serve as a sympathetic person with whom young people can raise sensitive and complicated issues about sexuality. The increased enrollment of children affected by and infected with HIV/AIDS has brought about the need to review general education curricula in terms of content, mode of delivery, and change in the role of teacher to teacher/counselor (Kelly, 2000).

Despite the efforts and achievements of Kyambogo University including HIV/AIDS information in the teacher training programs, there are areas that need to be changed and enhanced to adequately prepare teachers to become agents of change in the era of HIV/AIDS. Over 2 decades of living under the shadow of HIV/AIDS have elapsed without massive curricular innovation to effectively integrate HIV/AIDS throughout the teacher training programs.

Michael J. Kelly (2000) suggests three options for placing HIV/AIDS and reproductive health into the curriculum: (1) as a free-standing, separate, examinable subject; (2) as a segment of an existing carrier subject such as health education; and (3) as a cross-cutting issue to be addressed in all subjects. In the absence of a university policy, the inclusion of HIV/AIDS in teaching programs depends greatly on initiatives of individuals or departments.

Missed Opportunities

Considering Kelly's (2000) advice, many programs at Kyambogo University have missed opportunities to include HIV/AIDS in their curricula. In the curriculum for bachelor of arts, sciences, and vocational studies with education at Kyambogo University, the following core courses are taught: counseling and guidance (under educational psychology), foundations of education, curriculum studies, development studies, study and communication skills, and educational research and statistics (ITEK, 1999). The offering for primary teachers, Diploma in Primary Education, teaches similar subjects but includes special needs education (ITEK, 2000a).

The guidance and counseling for bachelor of education degree should prepare in-service and preservice teachers in the prevention of HIV/AIDS. However, this course focuses on general principles of guidance and counseling, with no particular reference to HIV/AIDS counseling by teachers.

Hence it does not adequately prepare teachers as counselors for HIV/ AIDS children and their parents.

Another course that has not been effectively utilized in HIV/AIDS education is developmental studies. Among the core courses of teacher training, developmental studies should provide an opportunity to address the issue of HIV/AIDS. Although one of the course lecturers admitted during an interview that HIV/AIDS issues are mentioned during some of the lectures, there is no documented reference to this topic in the existing curriculum (ITEK, 1999). HIV/AIDS is a health issue as well as a social problem. Teachers undertaking the course of developmental studies are missing an important opportunity to acquire skills to enable them to address HIV/AIDS issues despite the fact that HIV/AIDS is increasingly being recognized as a developmental issue. Stating it as goal six among the Millennium Developmental Goals, by the year 2015 Uganda has set the goal to have halted and begun to reverse the spread of HIV/AIDS (Tashobya & Ogwang, 2004).

Educational research and statistics, the capstone course in the existing curriculum, is yet another missed opportunity for empowering teachers on HIV/AIDS issues. This core course covers mostly general principles in conducting research. Students need increasing guidance as they conduct miniresearch projects and write academic papers in the area of HIV-related issues as part of their academic programs. The overall goal of training teachers is not only to empower them to teach, but also to develop AIDS-educated and AIDS-competent graduates who are adequately qualified to carry AIDS concerns into their subsequent life, to address AIDS issues in their professions, and to bring AIDS prevention to the attention of society (Kelly, 2001).

The diploma course in library and information science, a course which targets qualified teachers and other educators at various levels, has the objective of providing students with theoretical and practical skills in acquisition and processing of reading materials in effective and efficient dissemination of information (ITEK, 2000b). There should also be a course on preparing teachers in dissemination of information on important issues such as HIV/AIDS.

Teacher Training Curriculum Innovation in the Era of AIDS

Teachers who have graduated in the last 2 decades and those who will continue to join the profession as long as widespread HIV/AIDS continues are facing immense challenges. Teachers work very close to at-risk students on a daily basis. Many of these vulnerable students are living under economic hardships and have the daunting responsibility of heading households. Loss of parents may affect student behavior; thus teachers must be able to teach students with varying personalities and characteristics, along with those from complete or normal families.

In Uganda HIV/AIDS education has been integrated into the primary school curriculum, and the process is also underway at the secondary education subsector (Amone et al., 2003). Research has shown the need to empower teachers to handle the subject of AIDS effectively. Some teachers have expressed fears that doing so may crowd out important subjects and overcrowd the school timetable. Others have been concerned about the complexities involved in handling the subject, such as the level at which to introduce it (Amone et al., 2003).

Another underutilized area is the primary teachers college (PTC) curriculum. Assessment of PTC curriculum by preservice teachers who study it has revealed that most subjects covered have potential for providing knowledge, skills, and attitudes related to growing up and experiencing sexual maturation. However, discussions relating to HIV/AIDS have been skipped (Kamuli, 2000).

In-service training of teachers can be effective in helping teachers prepare youth in schools. The government of Uganda agrees that in-service training programs for teachers provide the most important exposure for teachers in the field to the rapid changes in technology and science regarding HIV/AIDS and to innovations in curricula and teaching methods (Government of Uganda, 1992).

The Africa Medical and Research Foundation (AMREF) (2001) assessed a project in Soroti in which teacher training was incorporated into a broader school district intervention. Teachers of students aged 13 to 14 were trained by a health educator on HIV and RH issues. Two years following the baseline survey, students whose teachers had received the training reported a significant decline both in number of instances of sexual intercourse in the past month and in the average number of sexual partners, compared to the control group. It was concluded that the quality of the implementation is probably more important than the detailed design of materials or curricula.

Guidance and counseling, which is a relatively new innovation in the education system in Uganda, has focused primarily on the appointment of senior women and senior men as teachers in schools (Hyde et al., 2002). However, the teachers have admitted lack of skills in counseling and guidance, especially in relation to HIV issues. In-depth interviews involving 12 patrons of school clubs in Uganda found that some female or male teachers did not possess adequate skills in counseling and guidance in relation to HIV/AIDS and other sexual reproductive health issues. The participants expressed the need to be facilitated to acquire better counseling and guidance skills (Amone et al., 2003).

The government of Uganda has realized that families, communities, and schools have a daunting but surmountable challenge in communicating about HIV/AIDS to young people. In early 2002, the President of Uganda proposed a strategy to improve communication on HIV/AIDS to young people: the Presidential Initiative on AIDS Strategy for Communication to Youth (PIASCY). With the already existing Universal Primary Education (UPE) program, which had increased enrollment of primary school children from 2 million (1997) to 7 million (2004), learners are constantly available for HIV/AIDS instruction (Amone et al., 2003). The main objectives of this Initiative focus on (1) increasing and sustaining HIV/AIDS education in school-going children and youth; (2) increasing the capacity of parents, teachers, and health service providers to engage in constructive deliberations with young people on HIV/AIDS; (3) strengthening the capacity of communities to implement HIV/AIDS prevention initiatives and assist young people in identifying and modifying behavior related to HIV/AIDS; and (4) training core personnel from different sectors on HIV/AIDS prevention among youths. The curriculum program, "Window of Hope," directly supports pupils of 5–13 years. The content is still under review to accommodate the technical and administrative interests of different groups (MOES, 2004).

Knowledge and Skills for the Current Generation of Teachers

Building the capacity for teachers to be counselors and agents of change in the area of sexual and reproductive health is a major undertaking. A teacher must reach beyond the conventional role of instruction as fact giving and become a personal change agent (Hyde et al., 2002). Teachers also need to know how to protect their own health and how to avoid putting any of their students at risk through their own behaviors. Teachers can act as role models, promoting school health, identifying students who need help, and providing accurate information. Teachers need skills and knowledge as well as support in communicating information effectively.

HIV/AIDS has created a particularly difficult challenge for the formal education system in Uganda due to the increasing number of orphans. This unique group has special needs including but not limited to insufficient resources to pay school dues, frequent absenteeism, and increased responsibilities for caring for others at home. Administrators and teachers have to respond to these needs in addition to other duties. These particular challenges have had profound implications for teacher training in the country.

Traditionally teachers have been expected to pass on knowledge to students and then examine the students to make sure they have achieved their objectives. In fact, the authors recall occasions when a teacher would merely read from lecture notes, expecting students to sit quietly and learn. This mimetic approach often restricts student learning and is challenged by Howard Gardner (1995):

> In what is called "mimetic" education, the teacher demonstrates the desired performance or behavior and the student duplicates it. . . . A contrasting tack in education has been termed "transformative" approach. In this approach, rather than modeling the desired behavior, the teacher serves as a coach or facilitator, trying to evoke certain qualities or understandings in the students. . . . The contrast between mimetic and transformative modes is clearly related to another, perhaps more familiar contrast—between an emphasis on basic skills and an emphasis on creativity. (p. 119)

Faced with the AIDS epidemic, communicating knowledge has become an increasing challenge for Kyambogo University in its preservice teacher preparation. The practicable implication of this HIV/AIDS preparation is that teachers must be ready to deal with the epidemic and assist in the process of instructional change throughout the education system.

High quality education should teach young people to interact in socially skilled and respectful ways: to practice positive, safe, health behaviors; to contribute ethically and responsibly to their peer group, family, school and community; and to posses basic competencies, work habits and values as a foundation for meaningful employment and engaged citizenship (Greenberg et al., 2003, pp. 466–467).

The teacher's work is not confined simply to transmitting information: knowledge must be stated in ways that promote problem-solving capabilities, allowing students to adopt perspectives through which they can link their solutions to broader issues.

Edmund J. King (1970) says that the real teacher leads people to reason. Teachers are personally improved by having their wits sharpened this way, and some of the rational attitudes thus developed will be communicated to pupils and students.

A teacher trained in the last 2 decades will be teaching a huge number of traumatized children who face multiple learning obstacles. According to Kelly (2000), the attitudinal and psychological problems faced by both children and adults call for establishment of an effective counseling program. Pupils and students are suffering bereavement and they are desperate for counseling and psychosocial support. A teacher trained today needs to assume the role of counselor as well as teacher; however the majority of teachers lack appropriate counseling skills. Planners therefore need to explore ways of modifying initial and in-service teacher development programs to include basic counselor training. Kelly also adds that, "All education programmes should attempt to provide compensation for what orphans have lost in life, providing them with security, stability, human warmth and opportunity for joy, gaiety and laughter" (p. 63).

A strong base of knowledge and skills is required for further specialization in specific curriculum or educational content. In Uganda, strategies of educating people on HIV/AIDS and reducing risks have already been implemented, but effectiveness will depend to a great extent on the skills of the educator (UNICEF, 1998). In training teachers to meet the needs of youth affected or infected by AIDS, additional areas of training should include instruction on corrective or strategic learning approaches, development of critical analytical communication systems, orientation to new approaches to the management of the epidemic, strategies for meeting the needs of vulnerable children, and requirements for developing psychosocial support environments in schools and surrounding communities. These extensions require that the teacher be prepared to go beyond the traditional teaching role, requiring more time and responsibility.

Curriculum reform of teacher training to accommodate HIV/AIDS requires training tutors—who become trainers of teachers in their respective institutions—to promote skills-based training which emphasizes counseling communication and life skills. The main goal of tertiary education, according to the 1992 draft *White Paper*, is to train senior technical, managerial, and professional personnel. The government has established the National Council for Higher Education in order to achieve this goal and has embarked on professional training and retraining programs for tutors at the tertiary level (Government of Uganda, 1992).

Constraints in Preparation of Teachers as Agents of Change

Improving the ability and skills of teachers to address the issue of RH and HIV/AIDS in their day-to-day work is a big task facing the education sector and the nation as a whole. The world is looking at the education sector as a logical entity to spread HIV/AIDS information and awareness since the schooling enterprise is already an organized infrastructure, which is cost effective and capable of reaching large audiences of young people. HIV/AIDS interventions in the education sector in the past have been targeting mainly learners other than teachers who are very significant as agents of change (Amone et al., 2003).

Teacher educators face several practical obstacles that can hinder effective outcomes. First, the teacher must reach beyond the conventional role of giving instructions and facts to become a personal agent of change

(Hyde et al., 2002). Present methods of teacher training do not prepare teachers adequately for this role.

Second, the MOES is still in the process of developing the education sector policy on HIV/AIDS, and consultations with different stakeholders are still in the formative stages (MOES, 2004a). Without clear and consistent guidelines, HIV/AIDS teacher preparation is left to different institutions, which may lack the capacity to carry it out effectively.

Limited resources and inadequate technical support constitute the third obstacle, complicating the task of preparing AIDS-competent teachers. Revising teacher training curriculum to include HIV/AIDS, then guiding and supervising the reform at the teacher training institutions is costly in money, time, and human resources, all of which may be unavailable when needed.

Fourth, many decision makers do not appreciate the interconnectedness and the interrelatedness between health and education, a major factor evident in planning not only in the private sector but also in government institutions. A young person's health status constitutes a major determinant of his or her educational achievement (National Health and Medical Research Council, 1996). The Education planners need to build the capacity of teachers as change agents in the area of RH and HIV/AIDS to promote health in schools for better education outcomes.

The lack of quality in-service training seminars is a fifth obstacle to developing HIV/AIDS competent teachers. However, according to Hyde et al. (2002), training of teachers as specialists in HIV/AIDS education is probably the best approach for providing qualified specialists because of financial concerns and because special skills and capabilities are called for. Furthermore, and not all teachers will be able to take on such a role.

Sixth, HIV/AIDS education has been regarded as an additional responsibility other than a policy issue. In the examination-driven education system, teaching and learning are geared at helping students pass a standardized exam so they can advance to the next level (MOES, 1989). Curriculum restructuring efforts—to incorporate HIV/AIDS prevention and treatment strategies—may face resistance from planners and recipients.

Seventh, according to Amone et al. (2003), there is no clear-cut budget line for addressing HIV/AIDS in the education sector. The sector is expected to depend primarily on the individual institutions and to plan accordingly. With limited resources in most of the institutions, HIV/AIDS education may not be considered a priority among institutional activities.

And finally, building teacher capacity to handle HIV/AIDS-specific curriculum reform without compromising instructional quality depends on the availability of sufficient numbers of qualified and trained teachers (MOES, 1989). The current lack of instruction materials and poor remuneration may adversely affect preparation of AIDS-competent teachers.

THE WAY FORWARD

There are benefits in adequately preparing teachers for educating Ugandan youth in the era of HIV/AIDS. Training and support must be provided to teachers to empower them to become effective in their role as educators. This chapter has demonstrated that HIV/AIDS teacher preparation is not an easy task, but a task that is achievable. The existing teacher training curriculum includes opportunities to incorporate the subject, and every opportunity possible should be utilized to ensure that no teacher leaves the training institutions without the necessary skills to address HIV/AIDS as necessary in her/his profession.

Preparation should address knowledge, attitudes and skills among the professional needs that will equip teachers to facilitate change and to support students and colleagues in RH and HIV/AIDS-related problems. It is easier for a teacher to market a product he or she is sure of and well informed about. Teachers of this generation should therefore be empowered to prevent apathy and frustration that can result from lack of adequate basic knowledge on HIV/AIDS, especially its psychosocial impacts at personal, community, and national levels.

In-service training to produce AIDS-competent teachers will multiply benefits since those trained will serve as resource people in schools and the community. Finally, it is worth noting that training HIV/AIDS competent teachers is a step in the right direction in the fight against HIV/AIDS in Uganda, assuming that training in HIV/AIDS communication skills can change a teacher at a personal level. Considering an estimated 900 teachers, in addition to the 2,000 teachers who graduate every academic year from Kyambogo University's internal and external programs (Kyambogo University, 2004a), a critical mass of young people may be saved from the risk of contracting HIV infection.

In order to achieve this goal, however, the MOES needs to work with teacher training planners toward a number of objectives. First, the MOES needs to encourage innovation within the existing curriculum, using all avenues possible to prepare HIV/AIDS-competent teachers for this generation and generations to come. Next, the government plays an integral role in encouraging teachers and tutors to continuously review their professional practices and knowledge. This will help obviate gaps in communicating RH and HIV/AIDS information in schools. Third, HIV/AIDS issues must become an integral part of teacher training in order to harmonize delivery of HIV/AIDS curriculum content and identify basic details of what should be covered and in what areas. This emphasis on HIV/AIDS training will help ensure that all opportunities are adequately and appropriately utilized including, but not limited to, educational psychology (guidance and counseling), gender, and developmental studies. Fourth, institutional policies should be developed to guide training of teachers in HIV/AIDS issues within the framework of the education sector's HIV/AIDS draft policy. A fifth initiative of the MOES should be to encourage research programs to identify the training needs to prepare teachers to address in schools the physical, social, and psychosocial aspects of HIV. And finally, the MOES should establish a regular forum (e.g., open days, seminars, workshops, public lectures, etc.) through which information relating to teacher training for educating the youth in the era of AIDS can be shared in order to continually improve approaches and outcomes.

REFERENCES

Africa Medical and Research Foundation (AMREF). (2001). *The effect of the Katakwi/Soroti school health and AIDS prevention project*. Kampala, Uganda: Author.

Amone, J., Bukuluki, P., Bongomin, M., & Oyabba, T. (2003). *Collaborative action research project on the impact of HIV/AIDS on the education sector in Uganda. Study one: Examining policy, leadership and advocacy responses in the sector*. Kampala, Uganda: MOES and IIEP/UNESCO.

Cogan, J., (2003). *Health education for all: A generic model for resource poor countries. Students Partnership Worldwide (SPW) concept paper*. London: SPW.

Gardner, H. (1995). *The unschooled mind: How children think and how schools should teach*. New York: Basic Books.

Government of Uganda. (1992). *Government white paper*. Kampala, Uganda: Author.

Greenberg, M. T., Weissberg, R. P., O'Brien, M. U., Zins, J. E., Fredericks, L., Resnik, H., & Elias, M. (2003). Enhancing school-based prevention and youth development through coordinated social, emotional, and academic learning. *American Psychologist, 58*(6/7), 466–474.

Hyde, K., Ekatan, A., Kiage, P., & Barasa, C. (2002). *The impact of HIV/AIDS informal schooling in Uganda: Summary report*. Brighton, UK: Centre for International Education, Brighton.

Institute of Teacher Education Kyambogo (ITEK). (1999). *Proposed professional studies curriculum for B.A. with education/B.S.C. with education/B.V.S. with education*. Kampala, Uganda: Faculty of Education, Kyambogo University.

ITEK. (2000a). A syllabus for a diploma in library and information—DLIS. Kampala, Uganda: Library Department, Faculty of Arts, Kyambogo University.

ITEK. (2000b). *Professional studies module, PS/1, 2, 3. Teacher education self-study materials for the Diploma in Education Primary External (DEPE) Programme.* Kampala, Uganda: Kyambogo University.

International Association of Universities (IAU). (2004). *Uganda: Education system.* Paris: UNESCO.

Kamal, D. (2002). *Accelerating the education sector response to HIV/AIDS in Africa: Projecting the impact of AIDS on the education system.* Paper presented at the Sub-Regional Seminar on Accelerating the Education Sector Response to HIV/AIDS in Mombasa, Kenya with Eritrea, Ethiopia, Uganda, Tanzania and Zambia.

Kamuli, E., & Katahoire, R. A. (2000). *Summary report on improving the teaching and management of growing up and sexual maturation in primary schools in Uganda.* Kampala, Uganda: Kyambogo University.

Kaweesa, K. D, (2002). *HIV/AIDS and the education sector: Uganda's Experience.* Paper presented at a Workshop for Principals of Primary Teachers Colleges and Technical/Vocational Institutions on HIV/AIDS and Girl's Education, Kampala, Uganda.

Kelly, M. J. (2000). *Planning for education in the context of HIV/AIDS* (Vol. 66). Paris: UNESCO.

Kelly, M. J. (2001). *Challenging the challenger: Understanding and expanding the responses of universities in Africa to HIV/AIDS.* Washington, DC: World Bank.

King, E. J. (1970). *The education of teachers: A comparative analysis.* London: Bartholomew Press.

Kyambogo University. (2002). *Bachelor of guidance and counseling degree programme.* Kampala, Uganda: Department of Psychology and Faculty of Education, Kyambogo University.

Kyambogo University. (2003). *Revised biology syllabus for national teachers colleges of Uganda.* Kampala, Uganda: Department of Biological Science and Faculty of Science, Kyambogo University.

Kyambogo University. (2004a). *Graduation ceremony handbook.* Kampala, Uganda: Author.

Kyambogo University. (2004b). *Proposed revised bachelor of adult and community education (BACE).* Kampala, Uganda: Department of Adult and Community Medicine and Faculty of Special Needs and Rehabilitation, Kyambogo University.

Malinga, F. (2000). Uganda: Designing communication and education programs to combat HIV/AIDS. *ADEA Newsletter, 12*(4), 13–14.

MOES. (1989). *Education for national development: Report of the Education Policy Review Commission.* Kampala, Uganda: Author.

MOES. (2004a). *Education sector policy on HIV/AIDS, Draft 2.* Kampala, Uganda: Author.

MOES. (2004b). *Presidential initiative on AIDS strategy for communication to youth: Helping pupils to stay safe. A handbook for teachers.* Kampala, Uganda: Author.

National Health and Medical Research Council. (1996). *Effective school health promotion: Towards health promoting schools.* Canberra: Common Wealth of Australia.

Ngobi, D. (2004). *Child participation in the development of coping strategies for children affected by HIV/AIDS: Uganda's experience*. London: Healthlink Worldwide.

Ssekamwa, J. C. (1997). *History and development of education in Uganda*. Kampala, Uganda: Fountain.

Tashobya, K. C, & Ogwang, O. P. (2004). *The effort to achieve the Millennium Development Goals in Uganda: Reaching for the sky?* Kampala, Uganda: Department of Health Sciences, Uganda Martyrs University.

Todaro, M. P. (2000). *Economic development in the third world*. Reading, MA: Addison Wesley.

UGA/97/P11. (1997–2000). *IEC in support of reproductive health in schools*. Kampala, Uganda: National Curriculum Development Centre, Kyambogo.

UNICEF. (1998). *Life skills for young Ugandans: Primary teachers' training manual*. Kampala, Uganda: Author.

PART III

NONFORMAL YOUTH AND CHILD HIV/AIDS EDUCATION PROGRAMS

CHAPTER 6

SOCIAL AND BEHAVIORAL DETERMINANTS OF HIV/AIDS EDUCATION PROGRAMS AMONG UGANDAN YOUTH

Delius Asiimwe and Richard Kibombo

INTRODUCTION

HIV/AIDS was first identified in Southwestern Uganda in 1982 and by 1985 the disease had reached epidemic levels. By December 2001, it was estimated that 947,552 deaths had resulted by AIDS-related causes. In 1991, a multisectoral approach was adopted and implemented by numerous government and private organizations. The goal of these efforts was to address essential prevention and control dimensions of HIV/AIDS, as well as increase the ability to manage the real and perceived consequences of the epidemic. This goal has facilitated a myriad of approaches resulting in a wide variety of prevention, care, support, and mitigation interventions. These efforts have been, and continue to be, championed by government institutions, local and international nongovernmental organizations (NGOs), faith-based organizations (FBOs), and the donor community.

Overcoming AIDS: Lessons Learned from Uganda, 105–123
105

These interventions have jointly helped in the abatement of the spread and incidence of the HIV/AIDS epidemic in Uganda. The Ministry of Health (MOH) HIV/AIDS Surveillance Report of 2002 indicated a decline of 11.5% in the weighted overall antenatal prevalence from 18.0% in 1992 to 6.5% in 2001. The decline in HIV prevalence in Uganda has been attributed to many factors, including high political commitment, a multisectoral approach, and high levels of awareness leading to a significant change in individual behavior. Individual behavior change has been identified as one of the primary goals in the National Strategic Framework for HIV/AIDS: Activities for Uganda, 2001–2006 (Government of Uganda [GOU]/Uganda AIDS Commission [UAC]/UNAIDS, 2000).

The three most common sexual and reproductive health (SRH) struggles that face Ugandan adolescents are STDs, HIV/AIDS, and unplanned pregnancies. Other socioeconomic factors that exacerbate SRH problems include poverty, drug and alcohol abuse, school drop out, lack of schooling, orphanhood, and gender socialization. Individual sexual behavior remains the primary defining risk factor for the variation of HIV/AIDS incidence and prevalence according to sex, geographical location, culture, and socioeconomic status. Sociocultural values and economic conditions underlie the nature of sexual interaction between individuals (Asiimwe, Kibombo, & Neema, 2003). In this chapter, we provide a broad overview of key nonformal youth and child HIV/AIDS education programs in Uganda. These program reviews cover several aspects such as the behavior targeted, program focus, population coverage, and the extent to which the programs achieve their stated objectives. Conclusions are presented on essential social and behavioral determinants of HIV/AIDS prevention and education among the youth and the implications these have on the reduction of HIV prevalence in Uganda.

HIV/AIDS educations programs in Uganda cluster within three broad categories of providers: government, faith-based, and local and international organizations and agencies. Many of these programs originated within a few years following the identification of the HIV/AIDS epidemic.

The following is a brief description of several of the more prominent and active HIV/AIDS programs currently found in Uganda. While they are not all of equal size, each makes an important and vital contribution to the immense effort underway to confront and solve the pressing and critical challenges presented by the HIV/AIDS epidemic in Uganda.

GOVERNMENT PROGRAMS

Government programs have been among the most widespread and internationally renowned approaches in Uganda's efforts to engage the HIV/

AIDS challenge. Many of these programs are joint efforts between the government and other well-established local and international organizations.

The School Health Education Project (SHEP)

From 1986 onwards, the School Health Education Project (SHEP) was initiated and implemented by the Ministry of Education and Sports (MOES) in collaboration with the MOH and other organizations and institutions. The project was set up as a peer education approach to HIV/AIDS prevention, targeting mainly students in secondary and tertiary institutions as well as out-of-school youth.

SHEP was one of the first government-led initiatives designed to focus directly on SRH problems, including an aggressive HIV/AIDS prevention component in schools. An evaluation of the SHEP project in 1994 indicated that while the program was quite successful in promoting knowledge, it did not have any measurable impact on behavior. This may have been partly due to the broad nature of the curriculum, which may have compromised the quantity and quality of specific information taught to the target groups. The issue of raising HIV/AIDS awareness and promoting behavior change, which was the primary objective of the project, was found to have insufficient emphasis (MOES, 2002).

One of the lessons learned from the SHEP initiative was that life skills for Ugandan youth are essential HIV/AIDS prevention and intervention strategies. A critical missing link in the SHEP intervention was identified as assisting children in translating knowledge into positive health behaviors. In the SHEP evaluation, and in subsequent evaluation efforts, critical life skills (identified as livelihood or vocational skills) include: (1) practical health related skills, for example boiling water before drinking, condom use, etc.; (2) physical skills; and (3) skills related to social behavior and interaction. The first two livelihood skills are knowledge based, whereas the last one is comprised of what people do with the previous two.

A limiting factor in creating and using skills-oriented curricula is teaching strategies that continue to be dominated by a traditional content and examination focus rather than a more holistic pupil-centered curriculum. This overly traditional focus has limited the ability of the education sector to utilize a more current curriculum inclusive of elements focusing on critical life skills and has thereby led to the creation of insufficient levels of critical social behavior and interaction skills among teachers and children.

In an effort related to SHEP, a wide variety of governmental, nongovernmental, and faith-based organizations were contracted to supplement

HIV/AIDS activities in secondary schools. These organizations included AIDS Care, Education and Training (ACET); Gulu Hospital; Waloko Kwo Project; Gulu Youth Development Agency (GYDA); Kampala Archdiocese Medical Office; Grassland Foundation; Baptist Student Ministry; Packwach AIDS Care; Straight Talk Foundation; and Agency for Cooperation and Research in Development (ACORD). Part of the support provided by the United Nations Development Programme (UNDP) was to improve the capacity and coverage of NGOs and FBOs and assist them to operate effectively in secondary school communities. Most of their approaches differed in content and style but the common theme of prevention remained the same.

Most of these organizations developed innovative program interventions that addressed life skills needed to empower adolescents to make correct decisions in preventing the further spread of HIV and AIDS. However, most if not all of these NGOs and organizations lacked a coordinated approach in both providing standardized information and reaching out to the same target group. Consequently, their potentially good work was fragmented and missed the chance to create the desired outcome: a critical mass of adolescents able to champion the crusade against HIV/AIDS, thus making these interventions self-sustaining in promoting positive behavior change (UNDP/UNESCO, 1997).

The Programme for Enhancing Adolescent Reproductive Life (PEARL)

Established in 1997, the Programme for Enhancing Adolescent Reproductive Life (PEARL) expanded to 13 districts of Uganda by 2000 at various renovated community centers. These community centers were used by adolescents for meetings, drama classes, seminars, and other reproductive health activities. The main services PEARL provided were in the areas of counseling and guiding youth. PEARL's twin objectives were to promote positive cultural practices that enhance adolescent reproductive life and to increase interpersonal communication between parents and children on reproductive health issues. The target audience for PEARL's services was 30% of all families in the 13 districts. PEARL also attempted to provide accessible, acceptable, and affordable reproductive health services for 15% of all adolescents in the PEARL operating districts and to advocate for the inclusion of the target groups' reproductive health problems in existing health units.

PEARL was therefore an effort to improve the quality of life among adolescents by, among other things, addressing SRH problems. The PEARL approach used renovated community centers as focal points where adolescents could come to receive SRH messages and services and also engage in social and economic activities that could enhance their lives. The primary target group for PEARL was out-of-school adolescent boys and girls between the ages of 10 and 24. Other target groups included community leaders, parents, religious leaders, and youth and adolescent organizations. However, throughout the life of PEARL, their data collection, management, processing, and utilization was poor at both the district and national levels. Poor data management limited the systematic monitoring and evaluation of PEARL activities and therefore did not allow for an adequate appraisal of the effectiveness of this extensive program in reaching its overall goals.

The Presidential Initiative on AIDS Strategy for Communication to Youth (PIASCY)

The Presidential Initiative on AIDS Strategy for Communication to Youth (PIASCY) is the most recent education program spearheaded by the MOES in response to the President of Uganda's call to find ways to improve communication on HIV and AIDS to young people. While PIASCY prefers focusing on parent-led efforts, the obstacles to that effort typically require other avenues of information dissemination. In contrast to parents, Uganda's approximately 125,000 primary school teachers are much more easily reached through their school supervisors. And, unlike many Ugandan parents, teachers generally all speak English. Teachers serve as parent-like role models at school and are ideally situated to help pupils understand their growing bodies and changing emotions. In addition, many pupils are orphans and teachers may be the only adults who ever talk to them about sexuality and safe social interactions. Through PIASCY, teachers are viewed as the most able and accessible people to help pupils abstain from early and unsafe sexual practices and to further encourage protective behavior to reduce the spread of HIV and other STDs and prevent pregnancy when students choose to engage in sexual activity.

When students entering puberty are approached by others for sex, they need strength, knowledge, and life skills to be able to resist and abstain. At this vulnerable stage of life, abstinence is a preferable and very positive choice. Abstinence is not just "not having sex," it involves actively thinking about sex and how to stay safe, expressing feelings about sex (saying no), and rejecting myths about sexual activity at a young age (MOES, 2004).

Unfortunately, PIASCY's principle strategy typically excludes children who are out of school. In addition, the English-based communication strategy assumes that children in school understand and discuss in English at a sufficiently high level of comprehension to participate in effective discussions regarding SRH activities. These two issues have limited the comprehensive effectiveness of the initiative.

FAITH-BASED PROGRAMS

Several FBOs have been providing educational services in Uganda since the middle of the nineteenth century, beginning first with Muslim missionaries, then with Christian Catholic and Protestant missionaries. Over the years, FBOs have also included health services to their followings and the population at large. These organizations have responded to the need for a response in the HIV/AIDS crisis with a number of substantial programs.

While many religious leaders have shunned the promotion of condom use as an effective method in the control of the spread of HIV/AIDS, others have embraced the government's "Abstinence, Be Faithful, and if not use a Condom (ABC)" strategy as the most effective approach in the fight against the pandemic. No Ugandan religion has an official policy position on the use of condoms and leaders can be found in each of Uganda's major religious faiths who advocate the use of condoms as a secondary method of prevention to abstinence and being faithful.

Catholic Church

In Uganda, the Catholic Church commands the largest following of any religious denomination, with about 44% of the country's population designated as Catholic. Traditionally, the Catholic Church has been involved in the provision of social services through its many missionary schools and health units, most of which are among the very best in the country. Using its comparatively vast resources, infrastructure, and following, the Catholic Church in Uganda has been one of the FBOs at the forefront in the fight against the HIV/AIDS pandemic. It has initiated and implemented a number of programs and interventions including the Behaviour Change Programme (BCP) and the Adolescent Sexual and Reproductive Health and Rights Programme.

The Catholic Church has a dedicated HIV/AIDS focal point office responsible for gathering and disseminating HIV/AIDS-related information in all Catholic Churches across the country. The Focal point office also facilitates the planning, implementation, monitoring, and evaluation of HIV/AIDS activities in all Ugandan Catholic dioceses. It also networks with the Uganda AIDS Commission (UAC) and other partners in the national HIV/AIDS response through a number of programs.

The Behaviour Change Programme (BCP)

The Behaviour Change Programme (BCP) is run by the Uganda Young Christian Students (YCS) movement under the Uganda Catholic Secretariat. The BCP was initiated in 1996 in response to the HIV/AIDS pandemic, which had by then affected in one way or another nearly all households in Uganda. The program was set up with the primary objective of promoting spiritual renewal and the redirection of moral conduct among the 13 to 25 year-olds, the age group most vulnerable to the HIV/AIDS scourge in Uganda. The program targets young persons that are still in school and was designed on the premise that young people often engage in risky sexual behaviors due to lack of proper guidance and support on matters of sex and sexuality. For two reasons, the BCP adopted a peer-based approach to induce and promote positive behavior change in this age group: (1) most students attend boarding schools and therefore spend very little time with their parents or guardians throughout most of the year; and (2) most youth relate better to their peers than older persons, including their parents. Thus, for the past 8 years, the BCP has recruited students to assume the role of "apostles of change" to fellow students in all of the Catholic dioceses in Uganda.

The main challenge of the BCP has been the continuous and unavoidable dropping out of "apostles of change" from the program, student drop out from school, and the completion or changing of schools by students. This continuous turnover, especially of the apostles of change, has necessitated the creation of new capacity through continuous recruitment and training. This is not only costly but raises questions of continuity, efficiency, and program impact.

The Adolescent Sexual and Reproductive Health (ASRH) and Rights Programme

This new program is funded by the United Nations Population Fund (UNFPA) and the African Youth Alliance (AYA). The program was designed in recognition of the fact that within the Catholic Church there are structural barriers that put young people at risk of SRH conditions and limit their access to SRH education and care in a systematic and organized approach. Among the major structural barriers is lack of integrated SRH education in the training curriculum of the clergy. Consequently, there is no systematic integration of SRH issues and guidance in typical pastoral and community work. There is also virtually no systematic linkage between Catholic Church-founded health centers and their educational systems. Low or no linkage is at least partly due to lack of guidelines and the negative attitudes of some of the leaders providing services to young people. Yet these conditions could provide opportunities to expand access to adolescent-friendly sexual and reproductive health education and care.

Another major structural barrier is the issue of the Catholic Church's canon law on marriage that permits girls to marry at the age of 14 and boys at the age of 16. This low age of marriage puts young people at greater risk of early sexual intercourse with attendant negative SRH conditions. This canon law is also contrary to the Constitution of Uganda that prohibits marriage of persons under the age of 18. Despite the many challenges posed by the HIV/AIDS pandemic, the ASRH advocacy program has recognized the need to instigate reforms within the Catholic Church. Reforms currently under review are possible changes to the canon law on age of marriage as well as revision of the training curriculum of the clergy so that they can optimally exploit the numerous opportunities they have to provide ASRH guidance during their community and pastoral work.

There is a great need to provide Catholic-sponsored ASRH services in order to expand access to young people in a manner and style that make them feel free to use both SRH information and services. Furthermore, the Catholic Church recognizes the need to allocate more resources and mobilize additional resources for ASRH programs.

Church of Uganda

The Church of Uganda commands almost an equal following to that of the Catholic Church, with about 40% of the population professing to belong to this Protestant faith. Thus, the Church of Uganda's major decisions and policies significantly influence the lives of many Ugandans.

Church Human Services Agency (CHUSA)

HIV/AIDS activities in the Church of Uganda are spearheaded by the Church Human Services Agency (CHUSA), which began its work in 1992. CHUSA is responsible for developing programs, coordinating HIV/AIDS activities, and advising Church leadership on HIV/AIDS-related issues.

Several individuals from the Church of Uganda have supported the ABC approach, including the use of condoms. For example, in one of CHUSA's AIDS documents of 2000, the director of CHUSA stated:

> The ABC of AIDS prevention is open to different people in different situations and it is based on personal informed decision. This teaching of ABC is

good and must be promoted and protected because abstinence, fidelity and condom use are independent options open to whoever wants to use them in the prevention of HIV infection.

Safeguarding Youth From AIDS (SYFA)

A UNICEF-Uganda initiative, SYFA has involved NGOs in HIV/AIDS-related activities supported to extend services to young people in various parts of the country. Under the Church of Uganda, the project was administered by CHUSA and implementation of activities started in 1993. The project's target population was children in the 5–15-year-old category who, at the time, were thought to be HIV/AIDS free. The project intended to reach this age group through team leaders of the Church of Uganda's youth organizations and the boys/girls brigades who were trained as peer educators. The CHUSA-SYFA project's main area of focus was to initiate and promote change in behaviors that increase the risk of HIV infection, such as involvement in sexual activity at an early age, having multiple sex partners, and inadequate care for STDs. Children were educated and sensitized through music and drama, as these were believed to be two of the most effective modes of communication with this age group.

The primary objectives of the CHUSA-SYFA project were to provide correct information on HIV/AIDS to youth in the various dioceses of the church, reduce the rate of STDs in sexually active adolescents, postpone the age of first sexual intercourse, reduce the number of sexual partners, and decrease the incidence of sexually risky behaviors. HIV/AIDS sensitization of the youth in the archdeaconries was to cover basic knowledge about HIV/AIDS and its prevention and consequences. In addition, life skills development was also promoted mostly through gardening activities. The gardening activities were aimed at combating poverty, which is considered one of the major factors contributing to the spread of HIV/AIDS (Ahimbisibwe & Asiimwe, 1995).

It should be noted that during the initial stages of CHUSA-SYFA, condom use as a preventative measure against HIV infection was not supported by the Church of Uganda and was therefore not promoted. This limited the options initially available for HIV/AIDS prevention, particularly among sexually-active adolescents. The program itself was being run during school days and hours which detracted from test-driven curriculum and was therefore not strongly supported by school management. The project's impact was further limited due to an inappropriate implementation design that conflicted with other nonacademic school activities. Lastly, in the initial stages of the program most parents were strongly opposed to having their children exposed to sex education during their early adolescent years; the program did not include a component for addressing the concerns and fears of parents.

Islam

As the first foreign religious group to come to Uganda in 1844, Muslims today make up approximately 15% of Uganda's population (U.S. Department of State, 2004). In the Islamic faith, ASRH programs and activities are spearheaded by the Population Committee of the Uganda Muslim Supreme Council (UMSC). This committee was established in 1996, with support from UNFPA, to address a number of concerns that were curtailing the involvement of the Muslim community in ASRH matters. The formation of this committee itself provoked opposition from a cross-section of the Muslim leadership who believed that the committee's real intention was to covertly work against the Islamic faith. Initial sensitization workshops held by the committee revealed that there was a lack of awareness about SRH issues at all levels and that certain SRH issues such as family planning were highly stigmatized. There was also failure to reconcile SRH issues and policies with the precepts of Islam, and the UMSC did not have any documented stand on SRH issues (UMSC/AYA, 1998).

Unfortunately, this situation does not seem to have changed much to date. While there is increased awareness about SRH issues, there remains a significant conceptual variance among the leaders of the Islamic faith about many SRH issues. Islamic tenets that govern sexual and reproductive behavior and health are not known to all Muslims in Uganda and have not been translated into standard policies that can guide the Muslim community on SRH issues and concerns (UMSC/AYA, 2003a; UMSC/AYA, 2003b). Thus, many SRH issues including early marriage, consent before marriage, preparation of intending spouses including voluntary counseling and testing (VCT) services and condom use, family planning, and use of modern contraceptives continue to be topics of concern within the Muslim community.

The Islamic Medical Association of Uganda (IMAU) was one of the first religious organizations to fight HIV not only among Muslim followers but also among all community members regardless of religious affiliation. IMAU was one of the first local organizations to have been funded by USAID, and subsequently by other large multilateral organizations including the World Health Organization and the UNDP. Recently recognized by UNAIDS as an example of best practices in the area of religion and the fight against HIV/AIDS, IMAU continues its grassroots prevention and treatment efforts within many Ugandan communities.

INTERNATIONAL ORGANIZATION PROGRAMS

Recognized globally for their positive influence and impact in most educational and humanitarian sectors, international organizations and agencies have also played a critical role in Uganda's engagement with the HIV/AIDS challenge. In many instances, these influences have taken the form of collaborative efforts, while others have been independent initiatives. In either form, these organizations and agencies have made an indispensable contribution. In this section, we outline UNICEF's collaborative HIV/AIDS efforts with the government of Uganda.

UNICEF

Since the beginning of the HIV/AIDS epidemic in Uganda, the UNICEF-Uganda collaboration has been part of government efforts to combat the spread of HIV/AIDS and mitigate its impact. The Government of Uganda-UNICEF (GOU-UNICEF) country-wide program is unique in that it is demand-driven rather than service-driven. The program focuses on involving people in diagnosing their own problems, deciding what action(s) need to be taken, and playing an active role in implementation. The three issues of self-diagnosis, decision, and implementation are considered critical for program ownership and sustainability.

Over the past 2 decades, a number of programs have been implemented under the ambit of the GOU-UNICEF country program. Two of the central programs in this regard are the Basic Education, Child Care and Protection, and Adolescent Development (BECCAD) and the Adolescent Development and HIV/AIDS Prevention Strategy.

GOU-UNICEF BECCAD Program

The GOU-UNICEF BECCAD program strategies and activities focused on three main areas: basic education, childcare and protection, and adolescent development. These three areas were initially implemented separately but were later merged to form one program under the structure of BECCAD. This unification grew out of the realization that all three programs were meant to address the same issues: the changing psychosocial, emotional, and cognitive developmental needs of a child from conception through birth, infancy, childhood, to adolescence.

The unified program objective of GOU-UNICEF BECCAD was to promote full cognitive and psychosocial development of children and adolescents within a supportive family and community environment. In particular, the family and community environment was meant to be conducive to education for all, prevention of HIV/AIDS, and adequate care and protection for children and adolescents from birth to adulthood.

Adolescent Development and HIV/AIDS Prevention Strategy Program

The primary objective of the Adolescent Development and HIV/AIDS Prevention Strategy program was to address the ASRH needs of children who were deemed to be most vulnerable to the risk of HIV/AIDS infection. The most vulnerable groups of children identified included out-of-school youth, children of illiterate parents, neglected and abused children, and girls without parental and community protection (GOU/ UNICEF, 1995). The program strategy was to provide support in the area of advocacy and policy formulation, health promotion, resource mobilization, and capacity building for adolescent-focused activities. At the family and community levels, the capacity of the family, the community, and schools were to be strengthened to promote safe sexual behavior among adolescents. In particular, the program sought to delay first sexual experience and to avoid premarital sexual activities.

All of the program goals and strategies were to be achieved through promotion of peer education and increased dialogue between parents and children. The program sought to instill in children, at an early stage, a feeling of responsibility and concern for their own health. In addition, adolescents were to be encouraged and assisted to develop programs which promote health seeking and safe sex behavior. Adolescents in the program were to develop their programs by seeking information and demanding services which address their ASRH needs directly. The program also aimed at promoting and strengthening counseling services for children and adolescents both in schools and in the community, and emphasized special problems such as disparities and vulnerabilities of female children.

At the service delivery and resource management level, the capacity of local governments was to be strengthened to promote safe sexual behavior among adolescents. This was done primarily through sensitizing and mobilizing public opinion and government decision-makers as well as by advocating for and facilitating the development of policies and plans for HIV/AIDS prevention among adolescents. Facilitators were trained in life skills, and paralegal training was supported to effectively deal with crimes of sex abuse which unduly exposes adolescents, especially girls, to HIV/ AIDS.

At the national level, support was given to advocate for and strengthen capacity to sustain activities promoting safe sexual behavior among adolescents. This was done through sensitizing and mobilizing government decision-makers and counterpart institutions, ministries, and NGOs in their advocacy and formulation of appropriate gender-sensitive policies on HIV/AIDS among children and adolescents. Assistance was provided to support the dissemination of gender-sensitive materials that promote safe sexual behaviors. Assistance was also provided to strengthen HIV/AIDS education in school curricula, such as the family life education and other life skills programs. Further assistance was provided to the UAC to carry out its coordinating role at the central and local government levels, especially for activities focusing on adolescents. Capacity was built, at all levels, to monitor performance of activities promoting safe sexual behavior among children and adolescents. This capacity focused on developing indicators and strengthening existing information management systems at the community, local, and central government levels (UNICEF, 1998).

SOCIAL AND BEHAVIORAL DETERMINANTS

Based on the prior discussion, it is apparent that HIV/AIDS interventions in Uganda take a variety of social and behavioral factors into account in their program design and implementation stages. Age, gender, peer influence, and the social environment in which young people live appear to be the major factors that most programs consider. In this section, we examine each of these variables as determinants for HIV/AIDS prevention (UNICEF, 1998).

Age

There is unanimous recognition of the fact that HIV/AIDS vulnerability and needs differ across age groups. Most HIV/AIDS interventions among young people have targeted the 6–14-year-old and 15–25-year-old age groups as distinct cohorts with specific HIV/AIDS-related needs and risks. The 6–14-year-old age group constitutes children who may not yet perceive their potential risk of HIV infection. Most children in this group seem aware of the existence of HIV/AIDS, either through school, the media, or by direct observance of their parents' and close relatives' HIV/AIDS-related illness and death. Most children infected during birth will have become symptomatic by this age and therefore have to deal with social stigmatization and curious questioning from their age and school mates. At the same time, 6–14-year-old children have to deal with uncertainty surrounding the health of their parents and relatives. These children are vulnerable to HIV infection mainly through sexual abuse and early marriages. School-going children, especially girls, are vulnerable to sexual abuse by some male teachers and administrators while most out-of-school children are either enrolled as child laborers or are married at an earlier age.

Given that the majority of 6–14-year-olds are enrolled in school, early interventions targeting this age group were implemented through school-based programs such as SHEP, the Health Education Network (HEN), and the Save the Youth from AIDS (SYFA) initiative. These programs focused on integrating HIV/AIDS in school activities and building the capacity of teachers to address issues related to HIV and AIDS. Currently, most HIV/AIDS interventions are trying to raise awareness in this age group about issues of sex, HIV/AIDS, dangers of engaging in early sex, body changes, as well as promoting dialogue with parents and teachers about these issues.

The 15–24-year-old age group includes adolescents and young adults, most of whom are not currently enrolled in school. HIV prevalence was, until the end of 2000, highest in this age group. Between 1992 and 1998, several innovative peer-support-based interventions were implemented mainly in secondary schools and tertiary institutions. The programs emphasized formation of AIDS challenge clubs, holding interschool debates on HIV/AIDS topics, providing youth-friendly information, education, and communication (IEC) materials, and training of peer leaders and counselors. During the late 1990s, additional programs such as PEARL, BECCAD, and the STF have been implemented. These programs generally seek to enhance youth skills in communication, sex negotiation, response to peer pressure, and development of rational and positive relationships with members of the opposite sex.

Gender

HIV prevalence varies widely between men and women in different age groups. In the age group of 25 and below, females are 2 to 3 times more likely to be infected than males. In the 15–19 year-old age group, females are 5 to 6 times more likely to be infected than males (MOH, 2000). The physical and contextual aspects of culture, power relations, and economics at domestic and national levels are among the major factors increasing the vulnerability of women to HIV infection. For example, girls are less likely to enroll in school, complete primary school, attend secondary education, or enter institutions of higher learning. A good number of girls are often forced into early marriages and have less power in sexual relationships. Because of their subordinated status, women often cannot insist on condom use or successfully resist sexual demands, especially from older men. Married women are generally unable to stop their husbands from having multiple sexual partners or from marrying other wives

(Neema, 2000). Wives are unable to refuse unprotected sex with their husbands, even when they know that the husband is HIV-positive or has engaged in multiple sexual relationships. There are also significant negative repercussions in sexual relationships from stereotyped roles that encourage submissiveness on the part of girls and aggressiveness on the part of boys (GOU/UAC/UNAIDS, 2000).

Several attempts to make HIV/AIDS programs in Uganda more gender sensitive have been instituted. These attempts include improving access to care and prevention services, involvement of women in advocacy, direct provision of HIV/AIDS services to women, and raising the visibility of women in political and socioeconomic affairs from the grassroots to the national level. In addition to general policy-wide activities, many contemporary HIV/AIDS programs, such as microenterprise development, school-based HIV/AIDS activities, and skills development, prioritize women in their design and implementation. The involvement of community-based institutions—like traditional birth attendants, traditional healers, religious leaders, and other civil society organizations in HIV/AIDS activities—has been another critical factor in improving access to HIV/AIDS services by women in Uganda.

Peer Influence

A third factor in the formation and change of behavior is peer influence. Because peer influence has proven to be a significant influence in behavior, it has become a major consideration in the design of most HIV/AIDS interventions targeting young people. The success of peer influence is based on the function of shared interests and beliefs that young people cherish. These cherished interests and beliefs form the basis of peer norms and values that enhance the attainment of common interests. Compliance to values and norms is critically monitored and provides an impetus for empathy and concern about others. In general, people living in communities—such as a school for young people or a rural village for adults—share information through a complex web of social networks. These networks include community groups, church activity groups, funeral gatherings, and various forms of interpersonal relationships. Many HIV/AIDS organizations have taken advantage of these strong community linkages and networks to provide HIV/AIDS-related services aimed at changing perceptions and practices regarding high-risk sexual behavior.

Youth programs, such as SHEP and PEARL described earlier in this chapter, are examples of organizations whose activities aim at changing individual behavior through peer education and influence. Peer groups comprising people living with HIV/AIDS have been used to offer support, counseling, and friendship. These programs and activities provide powerful evidence about the existence of HIV/AIDS and produce positive influences within communities. They also give hope to those already infected that it is possible to live a normal life. More so, peer influences and programs encourage those not yet affected to engage in safer sexual practices.

Social Environment

Another important determinant of successful intervention is the social environment in which young people live. Since behavior formation and change are both products of the individual's psychological and cognitive factors and interpersonal interactions, an enabling and supportive social environment is critical to the success of any behavioral intervention. Many HIV/AIDS programs targeting young people recognize that most young people live in social environments at home, school, or in the community that are not conducive for positive ASRH decisions.

For the most part, children do not receive adequate family life education in the home; cultural norms often prevent parents and other adults from discussing sex with children and youth. Religious leaders too often discourage the provision of ASRH information or services to adolescents. Consequently, in an effort to avoid conflict and breach long-established cultural norms, teachers and health workers are reluctant to provide adequate ASRH information and services to adolescents.

Many young people lack critical life skills. This is because most homes and schools do not create environments conducive for adolescents to develop these skills. Nonconducive environments result primarily from traditions which do not encourage children to express their own opinions, question the views of others, or make their own decisions. In this regard, a number of adolescent HIV/AIDS programs are attempting to change this situation by promoting open discussion of ASRH issues between teachers and parents and their pupils and children. Many programs attempt to stimulate active support for ASRH services among policy makers.

Challenges

Like other educational initiatives, HIV/AIDS programs often make a number of assumptions in their program planning and design stages regarding the school environment and teacher, parent, pupil, and peer factors. For example, in a school setting, a common fallacy is to assume that students have a uniform level of understanding of the messages and skills being presented to them. With so many types of schooling environments that exist throughout the country—such as urban and rural schools, universal primary education (UPE) middle-class public and private schools, and religious owned and operated schools—the quality of ASRH instruction likewise varies. Such variance among schools poses a serious methodological problem to effective teaching of attitudes and skills that would lead to behavioral change among adolescents attending schools. Most approaches to sex education in school settings do not take into consideration the limitations on program impact created by the heterogeneous cultural and religious backgrounds of student families, levels of understanding and languages of communication of students, different school environments (i.e., single sex, mixed-sex, day and boarding schools), or the surrounding environment (i.e., bars and movie theatres adjacent or nearby school premises).

Schools present an environment that is orderly, closely regulated, and make it possible for youth, peers, and teachers to share information. School assemblies collect a large number of students and pupils together in one setting. These gatherings represent convenient avenues to disseminate messages regarding HIV/AIDS. However, over a period of time, school assemblies are well known as check points for conformity with school rules, activities, and education standards. They are also places where punishments and reprimands are delivered to students. As a result, students tend to dislike school-wide assemblies. The very orderliness of schools in curricular structure and the rigid traditional nature and content of assemblies tend to limit their potential in raising awareness of critical HIV/AIDS knowledge that could help youth make better informed choices.

Many adolescent HIV/AIDS programs tend to focus exclusively on schools, excluding parents and community resources that have such a strong and lasting influence on shaping children's values and norms. Youth tend to engage in most of their risky behavior in the context of homesteads and communities rather than in tightly regulated schools. Most programs appear to assume that peer influence is found only between those students in the formal school setting, often ignoring substantial interaction that occurs between out-of-school and in-school adolescents. This is a critical oversight because most unplanned pregnancies for in-school girls usually result from sexual relations with out-of-school males.

CONCLUSION

In the modern era, the HIV/AIDS pandemic is perhaps the largest single test to Uganda's long-cherished social, cultural, and religious values and traditions. Since sexual intercourse is the primary means of HIV transmission in Uganda, change in sexual behavior has been and remains the major weapon in the fight against the HIV pandemic. However, initiating individual behavior change required nothing less than a sexual revolution and has necessitated discussing issues of sex and sexuality openly, something that hitherto has been regarded as taboo in most Ugandan cultures. This revolutionary discourse shift has been facilitated primarily through government, faith-based, and international HIV/AIDS prevention programs, along with promoting essential ASHR dialogue between children, their parents, and teachers.

Apart from the limitations imposed by scarce financial resources, the major challenge to HIV education programs, both faith-based and otherwise, are negative personal and cultural attitudes towards ASRH information and services. For example, there is widespread recognition that many young people engage in early sex and that there is a high prevalence of teenage pregnancies. In the face of these realities, some religious leaders and faiths still fervently oppose condom use to control the spread of HIV, acquiring other STDs, and in an effort to reduce the number of unplanned pregnancies. Furthermore, while most HIV/AIDS programs are making efforts to ensure that their interventions are culturally sensitive, the diverse nature of Uganda's deep-seated cultures, traditions, norms, and languages continue to present significant methodological challenges. Yet the success of these programs hinges heavily on being cognizant of these diverse factors, appropriately using those that reduce risk, and tactfully discouraging those which enhance high-risk behaviors.

REFERENCES

Ahimbisibwe, W. D. E., & Asiimwe, D. (1995). *An evaluation of Safeguard Youth from AIDS (SYFA) programme*. Kampala, Uganda: UNICEF/Uganda AIDS Commission.

Asiimwe D., Kibombo R., & Neema S. (2003). *Focus group discussion on social cultural factors impacting on HIV/AIDS in Uganda*. Kampala, Uganda: Makerere Institute of Social Research (MISR)/UNDP.

Government of Uganda (GOU)/UNICEF. (1995). *Life skills for young Ugandans, primary and secondary teachers' training manuals*. Kampala, Uganda: Authors.

GOU/Uganda AIDS Commission (UAC)/UNAIDS. (2000). *National strategic framework for HIV/AIDS: Activities in Uganda, 2000–2006*. Kampala, Uganda: Authors.

Ministry of Education and Sports (MOES). (2002). *Examination of best practices for HIV/AIDS reduction in the education sector: Draft report.* Kampala: Author.

MOES. (2004). *Presidential Initiative on AIDS Strategy for Communication to Youth: Handbook for primary school teachers.* Kampala, Uganda: Author.

Ministry of Health (MOH). (2000). *HIV/AIDS surveillance report, 1997–2000.* Kampala, Uganda: Author.

MOH. (2002). *HIV/AIDS surveillance report, 2002.* Kampala, Uganda: Author.

Neema, S. (2002). *The relationship between chronic poverty and health in Uganda: Evidence from the literature.* Kampala, Uganda: MISR.

Uganda Catholic Secretariat. (2003). *Advocacy strategic framework to promote adolescent sexual and reproductive health and rights in the Catholic Church.* Kampala, Uganda: Author.

Uganda Young Christian Students. (1998). *Behaviour change programme.* Kampala, Uganda: Authors.

UMSC/AYA. (1998). *Towards a happy and prosperous family: A reproductive health guide for the Muslim community in Uganda.* Kampala, Uganda: Author.

UMSC/AYA. (2003a). *Advocacy strategic framework for adolescent reproductive health project.* Kampal, Uganda: Author.

UMSC/AYA. (2003b). *Getting adolescent and reproductive health on the agenda.* Kampala, Uganda: Author.

UNDP. (2002). *Uganda human development report.* Kampala, Uganda: Author.

UNDP/UNESCO. (1997). *HIV/AIDS information, education and communication interventions in secondary schools: An assessment of effectiveness and impact of behaviour change activities on secondary school adolescents in Uganda.* Kampala, Uganda: Author.

UNICEF. (1998). *Government of Uganda: UNICEF Country Programme, 1995-2000: Country Progress Report.* Kampala, Uganda: Author

U.S. Department of State. (2004). *International religious freedom report.* Washington, DC: Bureau of Democracy, Human Rights and Labor.

CHAPTER 7

THE AIDS SUPPORT ORGANISATION (TASO)

ISSUES AND POTENTIAL FOR DEVELOPING COUNTRIES

**Alex Coutinho, Robert Ochai, Alex Mugume,
Lynda Kavuma, and John M. Collins**

HIV/AIDS is the leading cause of death in Sub-Saharan Africa, account-ing for 25% of all deaths. One in every seven members of the adult population is infected with HIV/AIDS (Björkman, 2002; Brown, 2004). Håkan Björkman (2002) reported that 5% of the adult population in Uganda is living with HIV/AIDS, and 55% of the population is living below the national poverty line. To address the HIV/AIDS epidemic, Uganda established the National AIDS Control Program in 1986, and in 1992 the government created the Uganda AIDS Commission to coor-dinate government, private, and civil efforts dealing with the virus (AMREF-Uganda, 2001). In the early 1990s the government of Uganda established a national task force on AIDS, which led to the creation of a multisectoral approach to dealing with the virus (UAC, 1993). The *National Strategic Framework for HIV/AIDS Activities for Uganda: 1998–*

Overcoming AIDS: Lessons Learned from Uganda, 125–150
Copyright © 2006 by Information Age Publishing
All rights of reproduction in any form reserved.

2002 emphasized the multisectoral approach developed by the task force (Government of Uganda (GOU)/Uganda AIDS Commission (UAC), 1997). The 1998 *Strategic Framework* asserted the government's commitment to a multisectoral approach and stated that individuals, community groups, different governmental agencies, nongovernmental organizations (NGOs), and community based organizations (CBOs) all have a collective responsibility in the prevention of, active response to, and management of the effects of AIDS. The *National Strategic Framework for HIV/AIDS Activities for Uganda: 2001–2006* (hereafter referred to as *Framework*) expands on this collective responsibility by calling for the creation and expansion of organizational capacity of both the government and nongovernmental sectors to address HIV/AIDS activities (GOU/UAC/UNAIDS, 2000).

In this chapter, we evaluate The AIDS Support Organisation (TASO), the largest indigenous NGO in the country of Uganda and the largest HIV/AIDS support organization in Sub-Saharan Africa. We examine the organization's objectives and ways the organization is meeting the needs identified by the *Framework*. We begin by presenting an overview of the *Framework* and its corresponding objectives. Next we look at TASO's role in the multisectoral approach outlined by the *Framework*. We then evaluate TASO's services and programs by examining how well TASO's four objectives help the organization meet the three objectives outlined in the *Framework*. The final section analyzes the strengths, weaknesses, opportunities, and threats (SWOT) of the organization.

THE NATIONAL STRATEGIC FRAMEWORK

The *Framework* was designed to minimize duplication of efforts in the fight against the spread of HIV/AIDS in Uganda, engender more focused interventions, and simplify monitoring and evaluation of HIV/AIDS (GOU/UAC/UNAIDS, 2000). In an attempt to position HIV/AIDS in the broader context of social and economic development within Uganda, the *Framework* for HIV/AIDS outlines three overarching objectives:

1.   Reduce HIV prevalence by 25% by the year 2006.
2.   Mitigate health and socioeconomic effects of HIV/AIDS at the individual, household, and community levels.
3.   Strengthen the national capacity to respond to the epidemic.

The *Framework* identifies public sector limitations to achieving these objectives, highlighting the need for partnerships with CBOs and

NGOs. According to Godfrey Bahiigwa (2003), the government of Uganda would be required to increase its spending on HIV/AIDS efforts by 83% if it were to combat the virus on its own (p. 20). However, the government recognizes the valuable human and financial resources that NGOs and CBOs contribute in the effort to combat the epidemic. The *Framework* also stresses the importance of a participatory approach functioning as a catalyst for increased ownership and responsibility of stakeholders in the process and recognizes the importance of including people who are infected/affected by the virus in the planning and decision-making process.

TASO'S ROLE IN THE MULTISECTORAL APPROACH

TASO was first organized in 1987 by 16 individuals who were infected or impacted by HIV/AIDS. The group met to provide psychological and social support to each other at a time when ignorance, discrimination, and high levels of stigma were associated with HIV/AIDS. Of the 16 founding members, eight have passed away (TASO, 2002; UNAIDS, 2001). TASO began by providing training workshops in hospitals to raise awareness of the needs of people living with HIV/AIDS (PWA).

TASO was founded on a desire to improve the quality of life for PWA and enable them to live positively with the disease. In 1987 there was no organized service or organization in Uganda that provided counseling, care, or support to PWA. TASO helped fill this enormous gap in responding to critical needs resulting from the HIV/AIDS epidemic (UNAIDS, 2001). Since its beginning with only 16 members, TASO has expanded and retained its reputation as the largest nongovernmental player in care and support for PWA in Uganda and Sub-Saharan Africa. TASO has steadily increased its client base by approximately 6,000 new clients every year (TASO, 2002).

TASO's vision statement identifies as its principal objective to help people live positively with HIV/AIDS. This statement refers not only to the physical well-being of PWA but also to their psychosocial well-being. The organization serves the needs of PWA and provides information to help communities understand, prevent, and treat HIV and AIDS.

People who are HIV positive become the client base of TASO and are given the knowledge and resources to live positively with the virus. Outreach programs help clients understand and work towards the following six goals: (1) accept their diagnosis and seek prompt and appropriate medical care, (2) practice safer sex to prevent the continued spread of the disease, (3) continue to earn an income and plan for their families' and dependants' livelihood, (4) seek counseling to help with the emotional and psychological effects of the disease, (5) maintain a balanced diet and ensure adequate sleep and exercise into a daily routine, and (6) continue with normal social activities while avoiding harmful habits such as drinking alcohol and smoking.

These outreach measures are attempts to provide simple lifestyle changes to help HIV/AIDS-infected clients live longer, healthier, and more productive lives with the disease. In this manner, TASO's organizational mission is to contribute to restoring hope and improving the quality of life of persons and communities affected by HIV/AIDS (TASO, 2002). Improving an individual's quality of life is not limited to diet and exercise. TASO takes a holistic approach by addressing HIV/AIDS issues at the personal, family, community, national, and international levels. At the personal level, TASO offers

> one-to-one counseling, which empowers the infected/affected person to make informed decisions, which improve the quality of life and facilitate the balance between rights and responsibilities of the individual. TASO attempts to provide sensitive and compassionate care while providing early diagnosis and treatment of opportunistic infections to help individuals live positively and die with dignity. (TASO, 2002, p. 6)

At the family level TASO provides

> counseling for the family members, which dispels their fears of contracting HIV through casual contact, facilitates care of the infected and affected persons and prepares the family for and supports them during bereavement and facilitates the provision of home nursing care and nutritional materials. (TASO, 2002, p. 6)

At the community level, TASO empowers the community through the provision of counseling services to help the community generate an appropriate response to the problems generated by HIV and facilitates community planned responses, evaluation of their responses, and the mobilization of resources. At the national and international levels TASO sensitizes the public about positive living through training appropriate personnel for service delivery and mobilizing resources for goal and objective achievement. TASO is also involved in several joint international efforts that strive towards the total defeat of HIV infection and disease. The core activities in which TASO is actively involved at these various levels include counseling services for individuals and families infected and/or affected by HIV/AIDS, medical services focusing on the treatment of opportunistic infections, social support that enhances practical positive living, training and capacity building of grassroots communities and districts in basic HIV/AIDS management, and AIDS education and advocacy for PWA.

In response to the *Framework*, the following four immediate objectives were designed to align TASO with the government of Uganda's objectives:

1. To continuously improve the quality, range, and coverage of TASO's HIV/AIDS prevention, care, and support services.

2. To continuously improve the competence of HIV/AIDS service providers through training, capacity building, and consultancies in HIV/AIDS for government institutions, CBOs, and NGOs including TASO personnel.

3. To continuously improve the existing social, political, and economic environment for PWA.

4. To develop and sustain the organizational capacity of TASO to carry out this strategy.

These objectives focus on improving TASO's efficiency and effectiveness in serving the needs of its clients. By aligning its objectives with the *Framework*, TASO believes that it will be able to better meet the needs of its clients while reducing the risk of duplicating services and wasting valuable resources. Further, TASO understands the importance of collaborating with other service providers as the demand continues to increase for AIDS-related services, since the structural and organizational capacity of TASO is not large enough to serve the entire HIV infected population in Uganda. Although TASO has numerous programs and multiple centers across the country, the organization understands that continual interaction and cooperation between CBOs, NGOs, and the government are essential to effectively deal with the HIV/AIDS epidemic.

To accomplish the many programs that TASO has developed, the organization has expanded significantly. Currently TASO has 11 distinct branches throughout the country and 10 mini-TASOs in regional or district hospitals that will open in the next 5 years.[1] The current coverage area has been restricted to the East Africa Highway, the primary east-west transit route (TASO, 2002). TASO currently provides direct services to 35 districts out of the 70 in the country and supports the remaining 35 districts indirectly through the training and capacity building of hospitals and CBOs involved in HIV/AIDS related care and support. TASO also has an international training center that offers training for HIV/AIDS service providers from both Uganda and abroad.

EVALUATING TASO'S SERVICES AND PROGRAMS

Information regarding the transmission and treatment of HIV/AIDS is continually being released as new discoveries are made regarding the disease. This requires continual in-service training of personnel to correct prior misconceptions and beliefs regarding the disease (Ondrusek, 2001). As the HIV/AIDS epidemic touches so many different facets of society in Uganda, and knowledge regarding the disease has dramatically changed since TASO was founded, we had to first determine what criteria to use to evaluate TASO. Michael Keeley (1978) argues that the effectiveness of an organization is measured by its ability to accomplish its official objectives. The first section of our analysis examines the level of alignment between TASO's objectives and the *Framework*. The second portion of our evaluation incorporates a SWOT analysis, which looks at the organization's strengths, weaknesses, opportunities, and threats.

Official Objective Analysis

In response to the three stated objectives of the *Framework*, TASO has developed four official objectives: (1) to continuously improve the quality, range, and coverage of TASO's HIV/AIDS prevention, care, and support services; (2) to continuously improve the competence of HIV/AIDS service providers through offering training, capacity building, and consultation and training for government institutions, CBOs, and NGOs including TASO personnel; (3) to continuously improve the existing social, political, and economic environment for PWA; and (4) to develop and sustain the organizational capacity of TASO to carry out this strategy (TASO, 2002, p. vii). The following sections provide an analysis of each of these objectives' alignment with the *Framework*.

Quality, Range, and Coverage of TASO's HIV/AIDS Services

In our evaluation of TASO's objective to improve the quality, range, and coverage of its HIV/AIDS prevention, care, and support services programs, we examine the number of clients served from 1997 to 2004 by the medical and counseling sessions. As portrayed in Table 7.1, the number of individuals who received counseling services from TASO has nearly quadrupled since 1997, increasing from 28,000 sessions to 100,000 sessions. The number of medical sessions from TASO has also quadrupled during this same time period, increasing from 50,000 sessions to 250,000 sessions. These efforts have required additional facilities, personnel, volunteers, and physical facilities, all of which require additional financial resources. These services have been limited to within 75 kilometers of each

Table 7.1.   Number of Clients Served By Year and By Service Area

Service Area	1997	1998	1999	2000	2001	2002	2003	2004
Counseling sessions	28,000	49,000	45,000	47,000	51,000	69,000	75,000	100,000
Medical sessions	50,000	57,000	63,000	66,000	79,000	117,000	164,000	250,000
Food supplementation	14,000	0	0	7,000	7,000	7,000	7,000	10,000
Schools scholarship/fees	300	300	150	120	510	1,100	1,400	1,400
Apprenticeship program	0	0	0	0	300	300	300	300
Drama performances	120	120	140	270	360	660	760	800
Number of people that have attended performances	50,000	50,000	70,000	90,000	100,000	120,000	150,000	180,000

of the 11 TASO centers. TASO's current effort is to create 10 mini-TASOs and establish regional directors to train, and work with district hospitals and other NGOs and CBOs in areas where TASO is currently not in operation. This will allow TASO to provide more medical and counseling services indirectly to PWA in the other 35 districts of the country.

Competence of HIV/AIDS Service Providers

In moving towards its objective to improve the competence of HIV/AIDS service providers, TASO has expanded its training capacities. For this part of our analysis we looked at the number of trainers trained or served as a result of TASO's training sessions between 1987 and 2003. The number of individuals trained increased from 5 a year in 1988 to 200 a year in 2003; likewise the number of counselors trained increased from 10 a year in 1987 to 260 a year in 2003. Additionally, community volunteers increased from 30 to 330 during this same time period. The outreach of these training programs has been significant as the number of people reached through the counseling and training programs has increased from 100 to 19,000 people a year. Although this is still a small segment of the target population, TASO is continually looking for new ways to reach out to individuals and communities.

One way TASO has adapted to increase its outreach services has been to train care providers of PWA. TASO medical workers observed that many PWA were being infected with opportunistic infections that could be easily treated at home. As many Ugandan hospitals are overcrowded,

TASO clients were waiting days to receive medical services. This led TASO to focus on training care providers of PWA on how to identify and treat opportunistic infections at home. This empowers care providers with the knowledge and skills to help prevent and treat opportunistic infections that plague HIV-infected individuals. This component of the training process has been identified by TASO as extremely effective in reducing the need for medical services by clients (TASO, 2002). For this reason, TASO has attempted to increase the number of individuals trained in opportunistic infections, increasing the number from 5 in 1988 to 140 in 2003 (see Table 7.2).

A service area that we feel is important to highlight because of the number of individuals trained is the area of outreach, particularly from 2002 to 2003. What factors could account for this significant increase from 9,000 to 19,000 individuals trained during this period? A corresponding trend was the decline in the number of community volunteers trained from 1999 to 2003. The number of trainers who received training quadrupled during the same time period and the number of counselors trained more than doubled. These trends lead us to believe that TASO's emphasis on providing training to nonvolunteer staff (i.e., counselors and trainers) is helping the organization to reach a larger proportion of the Ugandan population. Reasons why the number of community volunteers has decreased will be discussed more fully in the weakness section of the SWOT analysis. As for now, we note that community volunteers face unique challenges that make it difficult for them to have long-lasting impact and outreach. These are individuals who are nonpaid, service volunteers who must travel long distances to provide care and report there activities back to TASO. A scenario of high and frequent personnel turnover is perpetuated among community volunteers because there are limited reward mechanisms in place to ensure that volunteers remain with the organization for a long time and because most volunteers generally come from low socioeconomic status families. These factors combine to make the general outreach impact of community volunteers lower than that which is rendered by trainers and counselors. One connection that we do see is that the number of people reached through TASO's services increased substantially from 1999 to 2003, the same time period that saw a dramatic increase in the number of counselors and trainers. This finding leads us to conclude that TASO should prioritize its training efforts towards counselors and individual trainers as the organization continues to expand its outreach programs.

Improving the Social, Political, and Economic Environment for PWA

In evaluating the third objective, we studied the social support services that TASO provides. These consisted of food supplementation, school scholarships and fees, apprenticeship programs, and drama perfor-

Table 7.2. Number of Individuals Trained

Area	1987	1988	1989	1990	1991	1992	1993	1994	1995	1996	1997	1998	1999	2000	2001	2002	2003
Training of trainers	0	5	10	15	20	30	30	40	40	50	50	60	60	100	80	110	200
Counselors trained	10	20	40	60	80	80	80	100	100	100	80	90	100	150	180	220	260
Grassroots community volunteers	0	0	30	60	90	120	150	200	300	300	300	300	600	500	550	550	330
Outreach: People trained thru AIDS counseling and orientation workshops	0	100	200	400	500	700	700	700	700	700	800	1,000	1,500	2,000	3,000	9,000	19,000
Counselor supervisor trained	0	0	5	5	10	5	5	10	5	5	10	10	10	15	20	20	25
People trained in management of opportunistic infection	0	5	10	20	30	40	50	50	50	50	70	70	80	100	100	120	140

Table 7.3. Income Quintiles of TASO Clients

Income Percentile	1997		1998		1999		2000		2001		2002		2003	
	No.	%	No.	%	No.	%	No.	%	No.	%	No.	%	No.	%
Lowest 20th percentile	830	28	1,197	25	1,194	27	1,112	27	1,171	22	2,454	30	2,820	29
Second 20th percentile	904	30	1,132	24	769	18	884	22	1,002	19	1,438	18	1,527	16
Third 20th percentile	221	7	287	6	275	6	269	7	695	13	977	12	1,480	15
Fourth 20th percentile	792	27	1,757	37	1,597	37	1,211	30	1,810	34	2,307	28	2,471	26
Highest 20th percentile	227	8	360	8	518	12	563	14	627	12	1,011	12	1,367	14

mances, as shown in Table 7.1. In terms of social support services, the food supplementation has declined from 14,000 individuals served in 1997 to only 10,000 individuals in 2004. Food donations to TASO clients (from the World Food Programme [WFP]) stopped coming in 1997 due to other global emergencies at that time. TASO had to negotiate a new supplementation program that started with 7,000 clients in 2000 and increased to 10,000 in 2004 when WFP re-started food donations to TASO. The apprenticeship program has remained constant at 300 individuals from 2001 to 2004, while the drama performances have significantly increased. This has resulted in a substantial outreach to the public, as the performances now reach audiences of 180,000 people instead of the 50,000 they were reaching in 1997.

In addition, we looked at the income and education levels of TASOs clients, as seen in Tables 7.3 and 7.4. TASO's client base is highly diverse economically and educationally. As Anne Ruhweza Katahoire (2004) notes, the epidemic is impacting all segments of society in Uganda. The largest percentage of TASO's clients come from the poorest 40% of the population. In terms of education levels, it appears that many of the clients have attained very low levels of education. As was reflected by Table 7.3 and income groups, Table 7.4 shows the impact that HIV/AIDS is having on all segments of society.

As Katahoire (2004) noted, institutions of higher education are being impacted by the morbidity and absenteeism by faculty and students. The majority of TASO's clients have lower education levels, since 1997 nearly 60% of TASO clients have only completed primary school and since 2001 an increasing percentage approaching 30% have completed some secondary education. The remaining portion of TASO's clientele is evenly divided between completed secondary and completed tertiary. One thing that should be noted is that since 1999, the education levels of all clients have been rising. This phenomenon portrays the indifference HIV has on all people regardless of race, socioeconomic status, or education level. This also reflects the overall indifference and impact the virus has on the labor force, impacting highly skilled and trained individuals as well as the unskilled.

Organizational Capacity Building

The last objective established by TASO to align its operations with the *Framework* is connected with organizational capacity building. As demonstrated by the increase in medical and counseling services, as well as the drama performances, TASO has been growing dramatically over the last seven years. To staff the increasing number of centers, the number of full-time personnel has doubled since 1997, increasing from 300 to 600 full-time staff (see Table 7.5). The increase occurred mostly in 2004, as TASO

Table 7.4. Education Levels of TASO Clients

Education Level	1997 No.	%	1998 No.	%	1999 No.	%	2000 No.	%	2001 No.	%	2002 No.	%	2003 No.	%
Partial Primary	514	14	769	21	497	18	431	16	443	13	811	15	950	15
Completed Primary	1,642	46	1,438	39	1,335	48	1,239	48	1,512	45	2,320	41	2,416	38
Partial Secondary	268	8	370	10	294	10	354	14	760	22	1,596	28	1,822	29
Completed Secondary	976	27	961	26	283	10	216	8	228	7	300	5	521	8
Completed Tertiary	177	5	136	4	385	14	361	14	455	13	593	11	606	10

Table 7.5. Number and Type of Staff Working for TASO, 1997 to 2004

Staff	1997	1998	1999	2000	2001	2002	2003	2004
Full time personnel	300	300	350	350	350	350	350	600
Volunteer personnel	30	30	30	50	70	80	100	150

opened two new branches and attempted to increase its support to other districts. In addition, TASO has undergone organizational restructuring to increase organizational efficiency as well as outreach and training. The full-time personnel have been complemented by an increase in volunteer personnel, as the number of volunteers has increased from 30 to 150 between 1997 and 2004.[2]

TASO believes that its governance and management structure can support growth and change. TASO classifies its management structure as democratic with high involvement of PWA (TASO, 2002). Currently TASO is undergoing a process of organizational development and staff training as it begins to decentralize services to lower administrative levels. TASO's governance and management structure consists of a board of trustees, clients' council, center advisory committees, chairperson's advisory council, management committees, and donors meetings (see Figure 7.1). The board of trustees is the top policy and decision-making body of TASO; it provides the governance, policy guidance, and direction during the annual general meetings. The clients' council, which consists of client representatives from the different centers, acts as an advisory body to the Executive Director (ED) providing feedback on matters affecting clients. The center advisory committees are elected local leaders and community members who come together to contribute to the fight against HIV/AIDS in their communities. Theses groups provide local support and input into program directions and manage each center's implementation of activities; they are elected by the clients and registered members of TASO during annual general meetings. The chairperson's advisory council is a forum of all the chairpersons of the center advisory committees from the various centers. It provides the ED with feedback on management matters in relation to service delivery and client concerns. Various management committees at headquarters and centers are established to deal with issues with specific mandates and terms of reference. TASO holds quarterly donor meetings where the administrators and donors exchange open and frank opinions regarding the progress of projects, enabling TASO to keep on track and donors to stay abreast of the various programs.

Figure 7.1 outlines the organizational structure of TASO. The day-to-day running of TASO is under the direction of the ED, the deputy executive director, and a senior management team of six people. Each TASO center has its own management team guided by the center advisory committee and clients' council, as well as by headquarters through the ED. TASO uses both internal and external financial and auditing systems, as well as a monitoring and evaluation department to ensure transparency within the organization. To sustain its organizational capacity to carry out the *Framework*, TASO has expanded its operations and increased its operating budget. The 11 distinct branches and new mini-TASOs still do not

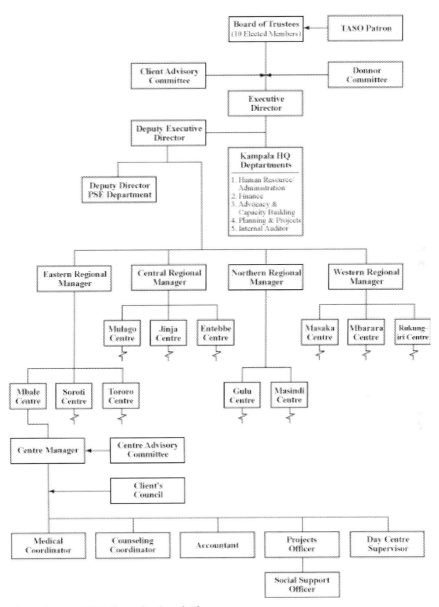

Figure 7.1.   TASO Organizational Chart.

cover all 70 districts of Uganda. However, to increase the coverage area TASO has introduced a regionalization project that dissects the country into four segments. Regional training coordinators work with district hospitals, CBOs, NGOs, and a regional structure that focuses on networking and increasing partnerships across the country to strengthen care and support activities. This process takes the form of advocacy, training, and subgranting to CBOs involved in HIV/AIDS counseling and care.

TASO's budget has grown significantly from the early years, when it was less than U.S.$1 million, to the mid-1990s, when it rose to approximately U.S.$3 million. From 1999 to 2002, TASO's budget increased to U.S.$4 million each year. In 2003 the amount increased to approximately U.S.$7 million annually, reflecting a 700% increase since the first years of the organization's establishment. The increase in financial resources has allowed TASO to expand and increase the number of programs and services offered, including the introduction of antiretroviral therapy (ART), and building of new TASO centers. The budget is comprised of nearly 95% from international donors, 2% from the government of Uganda, and 3% from local sources. According to the *TASO Strategic Plan* (2002) the general distribution of TASOs budget on an annual basis is typically divided as follows:

26% towards Medical Services
24% towards Counseling Services
5% towards Social Support Services
1% towards AIDS Education and Advocacy
20% towards training and building the capacity of other organizations
24% on administration (staff, stationery, vehicles, fuel, building, and maintenance)

As demonstrated by the breakdown of the budget, TASO expends one-fifth of its budget to train and increase capacities of other organizations. This subgranting aspect of TASO will become more important in the future as it attempts to increase the capacity of NGOs and CBOs in districts and regions that do not have TASO centers. With the potential of far greater returns in reaching PWA than the current medical, counseling, and training programs, TASO's subgranting programs will require additional monitoring and evaluation in the future.

TASO'S COMPARATIVE ADVANTAGE

TASO has distinguished itself in the care and support of PWA. Since 1987, TASO has had extensive experience in providing counseling, medical services, and social support to PWA. From this extensive experience, TASO has learned that involving PWA is essential for effective planning, implementation, and evaluation of its programs. PWA are important partners in TASO's decision making model, as they provide valuable knowledge and understanding to the needs of those affected by HIV/AIDS. This PWA human knowledge reservoir allows TASO to remain in touch with those impacted most by the disease. Thus, as noted in Figure 7.1, PWA are involved in all levels of decision making, keeping TASO in tune with the changing needs of PWA through the clients' councils. In addition, TASO has been leading the Sub-Saharan African region in HIV/AIDS counseling and training. TASO has developed extensive training and curriculum for a variety of scenarios, maintaining a highly skilled and knowledgeable workforce, and increasing the outreach ability of the organization. One of TASO's greatest strengths has been its ability to work in partnership with other organizations at the local, regional, national, and international levels.

TASO offers counseling services to PWA and their families at TASO clinics, in the homes of the clients, and in hospital wards. Due to limited governmental resources, there are no permanent counseling positions in government institutions, and the government relies on voluntary and nonprofit organizations such as TASO to provide this critical resource to PWA. These counseling services are provided to the individuals infected by HIV/AIDS, their caregivers, family, discordant couples, and children of infected parents.

TASO has worked to train counselors for other organizations to ensure effective counseling in all regions and districts of the country, as well as for individuals working in other Sub-Saharan African countries. One of the major gaps in services to PWA is the lack of trained and available counselors in government hospitals and clinics, often resulting in a deficiency of counseling services offered. TASO helps fill this gap by training counselors, including many who will eventually work in communities, hospitals, clinics, and districts where TASO is not currently located.

Home care, visitation, and complementary medical services for diagnosing and treating opportunistic infections are offered a minimum of 3 days a week at TASO clinics and in home visits. Some TASO centers also focus on pediatric clients and needs. Some TASO centers also focus on pediatric clients and needs. Because the Ugandan health system is overcrowded, many PWA must wait days to receive medical treatment from government hospitals and clinics. TASO works with trained community health workers to diagnose and treat opportunistic infections before they become life threatening. These medical services include training family caregivers in how to identify, prevent, and treat opportunistic infections.

For those clients who need more specialized medical care, TASO works in partnership with the government hospitals to secure beds.

To sensitize the public and promote positive attitudes towards people with HIV/AIDS and their families, TASO has established outreach programs of drama and performing groups composed of PWA who share their experiences with community members. Media campaigns are also carried out through radio and television programs that discuss the issues of HIV/AIDS and increase awareness of the effect of HIV/AIDS on individuals, families, and communities.

To minimize the social ills caused by HIV/AIDS, TASO provides material support to clients and their families. The social service component of the program has previously depended on external donor support, but TASO is currently trying to generate the internal resources to cover this service as well. As part of its social support services repertoire, TASO includes extensive child support, food assistance, training in new skills, and fellowship with other clients in day centers, as well as music, dance, and drama services. These services aim at helping clients to reintegrate into the socioeconomic life of the community and enable them to earn a living. The social services have been expanded to include scholarships to help children to attend formal education and vocational training, as well as an apprenticeship program that provides a skill to the children of PWA.

TASO has worked to build and support community-based efforts initiated to respond to the AIDS epidemic. The demand for HIV/AIDS-related counseling and medical services far exceeds TASO's present organizational capacity and physical infrastructure. In attempting to care for the masses, a decline in the quality of TASO's services has resulted. To offset this organizational overload, TASO helps build the capacity of other organizations involved with HIV/AIDS, and it networks and collaborates with other organizations to ensure that duplication of services is obviated. One attempt to reduce the strain on TASO clinics and direct services has been the training of community volunteers who in turn provide AIDS education, referrals, and basic care for PWA. In addition, TASO is heavily involved with regional AIDS committees and has pioneered attempts for greater involvement of people with HIV/AIDS (GIPA). GIPA empowers people who are directly infected with the virus to be part of the planning and decision-making process. As PWA are more acutely aware of their needs, their participation creates a sense of ownership. Through the collaboration of PWA and civil society organizations, such as TASO, stigmas and misconceptions are overcome, and PWA make valuable contributions to the creation of programs that more effectively meet their needs (Burkman, 2004; UNDP, 2004).

Factors Facilitating Success

Many factors have assisted TASO in achieving its official objectives. Due to increased global awareness of the epidemic, support has been sustained for many years from key donors in the form of basket funding.[3] In addition, the government of Uganda has been morally, politically, materially, and financially active in addressing the issues of HIV/AIDS, creating a supportive environment where TASO and other NGOs can function effectively. This has facilitated a sustained collaboration between service providers.

TASO has become a one-stop center through their integrated package of services for HIV/AIDS. This increases the number of services that a client can access at any one time from TASO's list of services. Results are also seen from a highly committed and hard-working group of staff and volunteers. The personnel have upheld principles of fiscal transparency and good governance, maintaining an innovative leadership position among NGOs offering HIV/AIDS services through effective partnership with clients in all activities and decision making.

Factors Limiting Success

Although TASO has made significant contributions to working with PWA in Uganda, the organization does have areas that can be improved. They are currently only reaching 30% of PWA with counseling service needs. Similarly, the outreach to orphaned children touches less than 10% of the total HIV/AIDS orphan population, signifying that more resources and greater outreach are needed. The limited number of PWA receiving services is a reflection of already stretched financial resources and an inadequate number of trained health workers available at local health clinics. The few qualified health workers who are available are overworked and do not receive needed additional technical training to provide up-to-date information and treatments to PWA.

Limited operational and program resources are compounded by the high levels of poverty, which prevents individuals from seeking appropriate and essential medical care and increases the risk of individuals contracting HIV. Although TASO has attempted to collaborate with other organizations, the lack of governmental resources at the district level has limited TASO's ability to implement joint programs, as district levels have weak planning and resource mobilization capacities. The high levels of poverty and inadequate resources at the district level significantly impacts community volunteers' ability to provide services to affected and infected individuals. These volunteers are unpaid and give freely of their time for

AIDS training and education programs, providing basic treatment and care for PWA in local communities. In addition, volunteers must travel long distances to bring in reports to TASO centers. These factors place heavy burdens on volunteers, leading to a high attrition rate. The armed conflicts in certain parts of Uganda have increased insecurity, displaced large numbers of people, and increased the incidences of rape, defilement, and the abduction of children.

As mentioned earlier, the HIV/AIDS epidemic is continually presenting new challenges to local NGOs involved in prevention, treatment, and mitigation efforts. NGOs must therefore continually adapt to the changing needs that arise from the disease. Additionally, organizations depend on donors for the majority of their funding, placing further restrictions and impingements on organizations. Bill Tassie, Vic Murray, and James Cutt (1998) identify the continuous challenges that NGOs encounter while interacting with donor agencies and stakeholders that have their individual and sometimes conflicting aid criteria. Although TASO functions on a basket funding system, it must still appeal to donors and demonstrate that it is meeting objectives, is cost effective, and is meeting certain levels of success. The vacillating environment in which NGOs function evolves over time, forcing organizations to adapt to new conditions or become extinct (Conti, 2002). As the largest indigenous nongovernmental organization in Uganda, TASO receives funding from governmental, multinational, intergovernmental, and international agencies. The dynamic environment surrounding the HIV/AIDS epidemic has forced TASO to think ahead and be proactive in providing HIV/AIDS services. On the other hand, the significant impact of the disease on multiple levels of society has forced TASO to be reactive, as it has been forced to deal with unforeseeable issues. The changing environment forces TASO to continually evaluate its strengths and weaknesses, while simultaneously assessing opportunities for future growth and potential threats to sustainable programs.

SWOT ANALYSIS

In this section we use a SWOT analysis to examine TASO's strengths, weaknesses, opportunity, and threats. The SWOT analysis is used to analyze an organizations ability to competitively function in its environment. It is also used to evaluate internal strengths and weaknesses of an organization while considering the corresponding opportunities and threats of the external environment. Albert Rizzo and Gerard Kim (2005) note that SWOT analysis has been used to provide a long-term examination of a business's position in the marketplace, but can also be used for any organization that has established objectives and missions.

Organizational Strengths

An organizational strength is any aspect: financial, physical, technical, or human that can help the organization to achieve its objectives. Having sufficient personnel is the most important resource at TASO, as it is a service delivery organization. The engagement of experienced staff dedicated to implementing program activities in the areas of medical, counseling, social support, and management in aid of PWA is the primary driving force to the survival of the organization. TASO has established a viable and reliable infrastructure for providing counseling, medical, and social support for PWA at the 11 established centers. A community volunteer and health workers' program that enhances the continuum of care at grassroots level reinforces this infrastructure.

TASO has established a functional monitoring and supervisory system to track performance both at the district and national level. Monitoring and evaluating are critical functions in maintaining quality assurance of services. Independent program midterm reviews are conducted by external experts, who evaluate the state of the programs and give direction to improve future interventions. The organization has evolved strict mechanisms to control resource utilization at the centers and at headquarters. An internal auditor monitors all centers and headquarters accounts to ensure compliance between program and fund allocations; annual external audits are carried out to provide an external perspective. TASO headquarters carries out quarterly management audits to ensure that center management complies with the policy framework and the organizational strategic interests. A comprehensive management information system at centers and headquarters has provided a wealth of data, which are analyzed to assist staff to make rational management and planning decisions. This system is also an excellent source of secondary data for research and evaluation of TASO services and monitoring of the PWA served by TASO.

Participatory planning and collaborative team-work among TASO staff, along with community involvement, have resulted in considerable success in preparing community interventions to promote both care and prevention programs. TASO has effectively networked with key stakeholders to achieve a range of programs, partnering with the Ministry of Health, local authority leaders, AIDS Information Center, Mildmay, blood bank, mission hospitals, Uganda AIDS Commission, Ministry of Finance and Economic Planning, Makerere University, Medical Research Council, Uganda Virus Research Institute, and the Regional AIDS Training Network. TASO has spearheaded advocacy for people with HIV/AIDS by giving people infected with the virus multiple entry points to voice to their interests and concerns. Functional clients' advisory councils exist at both board and district levels to ensure appropriate representation of PWA. Moreover, representatives of PWA are ex-officio members at the board of trustees and the center advisory committees.[4] Each of the 11 centers has a drama group consisting of 25 PWA. Their role is to promote HIV/AIDS education for care and prevention practices through song and drama, besides supporting each other.

TASO's programs primarily focus on improving the quality of life for PWA. According to the *TASO Strategic Plan* (2002), over 90% of the TASO clientele live in abject poverty and can hardly afford the basic needs for survival. Provision of medical care to manage opportunistic infections and counseling to address the psychosocial devastation has built the clients' confidence in services and forms a safety net for many PWA. Individuals living with HIV/AIDS who are able to take advantage of TASO's services are living longer, planning better for their posterity, and leading more productive lives. TASO has worked diligently to establish name-brand recognition. Perhaps its greatest strength is its reputation based on integrity and the desire to do all that is possible for PWA, their families, and communities.

Organizational Weaknesses

An organizational weakness is any problem or limitation that could inhibit the organization from achieving its objectives. TASO has been unable to consistently help clients establish sound income generation projects to offset the social and economic constraints of the disease. Another continuous struggle facing the organization has been its inability to generate adequate resources for AIDS orphans and vulnerable children. Similar to its struggle to create local means for people to secure income-generating projects, TASO has had minimal success raising local resources to cofinance its budget. A significant proportion of TASO's revenue derives from international donations. This raises questions of potential program sustainability should donors stop providing grants.

Thus far there has been inadequate production and provision of information, education, and communication (IEC) materials on HIV/AIDS for community volunteers, counselor trainees, training of trainers, and the general public. Neither has TASO fully utilized new research findings by respectable research organizations. While the training function in TASO is the mainstay of capacity building for TASO and other organizations, TASO has not sufficiently marketed this function and tends to respond reactively rather than proactively to national and regional training needs. Counselor trainers have not provided sufficient technical support to counselors at TASO centers; moreover there is no follow up mechanism for counselors trained by TASO who work in CBOs, NGOs, and government agencies for similar purposes.

Limited workspace in the Jinja and Mulago centers constrains the quality and extent of service delivery; the situation is currently most acute in Mulago. Capacity in these two centers already exceeds its limits when clients attend regular clinic days. In addition, staff stress is generated by the nature of work involved in counseling and medical services. Finally, there is no consistent follow up on clients referred to other organizations to assess the extent and quality of support provided there.

Opportunities for TASO

An opportunity is any aspect of the environment that creates a more favorable environment for an organization to provide its services more effectively or to achieve greater outreach and growth. In our opinion TASO's development and immediate objectives align well with the *Framework*. As a result of the *Framework* an increasing number of stakeholders are surfacing to help carry TASO's overhead and program-related expenses. The international community has also provided much needed technical and financial support. Examples of technical assistance include training staff members, organizing research and evaluation programs, and initiating and developing management information systems.

Good will and support from the Ministry of Health and other governmental agencies have been essential, especially during the late 1980s and early 1990s. Government hospitals have allocated buildings for TASO offices and land for construction of TASO premises. TASO has been a major partner with the Ministry of Health in the implementation of the STD/AIDS project, and it receives some financial assistance from the Ministry of Health annually. In conjunction with the Ministry of Health, TASO organizes medical workshops taught by respectable medical professionals from the Ministry of Health, who share experiences with TASO personnel. The Uganda Ministry of Health was recently selected to administer the multicountry AIDS project by the World Bank.[5] TASO expects to maintain its leadership role as a partner facilitator in capacity building of local and international AIDS service organizations.

Collaboration with grassroots organizations enables TASO to establish effective community programs that address practical problems at the local level and in remote rural regions. In addition, the presence of a strong and supportive political environment that promotes care and prevention efforts against HIV/AIDS and the recognition of TASO's services by the international community are both a challenge and an opportunity to continuously improve services in the organization for PWA. This collaborative partnership with TASO has created a mutually supportive and cost effective approach to working with PWA. The government's implementation of universal primary education (UPE) in 1996 meets some of the financial costs for orphans and vulnerable children. UPE reduces school fees, allowing parents to divert their already limited incomes to help with orphans, street children, and other vulnerable children.

The large number of PWA consistently seeking care services gives further credence for TASO service demands, especially in districts where no established centers exist. The national TB, family planning, and STD programs now in existence in all districts provide more partnership opportunities, and the TASO training center has potential to evolve into a more efficient training institution in the East and Central African Regions.

Potential Threats to the Organization

Threats are identified as elements of the environment that create obstacles or barriers that prevent an organization from effectively meetings its objectives. As a significant number of PWA live in abject poverty or are susceptible to become impoverished, issues of financial security for PWA and their families become a real issue (UNDP, 2004). Employment opportunities, food security, access to healthcare, and safe water are beyond the reach of these individuals. Though TASO attempts to address some of these concerns, it is not in a position to deal with all of the problems presented by these conditions. Many districts are not in a position to take on TASO programs because they are not adequately prepared either in human capacity or capital resources. In these areas, stigma, denial, and discrimination limit the extent to which people can come out for testing and receive subsequent support.

Voluntary service at the community level is hard to sustain given the many other pressing problems grassroots community workers have to address. Program sustainability under these circumstances is therefore potentially problematic. Another trend revolves around a feeling of complacency among the population that HIV is no longer as serious a problem as it used to be. This phenomenon creates a false environment of safety, increasing opportunities for the disease to proliferate among sexually active youth and other traditionally vulnerable groups.

There are still large subpopulations within Uganda that are highly susceptible to contracting the disease. The large numbers of orphans and vulnerable children require specialized counseling, material support, and education; transient populations such as those involved in large construction projects, internally displaced people, refuges, and rural to urban migrant populations living in suboptimal conditions are highly susceptible to contracting the disease. Many young unemployed women who live along major transportation routes and those who are migrating to Kampala through the process of urbanization become sex workers for survival. Some street children who have left their families because of varied social crises are themselves highly vulnerable to being abused sexually by unscrupulous men. Child abduction in parts of the country, particularly in Northern Uganda, has exposed many girls to premature pregnancies and risks of becoming infected with HIV. The long war crisis in this Northern Region has destabilized thousands of families, compelling them to be constantly on the move. Diaspora groups displaced by war are at a much higher risk of HIV exposure.

CONCLUSION

TASO is undergoing a period of rapid growth, where demand for its services has continued to increase. International donors continue to provide the needed resources to permit sustaining and expanding of TASO services. However, TASO has found it difficult to secure funding for some of its social support programs such as the scholarship and apprenticeship programs. These programs do not increase the integration of infected individuals into the socioeconomic system of society, but they do provide opportunities for education to the children and orphans of PWA. As HIV/AIDS continues to take the lives of the economically active and child-bearing population, additional social services will be needed to support the children of TASO's clients. As clients become more debilitated by the disease, greater financial strain will be placed on families, resulting in less education opportunity for their children. TASO has acknowledged the growing problem faced by PWA of how to provide educational opportunities for their children.

As the leading HIV/AIDS NGO in Uganda and one of the largest HIV/AIDS organizations in the world, TASO has established a precedence of collaboration and inclusion. This collaborative network has enabled judicious use of limited resources on projects that are being conducted by other organizations, and it is creating an environment where PWA can establish and exercise voice. TASO's policy to fight against the AIDS stigma has helped raise awareness and fight discrimination on a national and international level. Incorporating PWA and allowing them to share their knowledge, skills, and abilities contributes to curbing the HIV/AIDS epidemic.

NOTES

1. Mini-TASOs vary from the 11 traditional TASO centers since they are not staffed by TASO personnel. Established in district hospitals where current TASO centers are not located, Mini-TASOs provide counseling, medical care, and home visitations to HIV-infected individuals as a means to improve district hospital HIV/AIDS services. TASO does provide training services for mini-TASO volunteers and workers in the district hospitals.

2. The general volunteers identified in this section are different than the community volunteers. Where community volunteers are comprised of individuals who act as TASO's first line of defense in a triage-like role, the volunteers identified in this section are professionals (doctors, nurses, specialists, and counselors) that volunteer and work twice a week at the health clinics that TASO provides. Community volunteers act as community workers in carrying out AIDS education, referrals, and basic care for people with HIV/AIDS. Thus, unlike the professional volunteers, community volunteers are generally low-income members of the community who must divide their time between earning a living and engaging in HIV/AIDS work. Community volunteers receive no form of remuneration for their services.

3. According to the World Bank (2001) *basket funding* occurs when financial contributions are made by multiple donors to a common fund (basket) for a sectoral program based on a joint financial management framework agreed upon by the recipient organization and donors. When donors contribute directly to TASO, it enables the organization to establish programs and projects as it sees fit and in alignment with organizational objectives and already established programs. Reporting is provided on where money is allocated, but reduces the need for organizations to tailor reports to the stipulations of each donor. Basket funding is the least earmarked form of program aid. It is an on-budget contribution to the overall policy/organization. The basket can be managed by a multilateral institution, on the basis of a common donor financial management structure, or by the recipient organization. Typically the organization must demonstrate credibility and transparency, so that it can determine where funding is distributed according to its own rules, or rules agreed upon with the participating donors.

4. Ex-officio members have full voting and speaking rights. TASO has ensured that PWA are integral members of the administration and decision making process.

5. The World Bank has committed substantial IDA resources and leverages cofinancing on a country-by-country basis for African countries through the International Partnership against AIDS in Africa Program. The World Bank has already invested U.S.$1,088.2 million in flexible and rapid funding to 28 African countries and three regional programs. Uganda has received U.S.$47.5 million from the World Bank through 2004. The World Bank believes that many countries have not been able to reverse the prevalence rates in their countries regardless of having national strategies due to lack of financial resources. Any African country is eligible for the money as long as they meet the following criteria: (1) the country must have satisfactory evidence of a strategic approach to HIV/AIDS, developed in a participatory manner; (2) the country must have existence of a high-level HIV/

AIDS coordinating body, with broad representation of key stakeholders from all sectors, including PWA; (3) government commitment for rapid implementation arrangements, including channeling grant funds for HIV/ AIDS activities directly to communities, civil society, and the private sector; and (4) the country must have an agreement by the government to use multiple implementation agencies, especially NGOs and CBOs (World Bank, 2002).

REFERENCES

AMREF-Uganda. (2001). *Inventory of agencies with HIV/AIDS activities and HIV/ AIDS interventions in Uganda: A review of actors, interventions, achievements and constraints relating to the HIV/AIDS challenge in uganda*. Kampala, Uganda: African Medical and Research Foundation/Uganda AIDS Commission.

Bahiigwa, G. (2003). *Uganda's poverty eradication agenda: Measuring up to the Millennium Development Goals (MGDs)*. Kampala, Uganda: Economic Policy Research Centre.

Björkman, H. (2002). *HIV/AIDS and poverty reduction strategies: Policy note*. New York: UNDP.

Brown, M. (2004, July). Addressing HIV/AIDS challenges head-on. *Choices Supplement*, pp. 4–5.

Burkman, A. (2004, July). Realizing our victories. *Choices Supplement*, p. 7.

Conti, T. (2002). A road map through the fog of quality and organizational assessments. *Total Quality Management, 13*(8), 1057–1068.

Government of Uganda (GOU)/Uganda AIDS Commission (UAC). (1997). *The national strategic framework for HIV/ AIDS activities in Uganda 1998–2002*. Kampala, Uganda: Authors.

GOU/UAC/UNAIDS. (2000). *The national strategic framework for HIV/AIDS activities in Uganda: 2000–2006*. Kampala, Uganda: Authors.

Katahoire, A. R. (2004). *A review of key themes and issues emerging from literature on HIV/AIDS and higher education in Africa and Uganda in particular*. Paris: IIEP.

Keeley, M. (1978). A social-justice approach to organizational evaluation. *Administrative Science Quarterly, 23*(2), 272–292.

Ondrusek, A. (2001). Evaluating an HIV/AIDS book collection: Using a timeline approach. *Collection Management, 26*(1), 47–75.

Rizzo, A., & Kim, G. J. (2005). A SWOT analysis of the field of virtual reality rehabilitation and therapy. *Presence, 14*(2), 119–146.

TASO. (2002). *The AIDS Support Organisation: Strategic plan for the period 2003– 2007*. Kampala, Uganda: Author.

Tassie, B., Murray, V., & Cutt, J. (1998). Evaluating social service delivery: Fuzzy pictures of organizational effectiveness. *Voluntas: International Journal of Voluntary and Nonprofit Organizations, 9*(1), 59–79.

UAC. (1993). *The multi-sectoral approach to AIDS control in Uganda: Executive summary*. Kampala, Uganda: Author.

UNAIDS. (2001). *Uganda: HIV and AIDS-related discrimination, stigmatization and denial*. Geneva, Switzerland: Author.

UNDP. (2004). *Partners in human development: UNDP & civil society organizations.* Aarhus, Denmark: Phoenix Printing House.

World Bank. (2001). *Memorandum on the relationship between macro-oriented and sectoral program aid.* Washington, DC: United Nations and International Financial Institutions Department, Macroeconomic Analyses and Policies Division, World Bank.

World Bank. (2002). *Second multi-country HIV/AIDS program (MAP2) for Africa.* Washington, DC: Africa Regional Office, World Bank.

CHAPTER 8

EQUIPPING YOUTH WITH PREVENTION AND TREATMENT STRATEGIES

Literacy and HIV/AIDS Initiatives in Uganda and Five Other African Nations

Lynn R. Curtis

From 2001 to 2004, ProLiteracy Worldwide[1] (ProLiteracy), formerly Laubach Literacy International, completed the first phase of an HIV/AIDS prevention and treatment initiative in Uganda and five other African nations: Ethiopia, Kenya, Tanzania, South Africa, and Zimbabwe. The organization is currently in the process of sustaining and expanding this decade-long initiative for youth and adults. ProLiteracy, a nongovernmental education and action organization founded in 1955, is active in the United States and 56 countries in Asia, Africa, the Middle East, and Latin America. The global agency's Africa HIV/AIDS Initiative was started within a network of ProLiteracy's African literacy and community-action partner programs. These are independent local organizations that combine basic education and participant action in such

Overcoming AIDS: Lessons Learned from Uganda, 151–170
Copyright © 2006 by Information Age Publishing
All rights of reproduction in any form reserved.

areas as health, economic self-reliance, education, the environment, human rights, and peace. Responding to the concerns of their local members, leaders expressed a desire to initiate or strengthen HIV/AIDS efforts within the communities they serve. With this grassroots demand, the focus of the overall effort has been to provide training, materials development, and targeted financial support to enable these local education and action organizations to start, improve, or expand effective participatory, local-language HIV/AIDS treatment and prevention activities.

The initiative is being implemented through three distinct but related components or organizational types: community-based organizations (CBOs), schools, and churches. Data gathered from focus-group and individual interviews, pre and postintervention surveys, field reports, site visits, and observable accomplishments reveal findings specific to each of these three components. Results of the multicountry program regarding changes in knowledge, attitudes, beliefs, and awareness about HIV/AIDS will be presented later in this chapter.

PROGRAM OBJECTIVES AND GENERAL PROGRESS

One of the key objectives of the intervention program was to train leaders, facilitators, and teachers from existing grassroots education and community development organizations using health and AIDS materials and methods based on ProLiteracy's growing *Literacy Solutions* approach. This has resulted in the successful training of leaders and facilitators in the six African case countries mentioned above.

A second objective of the intervention was to enable youth and adults in local communities to gain access to new skills, information, and awareness in order to change behaviors and take concrete individual and group action steps to treat and prevent HIV/AIDS. These steps include avoiding high-risk behavior; teaching causes and prevention measures to family and friends; getting tested if a person suspects he or she has AIDS; seeking appropriate treatment options; accepting and providing physical, social, and emotional support to family and neighbors with HIV/AIDS; working with health-care workers to make treatment options available; working with neighbors to assist AIDS widows or orphans; and advancing sound nutrition, sanitation, hygiene, and health practices within the home and community. This second objective has resulted in a program with over 30,000 regular participants who have had or are currently undergoing HIV/AIDS training in the targeted communities.

In addition to disseminating ProLiteracy's existing health-literacy materials that already include a strong AIDS emphasis, a prototype AIDS-specific manual was developed for subsequent adaptation and local application throughout Africa. An English-language pilot version of the manual was completed and has been used as the basis for training and adaptation in all six countries. The manual was introduced in 2004 in five additional countries: Ghana, Niger, Cameroon, Lesotho, and Mali.

The initiative originally planned to establish a base of training, materials, and programs in six countries as a foundation for subsequent program improvement, expansion, and replication. With the training of teachers, leaders, and facilitators completed, and with leaders being exposed to the materials and methodology, existing groups now have programs in operation and momentum for expansion within their own networks. Additionally, the Ugandan Ministry of Education and Sports (MOES); the University of California, Los Angeles (UCLA); and Brigham Young University (BYU) have conducted a promising, complementary pilot study using ProLiteracy HIV/AIDS materials and training within 76 secondary schools. Beyond that, the Ministries of Health (MOH) in Uganda and Zimbabwe; the AIDS Network in Zimbabwe (including the Ministry of Education, the Centers for Disease Control, and several local church networks); the Lesotho Ecumenical Society for Development (LECUSDE) in Lesotho; the Meta Cultural and Development Association (MECUDA) in Cameroon; Literacy and Action International (LAI) in Ghana; the Rift Valley Children and Women's Development Association (RCWDA); the African Development Aid Association (ADAA); and a women-focused nongovernmental organization (NGO) called MAMA in Ethiopia, are all strong prospects to receive new or additional training during coming years.

The monitoring of progress and the evaluation of the impact of ProLiteracy's Africa HIV/AIDS Initiative has included quantitative performance indicators and a measurement of AIDS prevention and treatment effectiveness. The quantitative performance indicators include nearly all the broad numeric and schedule objectives for levels of program activity, participant enrollment, and participation in the various project sites.

The fact that goals for numbers enrolled and participating in classes and discussion groups and reading the materials are on-target is very encouraging, but that positive key benchmark does not necessarily establish the program's effectiveness in advancing HIV/AIDS prevention, treatment, and orphan care. To assess the actual impact within the constraints of a limited budget and relatively short time frame, several evaluation measures were and are being analyzed, including preliminary data gathered from focus groups and individual interviews, pre and postintervention surveys, field reports, site visits, and observable community action accomplishments. These measurement efforts reveal findings unique to specific program sites as well as general findings that apply to the overall efforts.

The initiative's quantifiable objectives were to recruit and train 778 leaders and facilitators within the six African case countries. Grassroots health and AIDS learning and action programs were to be established in more than 370 communities. In addition to disseminating ProLiteracy's existing health-literacy materials that already include a solid AIDS emphasis, a prototype AIDS-specific manual in English (*Overcoming AIDS: A Practical Guide for Prevention, Control and Treatment of HIV/AIDS* by W. James Jacob and the author) was developed for subsequent adaptation and local application throughout Africa. This manual has been translated and adapted into Oromifa, Amharic, Kiswahili, and Luganda, and additional translations in Zulu, Xhosa, Northern Sotho, Southern Sotho, Shona, and Mdebele are in progress. A foundation is now in place, and instruction is being provided that is enabling over 30,000 adults to participate in learning and action programs for HIV/AIDS prevention, treatment, and orphan care.

Underlying Assumptions, Methodology and Materials

ProLiteracy's global work with local education and action partner groups in a variety of areas, including the Africa HIV/AIDS Initiative, is based on a guiding belief that lasting solutions to problems of poverty, disease, and injustice come only when those most affected by these problems gain the literacy-based practices, information, and confidence to solve those problems. This participatory ideology is based on the theoretical framework of Frank Charles Laubach (1967), Paulo Freire (1971), and neo-Freirian practitioners, scholars, and policy makers (Curtis, 1990; Dyer & Choksi, 1998; Torres, 1998b).

Literacy for Social Change and Literacy Solutions

As a powerful component of its worldwide literacy and community action programs, ProLiteracy has developed a simple but highly effective tool to strengthen local program partners. This evolving tool, which is called *Literacy Solutions* (see Figure 8.1), includes a series of English-language, template manuals on learning and action themes that tend to be widely requested by learners in nearly all of the 56 countries where ProLiteracy is currently active.

With ProLiteracy training and support, grassroots organizations have translated these manuals into 29 languages and adapted their content

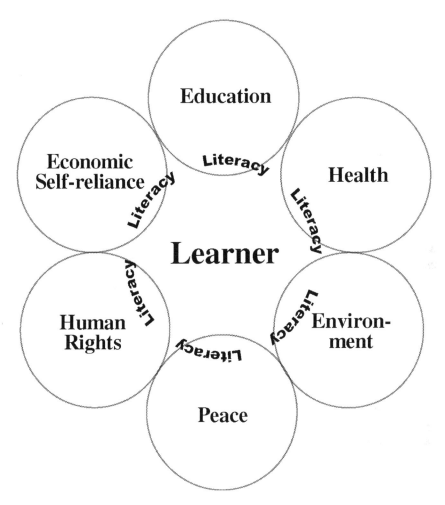

Figure 8.1.   Literacy Flower of International Development.

and appearance to reflect local circumstances. Through a highly participatory process, people not only learn reading and writing fundamentals,
but they also advance their capacity to work individually and collectively
to bring about desired family and community changes. This participatory
framework empowers both the learner and the teacher, a process that is
extremely necessary in sustainable education and social change programs
(Erickson, 1974; Samoff, 1999). While not entirely a learner-guided
approach, there is a careful balance between learner- and teacher-guided
empowerment, drawing from the local knowledge and expertise of the
participants (Curtis, 1996). The *Literacy Solutions* series is based on ProLi-

teracy's *Literacy for Social Change* methodology, which is a holistic instructional approach that accounts for the experiences, needs, preferences, and priorities of individual learners and their communities (see Figure 4.1).

The *Literacy for Social Change* methodology enables grassroots learners to access literacy-related skills, practices, information, and perspectives to bring about desired changes and improvements through a learning approach that integrates fundamental skills, cultural expression, critical thinking, and learner-initiated action (Curtis, 1990). Each manual in the series focuses on a particular developmental theme, such as health, economic self-reliance, or human rights, and each emphasizes participant discussion and reflection and learners' interest and priorities as the channels for improving individual, family, and community well-being.

Each manual in the *Literacy Solutions* series consists of a sequence of units that begin with a code (pictures or learning activities) that reflects realities from the learners' lives. These codes are typically developed locally and address relevant issues pertaining to a particular area of community development. In conjunction with these codes, learners generate a dialogue based on questions that guide them from observation to reflection to action. These layers of questions provide a structure that effectively communicates key ideas by allowing participants to generate the substance of the discussion based on their own experiences. As a result, learners exercise ownership of the ideas and internalize and apply important information readily.

Using this information, learners then design and implement action plans that address the development needs of their community. The plans include such activities as promoting human rights, starting health clinics, digging clean-water wells, forming microcredit and cooperative business ventures, overseeing reforestation projects, and a host of other participant-originated efforts. More significant than these observable projects, however, are the new skills, information, values, and insights that enable learners to continue development plans and efforts long after the outside agents are gone.

As part of the discussion and implementation of community action plans, participants also take part in literacy-learning activities. Basing their lessons on codes and using *Literacy for Social Change* techniques, facilitators help learners produce sentences and paragraphs relating to developmental themes that are then used in a range of reading and writing practice exercises. These literacy-learning activities are meaningful not only because they are based on the learners' own language and experience but also because they address the community's critical daily challenges, often going beyond the classroom to form a crucial part of solutions to shared concerns—including the HIV/AIDS epidemic.

Overcoming AIDS

ProLiteracy's primary vehicle to advance HIV/AIDS awareness, prevention, treatment, and orphan care is a manual in the *Literacy Solutions* series—*Overcoming AIDS*. This manual and its corresponding training component provide a framework of information, discussion questions, and techniques to stimulate critical understanding and to generate individual and group action.

The 25 *Literacy Solutions* codes and discussion topics in the *Overcoming AIDS* manual focus on key HIV/AIDS themes within four broad sections. The first section—*Talking about AIDS*—provides HIV/AIDS facts, discusses cultural issues, and teaches readers how to discuss AIDS in the home and community. The second section—*Protecting Yourself and Your Family*—covers a range of protection strategies and alternatives, such as abstinence, fidelity, condom use, and others. The third section—*Recognizing the Risks*—discusses individual and institutional practices that increase or reduce HIV risk. The final section—*Living with AIDS*—discusses attitudes and practices for accepting, supporting, and nurturing family, orphans, self, and others who may be HIV-positive. The understanding, attitudes, practices, and group action stimulated by participant-initiated learning and discussion of these codes provide a foundation for effective prevention, treatment, and orphan care.

OBSERVABLE OUTCOMES

At the outset of this program, levels of accurate knowledge and information about HIV/AIDS prevention and treatment, characteristics of people living with HIV/AIDS (PWA), and orphan care among youth and adults in participating communities were very low. This phenomenon was most pronounced among populations with lower education and reading levels. Leaders and members (students) of all participating CBOs, schools, and churches expressed an intense desire to participate in open, safe dialogue about HIV/AIDS. The first ProLiteracy session in each community generally tended to provoke a particularly intense emotional response of debate, tears, laughter, surprise, and so forth, accompanied by expressions of relief and enthusiasm for at last having a safe forum in which to learn about and discuss HIV/AIDS.

While not quite as intensely as during the first session, participants continued to demonstrate strong levels of interest and participation in and attendance at subsequent sessions. Further, participants expressed new awareness, knowledge, and skills related to avoiding high-risk behaviors and responded favorably to the literacy-based discussion process. As sessions continued, participants frequently articulated an intention to engage in new, more supportive behavior regarding people who are HIV-positive. Participants frequently proposed individual or group action to provide support or encouragement to people who are HIV-positive or to help AIDS orphans.

Participants also described improved communication/relationships emerging with key individuals, such as parents, children, extended family, neighbors, fellow students, teachers, and coworkers as a result of new HIV/AIDS conversations they were having in direct response to assignments coming from these sessions. It was further noted that ProLiteracy's provision of training, materials, technical assistance, and modest incentive grants generated accelerated organizational action and mobilized additional local resources.

AN EXAMINATION OF THE
THREE KEY PROGRAM COMPONENTS

As noted previously, ProLiteracy's HIV/AIDS program is being implemented through three related organizational components: community-based (CBO) programs, schools, and churches. A clearer understanding of the program and its scope and impact requires an examination of programmatic and evaluation activities within each of these three components.

Community-Based Organization (CBO) Component

CBOs are ideally positioned to take advantage of ProLiteracy's Africa HIV/AIDS Initiative. For the most part, the particular grassroots programs selected to pilot this project have already demonstrated knowledge of and a commitment to participatory education and action programs that can be tailored to the unique interests and needs of their neighborhood and village-based constituencies (Morisky, Ang, Coly, & Tiglao, 2004). Leaders have already identified HIV and AIDS as top priorities for community learning and action. Such CBO groups can make local decisions fairly rapidly and are positioned to adapt the materials to all emphasis areas of the program, including prevention, treatment, and orphan care.

While CBOs are structured to operate on an extremely cost-effective, largely volunteer basis, these groups typically do not have access to the larger public funding and infrastructure base of the public school or health system (Kelly et al., 2004). Although sometimes limited by their size and funding, the following CBOs have implemented ProLiteracy's curriculum successfully.

YWCA of Uganda

The YWCA of Uganda, which sponsors projects in 205 communities throughout the country, provides instruction in multiple languages, including Luganda, Lusoga, Runyoro/Rutooro, Runyankore/Rukiga, Atesot, Lunyole/Lusamia, Lugwe, Lumasaba, Lugbar, Alur, Luo, and English. Leaders from the YWCA were trained, and English instruction of the *Overcoming AIDS* curriculum began immediately. The manual was also translated/adapted into Luganda, the language of Kampala and the Central Region Districts of Uganda, and classes are currently being held.

In evaluation of the effectiveness of the curriculum, pre and post-launch surveys and focus-group interviews were conducted in six communities, three of which received the intervention and three of which were control sites that did not receive the intervention. With minor adaptation, these eight-page Luganda-language survey forms were similar to the questionnaires administered in the public-school component.

Operation Upgrade in South Africa

This Durban-based NGO sponsors community learning and action programs in communities throughout Kwazulu province. Languages of instruction include Zulu, Southern Sotho, Northern Sotho, Xhosa, and English. Leaders were trained, and English instruction began immediately. The manual is currently being translated/adapted into Zulu, the local language of Kwazulu Natal province, and classes in nine communities are now in place. An evaluation of the program was completed by conducting focus-group interviews in two participating communities.

Fifelela AIDS Project in South Africa

This CBO sponsors English- and Xhosa-language community learning and action programs in church, school, and community settings in Cape Town. Leaders were trained, and English instruction began immediately. The manual is being translated/adapted into Xhosa for classes in two neighborhoods to begin in May 2005.

Adult Literacy Organization of Zimbabwe (ALOZ)

Forty-five leaders and teachers completed training. Classes were initiated in 22 urban and rural communities in the areas of Harare and Bulawayo. The languages of instruction include Shona, Mdebele, and English. Informal interviews with administrators, teachers, and participants were conducted to evaluate the effectiveness of the curriculum.

YMCA of Tanzania

Leaders and teachers from nine participating communities completed training. The YMCA sponsors projects in communities throughout the Moshi Region of Tanzania. The language of instruction was Kiswahili, and informal interviews with teachers and participants were conducted to evaluate the curriculum.

Kenya Adult Learners Association (KALA)

Leaders and teachers from KALA member organizations, who sponsor projects in communities throughout Kenya, completed initial ProLiteracy training in 2003. Classes have since been implemented with materials translated into Kiswahili that have been adapted to the local context. Informal interviews and focus groups were held with external evaluators and local leaders and participants on several occasions to evaluate the program's success.

Engage Now in Ethiopia

Leaders and teachers from 17 participating communities in the Oromina District and communities near Addis Ababa completed ProLiteracy training and began classes with materials translated and adapted in Oromifa and Amharric. After the training and courses, informal interviews and focus-group discussions with leaders were held to evaluate the program.

CBO Component: Unique Findings and Analysis

Findings at this stage strongly suggest that CBO interventions significantly increase participant information, awareness, and intent, leading to attitudes and behaviors that reduce the risk of HIV infection and increase levels of participation in the positive treatment of and response to AIDS sufferers and AIDS orphans. Beyond this key general conclusion, the following findings emerged that are unique to the CBO component.

First, by nature of their structure and mission, CBO programs in this initiative tended to be more readily positioned to initiate proactive treatment efforts than their school and church counterparts. For example, Operation Upgrade in South Africa initiated efforts to seek out, feed, and provide hospice care to dying AIDS victims. ALOZ in Zimbabwe provides nutrition and healthy-living counseling and instruction for families with HIV-positive members. YWCA-Uganda complements its AIDS instruction with microfinance and small-business support; for HIV-infected individuals, this means the capacity to sustain a healthy lifestyle, and for those not infected, particularly young women, this effort offers financial alternatives to high-risk prostitution.

Second, CBOs in this initiative are achieving extensive results with extremely limited shoestring budgets augmented by grassroots volunteer and in-kind resources. CBOs often have a unique ability to implement nationwide programs without having to go through unnecessary governmental bureaucracy. And finally, given the widespread fear and concern about HIV and AIDS at the grassroots level, the issues revolving around the disease have recently become extremely high priority for the grassroots education and action organizations participating in this initiative.

School Component

Programs are being conducted within middle and secondary schools to advance knowledge and change behavior leading to HIV/AIDS awareness, prevention, and openness to support, as well as treatment of AIDS orphans and HIV-positive family members and neighbors. Participants include students from forms 1 to 6 (equivalent to grades 6 to 12 in the United States). Initial pilot efforts were conducted in Uganda and Zimbabwe.

A unique strength of the school program is that the public schools represent an established widespread delivery system in all countries and can potentially mobilize large-scale governmental resources (Torres, 1998a). Further, teen students represent a prime population at risk for HIV infection.[2] Although students can have tremendous influence on their peers and families, they and their schools typically lack the authority to initiate community action measures outside the school population, particularly those related to areas of treatment and orphan care. Accordingly, school-based programs tend to emphasize prevention, as opposed to treatment and orphan care, more than the adult-focused CBO and church-based programs.

Uganda MOES

Representatives of a collaboration of the Ugandan MOES, UCLA, and BYU trained teachers and administrators to use the *Overcoming AIDS* manual and intervention program. Projects were initiated in a stratified random sample of 76 urban and rural schools throughout Uganda, including Kampala (see chapter 4). On average, classes were conducted on a twice-weekly basis throughout the duration of the program. In-depth, qualitative interviews were conducted with 108 administrators, teachers, students, and parents of students who responded to open-ended questions about the impact of the program regarding lessons learned, new insights, intended behaviors, and so forth. Pre and postintervention surveys were conducted to determine changes in respondents' knowledge, attitudes, intentions, and skills related to HIV/AIDS behavior.

School Programs in Zimbabwe

ProLiteracy representatives trained leaders of the Deseret International Foundation, who have developed an expanded curriculum that incorporates much of the *Overcoming AIDS* manual and includes a specific emphasis on organizing *Youth Alive* clubs led by peer student leaders. Full programs were implemented in four schools among secondary students from the same grade levels as those used in Uganda. Approximately 2,200 students participated. Focus interviews were completed with administrators, teachers, and peer student leaders who responded to open-ended questions regarding the impact of lessons learned, new insights, and intended behaviors of the program.

School Component: Unique Findings and Analysis

Findings suggest that school-based intervention, like the CBO interventions, significantly increases participant information, awareness, and positive intent, leading to attitudes and behaviors that reduce the risk of HIV/AIDS infection and increase levels of participation in the positive treatment of and response to AIDS sufferers and AIDS orphans. Beyond this key general conclusion, the following findings emerged that are specific and unique to the school component.

Although not always part of the official secondary education curriculum or syllabus for each subject, head teachers generally welcomed open dialogue associated with the AIDS epidemic. In the school programs, the only negative responses, which were few, came as a result of the limited time of already overburdened administrators and teachers. Students, for the most part, showed great interest in attending and participating in HIV/AIDS discussions, and the topic often brought to the surface many emotions, memories, and firsthand experiences all the participants had had with friends and kin who had suffered from the disease.

Even though all participants in this study strongly support the need to include HIV/AIDS as part of the regular examinable curriculum, a preliminary analysis of the national secondary education curriculum among secondary schools shows that many administrators, teachers, and students are unaware that the respective Ministries of Education do not require schools to teach students about HIV/AIDS as part of the regular curriculum in all applicable subjects. Efforts are being made in Uganda to bridge this gap, but it will take time to integrate these discussions into every subject.

Many teachers and administrators expressed frustration relative to the HIV/AIDS issue. While instructors are positive regarding the curriculum and its impact on students, they feel strong constraints from selected funding sources, parents, and officials who are highly concerned that the schools need to prepare students for college or vocational advancement. This project's AIDS curriculum, however needed and worthwhile, does not necessarily improve test scores that will be scrutinized by parents and officials and, as such, represents a potential distraction from the mandated, testing-based requirements that teachers and administrators are facing. As this effort continues to expand and gain popular recognition, there will need to be a parallel level of political policy change and funding support instituted at the regional and national levels. The growing success of this effort will be a key tool in mobilizing this broader level of support.

Church Component

Throughout Sub-Saharan Africa, churches play a very powerful social role as educators, influencers of public opinion, and mobilizers of community action. An effective church-based program can reach many significant audiences that other programs cannot.

Relative to AIDS education, the role of churches has recently taken on increasing importance. Many local congregations and leaders have responded very negatively to the strong emphasis on the distribution and use of condoms as the predominant means of prevention and social response. Many churches have started to aggressively attack the condom strategy with two arguments. First, they argue that promoting condoms encourages greater promiscuity, especially among the high-risk young adult populations, and thus encourages the spread of AIDS. This may in fact be a valid argument, since some regions that have achieved the highest condom usage rates are also achieving the highest HIV infection growth rates (Savage, 1999; Wolitski & Branson, 2002; Mwizarubi, Mwaijonga, Laukamm-Josten, Lwihula, Outwater, & Nyamwaya, 1991). Second, they argue that condoms are faulty and have leaks, and they do not provide reliable HIV protection. They maintain that abstinence is the only option. Medically, this argument is not really correct; condoms, when used properly and consistently, have proved to be highly effective in preventing gonorrhea/Chlamydia infections (Warner et al., 2005). Unfortunately, they frequently are not used properly or consistently. There is need for education on proper, consistent condom use. The emerging church message of abstinence before marriage and faithfulness to one's spouse after marriage may be extremely helpful for youth prepared to abstain or for faithful marital partners in monogamous relationships. But for others it further stigmatizes the issue and can cause people who are sexually active with multiple partners to give up on using condoms. If churches can present a balanced message that encourages dialogue and support for victims and allows for the proven ABC strategy—*Abstain, Be faithful* in marriage, and, if needed, use *Condoms*—they can be an extremely powerful and unique source of destigmatizing education for HIV/AIDS prevention, treatment, and orphan care. However, like CBO programs, churches typically do not have access to the larger public funding and infrastructure base of the public school or health system.

South Africa: The Church of Jesus Christ of Latter-day Saints in Johannesburg and Pretoria Areas, and the Baptist Church in the Durban Area

The Church of Jesus Christ of Latter-day Saints in the Johannesburg area adapted the ProLiteracy manual and training to create *The Gospel and HIV/AIDS*, a Bible-based discussion and action guide that they pilot-tested with 24 congregations in the Johannesburg and Pretoria areas. Initial success of this pilot effort has recently generated a region-wide launch of the program in church congregations throughout eastern and southern Africa. The Baptist Church leaders in the Durban area received ProLiteracy training, and two pilot congregations began classes. In evaluation of ProLiteracy's church-centered intervention program with both churches' instruction manuals, pre and postquestionnaires were conducted with leaders and participants, and focus-group evaluation sessions were conducted with teachers and members of participating congregations. Findings indicate a significant knowledge increase and a more open dialogue established between church leaders and congregation members about the sensitive issues associated with HIV and AIDS.

Zimbabwe Council of Churches in Partnership With the Deseret International Foundation

ProLiteracy representatives trained Deseret International Foundation leaders, who in turn trained leaders from Zimbabwe Council of Churches congregations (primarily Anglican and Methodist) throughout the Bulawayo area. To date, nine congregations have established classes. In-progress evaluations of this program have included a series of informal interviews and focus-group discussions with leaders and participants.

Church Component: Unique Findings and Analysis

Findings at this stage strongly coincide with the school-based and CBO intervention findings. Beyond this general analysis, the following findings emerged that are unique to the church-based component. First, each of the churches participating in this project adapted the content, methodology, and format of ProLiteracy's *Overcoming AIDS* manual to correspond to the terminology and forms of their respective denominations. Leaders and participants reported that this adaptation allowed for more open and safe discussion of sensitive HIV/AIDS issues. Second, participants expressed satisfaction at being able to discuss previously taboo AIDS issues within their church settings with people who have similar beliefs, and they also felt safer getting important but potentially threatening information from people they trust.

OVERALL FINDINGS AND ANALYSIS

As noted at the beginning of the chapter, numerous observations were substantiated through the interventions conducted by the CBOs, schools, and churches. In this section, I will summarize 10 of these observations.

First, the overall levels of accurate knowledge and information about HIV/AIDS prevention, treatment, and orphan care among adults and youth in participating communities tend to be relatively low. This phenomenon is most pronounced among populations with lower education and reading levels. Participants in urban areas tended to demonstrate higher levels of knowledge and awareness than those in rural areas, and levels of knowledge were lowest among the oldest and youngest segments of the participant populations. However, pretest surveys, focus-group discussions, and informal interviews indicated that prior to participation in the ProLiteracy program, the majority of participants—rural and urban, young, middle-aged, and old, including many leaders—expressed levels of knowledge, attitudes, and intentions to improve that suggested the majority of participants were at risk of behavior that would lead to HIV infection. There were widespread misconceptions about the causes of AIDS and its modes of transmission, as well as unfounded beliefs about having contact with HIV-infected individuals. Individuals had difficulty connecting their own intense but generalized fears about AIDS with specific risk attitudes and behaviors in their own lives.

A second observation dealing with leaders and participants (students) from all participating CBOs, schools, and churches indicated an intense need and desire to participate in open, safe dialogue about HIV and AIDS. In virtually every setting where the classes were offered, there was an enthusiastic response and high attendance.

Third, the first ProLiteracy session generally tended to provoke particularly intense emotional responses of debate, tears, laughter, surprise, etc., accompanied by expressions of relief and enthusiasm for at last having a safe forum in which to learn and discuss HIV/AIDS. Participants expressed feelings of pent-up frustration, fear, confusion, and sadness, particularly during the first session. They reported feelings of anticipation, excitement, and sometimes anxiety before the class began. As the discussion continued, people began to express relief and enthusiasm for continuing the process. Leaders noted high levels of outspoken participation and dialogue. Many participants shared intimate personal perspectives and experiences. In a few highly charged sessions, some individuals actually "came out of the closet" by announcing that they had tested positive for HIV. These announcements were followed by support in the form of hugs and touching. Such demonstrative physical contact provided a dramatic, visible counter to participants' fears and reluctance to have contact with those who are HIV positive.

While generally not quite as intense as the first session, a fourth observation highlighted participants' persistence in expressing and demonstrating strong levels of interest, participation, and attendance at subsequent sessions. Eager to find ways to continue to discuss HIV/AIDS issues, many participating organizations committed to maintaining this dialogue as part of their regular activities.

Fifth, participants generally expressed new awareness, knowledge, and skills related to avoiding high-risk behavior. Participants responded favorably to the literacy-based discussion process. In many different ways, participants and leaders demonstrated that they had acquired new insights and intended to avoid high-risk behavior. Not only did the surveys, focus groups, and informal interviews support this conclusion, but in the discussion groups themselves, there were repeated statements of new understanding, intent, and commitment to avoid high-risk behavior. Some of the most powerful statements were in the form of informal participant initiatives that emerged from the discussions, such as "in-your-face" calls for abstinence by teen female participants to their male peers, families committing to start home AIDS discussion circles, people publicly committing to go get tested, and parents discussing ways to keep their daughters away from prostitution.

The sixth observation came about as sessions continued: participants frequently articulated statements regarding intentions to engage in new, more supportive behavior regarding people who are HIV-positive. This dimension of the discussions came as many people expressed "ah-hah" moments of insight about the scope of the problem and their own denial and fears surrounding the issue. People talked about feeling bad about family members and neighbors that they had shunned or ignored in the past, they discussed a new willingness to consider touching people they know who are HIV positive, they stated a desire to be more supportive and friendly with those they suspect might be HIV-positive, and they expressed various other personal manifestations of support or empathy.

Seventh, participants often proposed individual or group action to provide support or encouragement to PWA or to help AIDS orphans. Beyond the more personal expressions of intent noted above, many participants and groups of participants actually planned and organized concrete steps to provide support. This was particularly true among CBOs and church-based groups. For example, many subgroups were organized to visit or volunteer at local orphanages. Two subgroups organized neighborhood information and referral efforts to gather information about HIV/AIDS-related needs, including resources for testing, clinics, counseling, and so forth, in their areas. Information flyers about testing were created. Building on the momentum of interest and motivation, some of the CBOs and church groups were able to initiate or strengthen HIV/AIDS treatment programs within their institutions, such as home visiting programs, support for extended-family orphan care providers, healthy-living supplemental programs for HIV-positive persons (nutrition, income generation, hospice, clinics/antiretroviral medications, preparation for the children of dying parents, etc.), and expanded education efforts.

Eighth, reporting on assignments accepted and commitments made at previous discussion sessions, many participants described successful as well as disappointing experiences of speaking with spouses, children, extended family, fellow students, friends, and neighbors about the information they had learned in earlier sessions. In some cases, they were received with hostility or indifference, but more often they reported a positive initial experience. Most participants wanted to continue these out-of-class discussions. Some said starting the conversations was the hardest and most awkward part, but they were generally glad that they had done so. A few even reported changed behavior as a result of these out-of-class conversations, such as a family member going to be tested or an at-risk husband (sexually active before their recent marriage) starting to use a condom.

Ninth, participants often described improved communication and relationships emerging with key individuals like parents, children, extended family, neighbors, fellow students, teachers, and coworkers as a result of new HIV/AIDS conversations they were having in direct response to assignments coming from these sessions. Those describing conversations about HIV/AIDS with significant people in their lives also frequently noted that the conversations had lead to strengthened closeness and unity in their relationships and communication at home or with these key people.

And finally, ProLiteracy's Africa HIV/AIDS Initiative generated accelerated organizational action and mobilized additional local resources. Initial exposure to ProLiteracy's materials, training, and incentive grants generated an enthusiastic, active organizational response and stimulated all participating organizations to launch expanded and improved HIV/AIDS programs. In the process, they mobilized more additional programmatic resources for prevention and treatment than originally planned.

CHALLENGES ENCOUNTERED AND THE WAY FORWARD

The overwhelming dimensions of the AIDS epidemic in Africa—skyrocketing infection and death numbers; entrenched, multiple high-risk conditions and behaviors; tragic suffering; incredibly scarce resources; and widespread denial, lack of awareness, and stigmatization—can either motivate increased response or discourage and immobilize action. This is equally true for the individuals and programs affected by this initiative. There is so much to be done with so few resources.

These realities generate the defining challenges and opportunities inherent in this initiative. On the negative side, numbers of participants—though impressive and rapidly growing—represent a drop in the vast Africa-AIDS bucket. Even with more information and commitment, the availability of treatment resources for individuals (clinics, testing, orphan care, income, and medicines) is painfully limited. Program budgets for all the participating and potential program partners are stretched to bare-bones levels; general fears and stigmas and government-level dysfunction and indifference abound.

Ironically these very same challenges give this initiative its greatest strength. The high demand and enthusiasm for the program is based on the lack of existing alternative programs. For every ProLiteracy dollar invested, an average of approximately five more dollars from local and other sources is leveraged. Attendance is high, participation is high, and participants, volunteers, and leaders are eager to expend the energy to make HIV/AIDS programs thrive and grow. Leaders find creative ways to stretch cash and material resources, mobilize volunteer involvement, and keep the programs moving. Methods and materials are proving to be effective, but their effectiveness is greatly magnified by the high level of need, interest, and potential participation in this issue. While not every single participant will complete the program or change their high-risk behavior, findings at this point suggest that a majority will. And the number of individuals eager to participate, and the number of school, church, and CBO leaders eager to take advantage of the materials and training, greatly compensates for the limited attrition. Leaders and participants have shown a willingness to overcome great difficulties to make this effort work. Limited external resources invested have the potential to travel a tremendous distance. In spite of daunting obstacles and limitations, and with continued funding, programs and individuals can find ways to make individual advancement and program expansion a continuing reality.

NOTES

1. ProLiteracy Worldwide is the world's oldest and largest nongovernmental literacy organization and is headquartered in Syracuse, New York. Many of the funds associated with this study came from the Pfizer and Deseret International Foundations.

2. Although students in Sub-Saharan African secondary schools are generally in their teenage years, the range of student ages can be from 12 to 26 years. There are several reasons for this large variance, including students who are held back because they did not pass the leaving examinations, lack of sufficient financial support to completed formal education within a continuous 6 year period, and lack of parental support. AIDS orphans generally encounter one or all of these challenges, thus highlighting the negative synergistic challenges associated with orphanhood and obtaining an education.

REFERENCES

Curtis, L. R. (1990). *Literacy for social change*. Syracuse, NY: New Readers Press.

Curtis, L. R. (1996). *Picturing change*. Syracuse, NY: New Readers Press.

Dyer, C., & Choksi, A. (1998). Education is like wearing glasses: Nomads' views of literacy and empowerment. *Journal of International Educational Development, 18*(5), 405–413.

Erickson, S. C. (1974). *Motivation for learning*. Ann Arbor, MI: The University of Michigan Press.

Freire, P. (1971). *Pedagogy of the oppressed*. New York: Continuum.

Freire, P. (1998). *Politics and education*. Los Angeles: UCLA Latin American Center.

Kelly, J. A., Somlai, A. M., Benotsch, E. G., McAuliffe, T. L., Amirkhanian, Y. A., Brown, K. D., et al. (2004). Distance communication transfer of HIV prevention interventions to service providers. *Science, 305*(5692), 1953–1955.

Laubach, F. C. (1967). *Thirty years with the silent billion*. Westwood, NJ: Revell.

Morisky, D. E., Ang, A., Coly, A., Tiglao, T. V. (2004). A model HIV/AIDS risk reduction program in the Philippines: A comprehensive community-based approach through participatory action research. *Health Promotion International, 19*(1), 69–76.

Mwizarubi, B. K., Mwaijonga, C. L., Laukamm-Josten, U., Lwihula, G., Outwater, A., & Nyamwaya, D. (1991). *HIV/AIDS education and condom promotion for truck drivers, their assistants, and sex partners in Tanzania*. Paper presented at the 7th International AIDS Conference on AIDS Abstracts, WD4017.

Samoff, J. (1999). Education sector analysis in Africa: Limited national control and even less national ownership. *Journal of International Educational Development, 19*, 249–272.

Savage, D. (1999, July). Bucking the condomocracy. *OUT*, p. 34.

Torres, C. A. (1998a). *Democracy, education, and multiculturalism*. Lanham, MD: Rowman & Littlefield.

Torres, C. A. (1998b). Introduction: The political pedagogy of Paulo Freire. In P. Freire (Ed.), *Politics and education* (pp. 1–16). Los Angeles: UCLA Latin American Center.

Warner, L., Macaluso, M., Austin, H. D., Kleinbaum, D. K., Artz, L., Fleenor, M. E., Brill, I., Newman, D. R., & Hook, E. W. (2005). Third application of the case-crossover design to reduce unmeasured confounding in studies of condom effectiveness. *American Journal of Epidemiology, 161*(8), 765–73.

Wolitski, R. J., & Branson, B. M. (2002). "Gray area behaviors" and partner selection strategies: Working toward a comprehensive approach to reducing the sexual transmission of HIV. In A. O'Leary (Ed.), *Beyond condoms: Alternative approaches to HIV prevention* (pp. 173–197). New York: Kluwer Academic/Plenum.

CHAPTER 9

SUCCESSFUL STRATEGIES IN HIV/AIDS PREVENTION

The Case of the Uganda Youth Anti-AIDS Association, 1992-2004

Sande Ndimwibo and Julie M. Hite

Since the government of Uganda introduced HIV/AIDS prevention campaigns on a national level in 1986, and established the AIDS Control Program in 1987 (Okware, Opio, Musinguzi, & Waibale, 2001), direct and open strategies have been employed in Uganda to achieve the successful curbing of the HIV/AIDS epidemic within this East African nation (UNAIDS, 1995). Both formal and nonformal education programs have clearly and intentionally been the main vehicles for accomplishing critical HIV/AIDS prevention strategies (Mirembe, 2002). Working in concert with formal educational programs, private, and community-based organizations (CBO) have also worked tirelessly with the goal of HIV/AIDS awareness and prevention. Of these organizations, the Uganda Youth Anti-AIDS Association (UYAAS) represents a model program that has contributed in many significant ways toward HIV/AIDS prevention.

Overcoming AIDS: Lessons Learned from Uganda, 171–187
Copyright © 2006 by Information Age Publishing
All rights of reproduction in any form reserved.

The purpose of this chapter is to describe the vision, structure, strategies, and successes of the UYAAS and then to explore and explain possible reasons for their success and to generate potential implications for other HIV/AIDS prevention programs, both in Uganda and in other affected nations.

HIV/AIDS SITUATION AMONG YOUNG PEOPLE IN UGANDA

Despite the national and local strategies to reduce HIV/AIDS prevalence rates in Sub-Saharan Africa, the HIV/AIDS epidemic continues to threaten political, social, and economic development in this area (Piot, 2001). With a population surpassing 26.6 million at the end of 2003, UNAIDS and the World Health Organization (WHO) (2004) estimate that as many as 1.9 million people (7.2%) may be infected with HIV, whether or not they have developed symptoms of AIDS. The vast majority of HIV infections occur in the population segment between ages 15 and 49. Half of these new HIV/AIDS infections occur in young people ages 12–24. Actual HIV infection rates in the 15–24 year age range vary between 3.7% –5.6% among females and 2.0%–2.4% among males. Thus, between ages 12 and 24, females are becoming infected at a higher rate than their male counterparts. However, after age 24, males are more at risk of becoming infected with HIV than are females (Ministry of Health, MOH, 2001).

Young people's vulnerability to HIV/AIDS infection is further aggravated by entrenched poverty, neglect of girls, and other cultural or traditional norms and gender-biased beliefs (Obbo, 1995; Parker, Barbosa, & Aggleton, 2000; United Nations, 2001). Like many African countries, Uganda still has an extremely high number of youth who become sexually active at an early age (between ages 15 and 19), although in Uganda the percentage of sexually experienced youth decreased between 1989 and 1995 (UNAIDS, 1995). This cultural situation, combined with the higher rates of actual infection for young girls, suggests that girls are at a higher risk of HIV/AIDS infection, as well as other reproductive health problems, than their male counterparts (Malinga, 2000). In Uganda, children with special needs—such as orphans, street children, and children with disabilities—are also very vulnerable to HIV/AIDS infections (Jacob, Smith, Hite, & Cheng, 2004; UNAIDS/UNICEF/USAID, 2004). These children are even less able to protect themselves against HIV than are children who are physically and mentally able and who live in more secure circumstances.

HIV/AIDS clearly affects the lives of young people in Uganda, and these young people—particularly girls and those with special needs—are in great need of reproductive health and HIV/AIDS information and education. However, in order to achieve the highest benefit, the youth must put this information and education into practice. Uganda's national policy for fighting AIDS has been to give it a human face and to expose it openly and directly as a total enemy. As a result of this national openness, Uganda has achieved a very high degree of HIV/AIDS awareness. UYAAS is a model example of an organization that helps protect the youth of Uganda by providing education and by facilitating behavioral change as the youth put education into practice.

UGANDA YOUTH ANTI-AIDS ASSOCIATION

In its response to the adolescent reproductive heath and HIV/AIDS epidemic, UYAAS is one of the pioneering AIDS-fighting organizations in Uganda. Formed in 1991, UYAAS is a nongovernmental organization (NGO) that was registered in 1992 with the Ministry of Internal Affairs' NGO Board under the NGO Statute of 1989.

UYAAS has developed and communicated a clear vision and mission along with specific strategies to accomplish their mission of responding to the HIV/AIDS epidemic. As a result, they have experienced many successes in the fight against HIV/AIDS. The vision of UYAAS is the improvement of the reproductive health status of the youth in Uganda through limiting the further spread of HIV/AIDS and other sexually transmitted diseases (STD). Within this vision, their mission is to involve all youth in the fight against HIV/AIDS and STDs through school- and community-based educational efforts that focus on youth ages 10–24 in school and youth ages 18–30 out of school, especially in rural areas.

Since 1992, UYAAS has been a positive force for directly influencing the improvement of reproductive health for youth, particularly through involving youth in their educational efforts in order to effect behavioral change. The involvement of youth in HIV/AIDS education is a crucial element in behavioral change (Olson & Wilkins, 2001; Stoneburner & Low-Beer, 2004). Uganda's promotion of prevention programs has resulted in an HIV prevalence decrease from 1993 to the present (Jacob et al., 2004; UNAIDS/WHO, 2004) that is more than would be expected from natural causes alone and is most prevalent among young age groups. This suggests that efforts to reach the youth through education may indeed be influencing behavioral change (Bennell, Hyde, & Swainson, 2002; Blanc, 2000). In the past 14 years, UYAAS has gained vast experience in working directly with young people on educational and behavioral issues concerning HIV/AIDS, STDs, and adolescent reproductive health in general. As a result, they have enjoyed tremendous growth in the number of youth that they have reached through their strategies and programs. In each of the

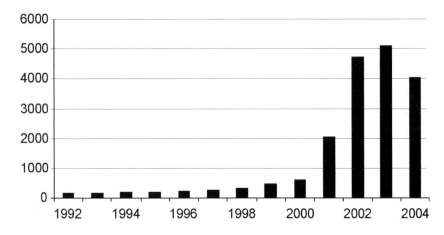

Figure 9.1.   Number of youth reached through UYAAS Training programs in 10 Districts, 1992–2004.

past 3 years, since 2002, over 4,000 youth participated in UYAAS programs, compared with some 200 people when the organization first began in the early 1990s (see Figure 9.1).

UYAAS is managed by a board of seven members, including the executive director (see Figure 9.2). The board is the governing and policy-making body of UYAAS and, as such, monitors the implementation and performance of the organization's project activities. UYAAS has 28 full-time staff members and 180 district- or community-based volunteers. The UYAAS offices in Kampala coordinates and implement national HIV/AIDS, STD, and adolescent reproductive health (ARH) activities. Through their expansion program, they now reach 14 of 70 districts in Uganda, including Kampala, Jinja, Iganga, Kamuli, Bugiri, Mayuge, Busia, Mpigi, Wakiso, and Pallisa, and they have made recent expansions to the Masindi, Hoima, Kaliro, and Budaka Districts.

UYAAS STRATEGIES FOR IMPROVING THE REPRODUCTIVE HEALTH OF YOUTH

To accomplish their mission, the core strategy of UYAAS is the direct involvement of youth in the improvement of the reproductive health status of Ugandan youth. This strategy has been designed to overcome several obstacles that threaten the future sustainability of UYAAS programs: donor and government commitment to HIV/AIDS programs; effective government policies, including the provision of antiretrovirals (ARVs);

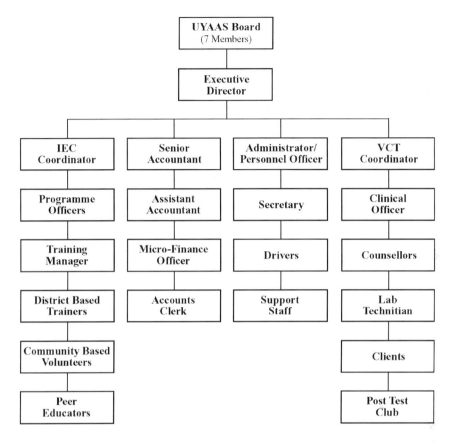

Figure 9.2.   UYAAS Organizational Chart.

poverty; resource mobilization; strengthening of care and support services; accountability through internal and external program evaluations;
and maintaining rapport with clients. They have developed efficient and
effective approaches at multiple levels for reaching youth and those who
directly influence youth, and they employ a variety of strategies that target the improvement of adolescent reproductive health in both rural and
urban areas.

UYAAS is highly active, well connected, and willing to participate at
the individual, school, community, district, national, and international
levels. Their strategy is simultaneously wide-reaching and yet also focused
on improving the lives of individual youth. The key elements of UYAAS's
strategy are as follows: (1) building a broad national and international
network, (2) maintaining an active research agenda, (3) involving youth
through national mass media, (4) delivering educational and technical

support, (5) providing voluntary counseling and testing services, (6) reaching out to youth through community services, (7) facilitating peer education among youth through schools, and (8) producing and distributing educational materials.

Building a Broad National and International Network

One of the most important strategic factors in UYAAS's success has been the development of a broad collaborative network with national and international agencies. Such partnership building in the fight against HIV/AIDS is encouraged by the Uganda AIDS Commission (Okware et al., 2001). Participation, cooperation, and collaboration with these agencies has enabled UYAAS to increase both their influence and their effectiveness in the challenging task of improving the reproductive heath status of youth in Uganda. In addition, these network relationships have provided UYAAS with access to resources, information, and influence that would otherwise be unavailable to them (Hite & Hesterly, 2001). For example, since their inception in 1992, this network (see Table 9.1) of national and international agencies has provided UYAAS with necessary financial support and technical assistance to accomplish their strategies and carry out their programs.

At the international level, UYAAS has been involved with many organizations that are also focused on addressing HIV/AIDS and reproductive health issues. They represented Uganda in the Global Festival of Youth, Solidarity, and the Fight Against AIDS organized by SOLIDARITE SIDA in Paris, France. They have participated in international conferences on such issues as adolescent reproductive health, HIV/AIDS, youth-friendly services, STDs, and communication. In addition, UYAAS coordinated an international conference on promoting and protecting the rights of street children, which was funded by the Consortium for Street Children (CSC) based in the United Kingdom.

At the national level, UYAAS has worked on many projects in coordination with the Uganda Ministry of Health and the Uganda Ministry of Education and Sports to accomplish their joint goals of increasing HIV/AIDS awareness. They also participated in the national-level HIV/AIDS and STD planning and workshops for the World AIDS Campaigns, the Joint Multi-Sectoral Planning Forum for HIV/AIDS in Uganda, and other organizations. UYAAS is a member of the National Task Force for the Presidential Initiative on AIDS Communication Strategy to the Youth (PIASCY) and is one of several PIASCY National Facilitators. UYAAS also actively participated in writing the PIASCY Primary Teachers Hand Book

**Table 9.1.   Members of UYAAS's National and
International Network of Financial and Technical Support**

AIDS Control Project
AIDS Information Centre
Canada Fund Uganda (CIDA)
Center for AIDS Intervention Research (USA)
Elton John AIDS Foundation
Family Planning Association of Uganda
French Embassy
Friends of Africa Foundation (UK)
National Council for International Health
Pacific Institute of Women in Health (USA)
Program for Appropriate Technology in Health (PATH–Kenya)
Program for Appropriate Technology in Health (PATH–USA)
Shell Uganda
Talent Calls
The AIDS Support Organisation (TASO)
Uganda AIDS Commission
Uganda AIDS Control Project (UACP)
Uganda Association for Women Doctors
Uganda Ministry of Education and Sports
Uganda Ministry of Health
Uganda Reproductive Health Bureau
Joint United Nations Programme on HIV/AIDS (UNAIDS)
Vronestein Foundation (The Netherlands)

and has cochaired other national groups on HIV/AIDS and STDs. In addition, UYAAS is a lead Ugandan agency for the implementation of the Global Fund to Fight AIDS, Tuberculosis and Malaria. In this role, UYAAS coordinates the efforts of CBOs and NGOs working with young people in and out of school in the districts of Jinja, Iganga, Kamuli, Mayuge, Bugiri, and Busia.

The national and international network that UYAAS has developed creates effective partnerships that strategically facilitates UYAAS's success in improving the reproductive health of youth in Uganda. This collaborative approach has magnified the ability of UYAAS to reach out to the youth in Uganda, enabling them to provide support and education to other organizations and to contribute to the larger national and international efforts in addressing this crucial challenge.

Maintaining an Active Research Agenda

Another element of UYAAS's strategy is to maintain an active research agenda that seeks to understand and change the behaviors of youth in relation to their reproductive health. UYAAS has managed research projects for various national bodies such as the Uganda Ministry of Education and Sports. They are also actively involved in HIV/AIDS research with such entities as the Global AIDS Intervention Network (GAIN 2001/2002), in which they are studying the role of popular opinion leaders on influencing behavioral change among HIV/AIDS-vulnerable groups. Representatives of UYAAS have presented many papers and research reports at international conferences (see Table 9.2).

This active research agenda allows UYAAS to remain at the forefront of creating new knowledge and acquiring new knowledge from others. Such active participation in the larger research community enables UYAAS to incorporate current research findings into its various program activities as it serves individuals, members of local communities, and those in the national and international arena.

Involving Youth Through National Mass Media

Building off of Uganda's national strategy of openness and increasing awareness regarding adolescent reproductive health, UYAAS has taken advantage of mass media opportunities to reach large numbers of Ugandan youth. Through the use of electronic mass media, UYAAS has increased its ability to reach a wider population both within its area of operation and beyond. For example, since 1994, UYAAS has presented a number of talk show-style radio programs aimed at increasing awareness and education of HIV/AIDS, STDs, and other reproductive health issues among Ugandan youth. The radio shows target young people both in and out of school, but especially aim to reach youth who are not in school through nonformal education programs.

Given that UYAAS expects that young people's behavior can change, they designed radio youth talk show programs to help influence positive behavioral change through empowering youth to make informed decisions and set good priorities. The radio programs are aimed at openly discussing issues of relationships, sexuality, HIV/AIDS, STDs, family planning, behavioral change, abstinence, voluntary counseling and testing (VCT), preventing mother-to-child transmission, and many other HIV/AIDS-related health concerns. The talk shows are open, live telephone programs that are presented and hosted by a medical doctor. To increase their impact, the shows are conducted in several local languages to accommodate literate and illiterate, old and young, rural and urban listeners. Young people from different areas of Uganda listen and ask questions that the medical doctor then answers on the air. Those who do not have telephone facilities are encouraged to write to the medical doctor at the radio talk show or to the UYAAS office, and their questions and con-

Table 9.2   Review of UYAAS Research Presentations

1995   "The HIV/AIDS Pandemic—A Global Overview." East and Central Student Conferences on Health Education and HIV/AIDS, Kampala, Uganda.

1997   "Critical Issues Facing Adolescent/Parents." Regional Congress of Psychology Interfacing the Science and Practices, Mexico.

1997   "How School-Based Population Programs Can Succeed in Changing Behaviours of Youth." Africa Forum on Adolescent Reproductive Health, Addis Ababa, Ethiopia.

1998   "Adolescent Sexual Behavioural Knowledge Beliefs and Attitudes." National Council for International Health—25th Anniversary, June 1998, Marriott Hotel, Arlington, Virginia

1998   "STD/AIDS and Its Impact on Young People." Pediatric and Adolescent Gynecology Conference, Florida.

2002   "Best Practices in HIV/AIDS Control among Youth in and out of School in Uganda: A Case Study of Uganda Youth Anti-AIDS Association." Global AIDS Intervention Network (GAIN) Conference, May 11–13, 2002, Amsterdam, The Netherlands.

2002   "Examination of Best Practices in the Reduction of HIV/AIDS in the Education Sector in Uganda." Third National AIDS Conference and First HIV/AIDS Partnership Forum, October 28–30, 2002, International Conference Center, Kampala, Uganda.

2002   "Research Study on Popular Opinion Leaders on Influencing Behavioral Change among HIV/AIDS Vulnerable Groups." Medical College of Wisconsin, Milwaukee, Wisconsin, USA.

2002   "Street Children/Youth and HIV/AIDS in Uganda." East and Southern Africa Civil Society Forum on Promoting and Protecting the Rights of Street Children, Nairobi, Kenya.

2004   "Reviewing the MOES HIV/AIDS Action Plan 2003–2006." Stakeholders Workshop, June 23–24, 2004, Hotel Africana, Kampala, Uganda.

2004   "Another Weapon of Mass Destruction—HIV/AIDS: What Is the Way Forward for the Youth Who Are the Majority Victims?" The National Youth Conference, August 13, 2004, Speak Resort, Munyonyo, Uganda.

cerns are answered in the subsequent programs. Over a decade since UYASS first broadcasted talk shows on the radio, more than 10,000 young people have participated in the programs. As a result of the talk shows, over 30% of the young people that participated were referred for VCT services and 15% were referred for further STD treatment.

As well as reaching out to youth, the radio programs also reach parents and other members of the local communities. As a result, the program enhances open communication, discussion, and interaction between parents and their children, particularly in terms of talking about HIV/AIDS and other reproductive health issues and concerns.

Continuing their strategy of using national mass media, UYAAS is also planning in the near future to begin publication of *Youth Link*, a national-level quarterly newsletter for young people that is both developed and produced by young people themselves. This newsletter will further facilitate UYAAS's aim of increasing awareness and education of adolescent reproductive health issues.

Delivering Education, Training, and Technical Support

UYAAS also provides technical support and education for its network partners at the district and national levels who focus on HIV/AIDS and individuals' capacity to maintain their own reproductive health. Their goal to build community, district, and national capacity is a critical piece in the larger picture of addressing the HIV/AIDS epidemic (Population Council, 2001). They have provided training to CBOs, NGOs, and other national-level groups, including the Uganda Reproductive Health Bureau, Uganda Youth Council, CASEDEV, Omega Development Association, Pearl Uganda, Pentecostal Churches Finish AIDS Project (Mpigi), Banda Community Development Association, Uganda Association for Social Economic Progress, and the Christian Children's Fund.

In addition to national-level groups, UYAAS also provides technical support and education at the district level, where they continue to focus on HIV/AIDS and reproductive health capacity building. They are also involved in district-level planning for HIV/AIDS strategies. For example, UYAAS is currently one of the organizations on the committee for developing a training manual on youth involvement in prevention of STDs and HIV/AIDS in the Kampala District. In addition, UYAAS has also been invited by school administrators in several districts to give keynote addresses and present papers on HIV/AIDS and adolescent reproductive health for conferences, school days, parties, and other functions. Examples of district-level groups that UYAAS has served include the Rubaga Youth Development Association, the Community Education Foundation (CEF) in Hoima, Bugiri Rural Development Association, Iganga Youth Development Agency, Community Action for Development (CCAD)–Kawempe, Pallisa Youth Anti-AIDS Project, Kiboga Integrated Development Initiative (KIDI), and the Uganda Muslim Bugiri Development Association.

One very successful strategy of UYAAS involves training peer educators and local community leaders for various districts, communities, schools, and youth groups. For example, the Training of Trainers (TOT) program was adopted by UYAAS in 1992 to expand the districts' capacity to provide HIV/AIDS and reproductive health education by training community-based volunteers (made up of teachers, local leaders, and church leaders) to be trainers with each district. The volunteer training sessions are mainly participatory and thus enable participants to share experiences on issues such as adolescent health and development, sexuality, life-planning skills, HIV/AIDS and STDs, family planning, reproductive anatomy and physiology, and behavioral change. This training is aimed at strengthening the capacity of the trainers and promoting their excellence and innovativeness. The training also empowers them with skills that will enable them to design and conduct workshops for peer educators among both the in- and out-of-school youth. Since 1992, over 2,800 district-level community-based volunteers have been trained. These trainers have, in turn, educated over 40,000 people on HIV/AIDS care and prevention. Clearly, the TOT strategy allows UYAAS to increase their services and to reach more young people within UYAAS outreach communities as a result of decentralization from the national to the community level (Okware et al., 2001). As such, TOT spreads UYAAS's influence to the lives of individual young people by educating, empowering, and preparing trainers such as community and church leaders at the community level who work directly with the youth.

UYAAS plans to expand its educational initiatives over the next 5 years by implementing several additional programs. Working closely with the Ministry of Education and Sports (MOES), UYAAS will help in the integration process of HIV/AIDS education in the national curriculum. It will also play a leading role in setting up information and technology programs for school-based anti-AIDS club members. Together with the leadership of many school-based anti-AIDS clubs, UYAAS has agreed to establish income generating activities with the goal of getting larger numbers of youth to participate in the anti-AIDS campaign. Finally, UYAAS plans to focus on training 7,650 teachers in 170 schools as anti-AIDS change agents.

Providing Voluntary Counseling and Testing (VCT) Services

Since 1992, UYAAS has provided counseling services to over 4,000 youth both in and out of school. Over 2,500 of these youth were then referred to other reproductive health service providers. In February 2004, UYAAS launched their own voluntary counseling and HIV testing (VCT) services at their center in Mengo. The purpose of VCT is to provide early knowledge to participants on their serostatus, which will in turn help mitigate HIV/AIDS dissemination among the young people.

VCT is a powerful tool for behavioral change with respect to HIV/AIDS prevention. Personalizing risk for HIV infection through VCT is critical in encouraging changes in the behavioral attitudes and intentions of youth in order to reduce or eliminate their risk of exposure to HIV/AIDS. VCT also helps youth make informed decisions regarding relationships and childbearing, prepares them to access care and support, and restores the hope of youth who suspect or know that they are infected with HIV/AIDS. In the first 6 months of the VCT project, UYAAS has counselled and tested over 500 youths both in and out of school. While most of the organization's VCT efforts have traditionally targeted youth in urban centers, UYAAS plans to offer more VCT services over the next 5 years expanding particularly into the more rural regions of the country. One way UYAAS plans to reach distant regions in the country is through the establishment of a mobile VCT program that can travel to various rural regions on a periodic basis.

Reaching Out to Youth Through Community Services

UYAAS reaches out to local youth by mobilizing communities. In particular, their community efforts focus on out-of-school youth in order to more directly influence them in terms of increasing awareness and education of HIV/AIDS and other reproductive health issues. In addition to their TOT program, UYAAS's community services include outreach seminars, microfinance credit, and condom distribution.

Outreach seminars have been an important strategy of UYAAS in serving communities. Since 1992 UYAAS has conducted over 500 community outreach seminars and over 90,000 youth have been reached through this education medium. The seminars are aimed at reaching out to youth in nonformal education settings, parents, local and church leaders, people with disabilities, young women, and displaced youth in refuge camps. Impact of the seminars includes disseminating HIV/AIDS-related information so that youth are better prepared to protect themselves from the disease. In addition, community outreach seminars respond to individual and community sexual and reproductive health needs by visiting homes and communities primarily in rural villages and slum areas.

In addition to serving communities through outreach seminars, UYAAS works in collaboration with the Council for Economic Empowerment of Women in Africa (CEEWA) to manage their Micro-Finance Credit Project. This project benefits and supports women, particularly widows, living with HIV/AIDS and affected families. The CEEWA Project provides women with microfinance credit opportunities to improve their living or health conditions, acquire basic business skills, make and manage investments, start-up income generating activities, meet their basic needs, reduce poverty at the household level, and support families and AIDS-orphaned children. This financial support directly affects youth living in these families as well as young people who are struggling to support siblings or other members of their immediate families. For example, clients of the Micro-Finance Credit Project are involved in such ventures as retail business, market vending, petty trade, brick making, piggery projects, baking, heifer projects, tailoring, horticulture, local charcoal-stove making, and school canteens,[1] just to name a few. Over 500 of these clients across many communities in Uganda have been trained in business and equipped with entrepreneurship skills. Preliminary findings from this project indicate that over 50% of all clients have been able to carry out successful business ventures and indicated that their livelihoods have improved as a result of UYAAS support.

A third community-service strategy is UYAAS's involvement in condom procurement and distribution. Since 1993, more than 3,000 cartons of condoms have been procured and distributed to young people in the project areas.[2] Condom promotion and distribution as a preventive strategy has been recommended by the Uganda Ministry of Health AIDS Control Project to reduce infection rates of HIV/AIDS and STDs among young people who are sexually active. A 1995 survey in Uganda indicated condom use did increase in Uganda dramatically between 1989 and 1995 (UNAIDS, 1995). UYAAS regards the enhancement of the practice of safe sex, the reduction of the HIV/AIDS risks, and the reduction of unplanned pregnancies among the young people of Uganda as one of its most important priorities and activities.

Facilitating Peer Education Among Youth Through Schools

One of the most effective strategies for directly influencing in-school youth regarding their reproductive health is facilitating peer education, which can be effectively accomplished in school environments (DiClemente, 1997; Elford, Bolding, Maguire, & Sheer, 2000; Murdock, Garbharran, Edwards, Smith, Lutchmiah, & Mkhize, 2003). UYAAS's peer education program is run by the schools' local community-based trainers, illustrating the leveraging effect of the UYAAS training programs.

Since 1992, UYAAS's community-based trainers have trained over 18,000 youth in over 400 schools in 10 districts as peer educators. This peer educator training is aimed at equipping young people with appropriate and accurate skills and knowledge regarding HIV/AIDS and reproductive health. As peer educators, these students are then in a position to educate and inform their classmates about issues concerning HIV/AIDS, STDs, and reproductive health in general. Peer education and the involvement of youth in HIV/AIDS education is one of the most vital strategies for affecting behavioral change in youth (Mirembe, 2002; Murdock et al., 2003).

After each peer education workshop, school-based anti-AIDS clubs are formed to support UYAAS's efforts and sustain the anti-AIDS campaign. Since 2002, UYAAS has established and supported over 80 school-based anti-AIDS clubs in Uganda. UYAAS extends microcredit funds to help facilitate income-generating activities and also sets up information and technology programs for these clubs. The clubs engage in extracurricular activities such as sports, drama, games, drawing, and holding regular focus-group discussions on HIV/AIDS and other health-related issues.

In addition to peer education for students in schools, the UYAAS also offers a program for Training of School Teachers as Change Agents (TOT/CA). This training educates and empowers teachers to act as change agents in their schools by addressing HIV/AIDS, STDs, and other adolescent reproductive health challenges. In the first 10 months of this program—which began in November 2003—about 450 school teachers have already been trained. The training is aimed at empowering teachers with knowledge and information on how to deal with HIV/AIDS challenges in schools. These teachers are trained and expected to pass on appropriate and factual information to the students, engage youth in constructive discussions, offer youth-friendly services, and influence positive behavioral changes. Where teachers are sometimes regarded as an obstacle in teaching students about HIV/AIDS prevention methods and behavior change strategies, the TOT/CA program is particularly important. Teachers have been blamed for defilement, sexual abuse, and rape of young girls, as well as for fornication and adultery. At the end of each TOT/CA workshop, a UYAAS Teachers Change Agent Club is formed to support the training efforts. Club members are encouraged to design and conduct training for peer educators and provide community outreach seminars in their respective schools and communities. Through TOT/CA training, teachers increase their capabilities to encourage behavioral change among the youth in particular, as well as among the wider community in general. TOT/CA training is an example of UYAAS's goal to increase the awareness of HIV/AIDS issues and to build community capacity to address these challenges.

Producing and Distributing Educational Materials

To supplement their various strategies and programs, UYAAS is actively involved in the production and distribution of educational materials related to HIV/AIDS and other reproductive health issues. These reading materials reinforce training and supplement UYAAS efforts in the HIV/AIDS work through responding to the needs of young people, filling in gaps with accurate information, and dispelling myths and misconceptions regarding HIV/AIDS, STDs, and other reproductive health concerns. Since 1995, UYAAS has developed, produced, and distributed over 1.2 million pieces of information, education, and communication (IEC) materials in a variety of forms, such as brochures, booklets, leaflets, posters, stickers, newsletters and peer educators cards. Using their production base, UYAAS will also support and facilitate the upcoming publication of the *Youth Link* newsletter.

The purpose for producing IEC materials aims at ensuring that young people—both in and out of school—have access to HIV/AIDS-related information and thus can become more informed and less vulnerable to HIV infection. These materials and information are age appropriate, youth friendly, factual, and relevant to the youths' actual situations and life challenges.

IMPLICATIONS OF UYAAS SUCCESS FOR HIV/AIDS ORGANIZATIONS

UYAAS success is directly attributable to their clear vision, which they have communicated effectively to a broad base of national and international stakeholders. Their multipronged strategies are organized well, complement each other, and align effectively with their vision. Taking advantage of Uganda's national vision and strategy of openness and increasing awareness of HIV/AIDS, UYAAS has been able to tap into a larger network of people and agencies that also have an intense interest in and energy for addressing these problems. The national and international network UYAAS has developed has allowed them to access resources beyond their own resources; engage in an active research agenda; and provide influence, education, training, and technical support at the school, community, district, and national levels. They have worked hand-in-hand as partners in Ugandan national efforts to address the HIV/AIDS epidemic.

By working at multiple levels simultaneously—with an emphasis on decentralization—UYAAS has been able to increase their services, leverage their efforts, and create a snowball effect by training the trainers who then train the peer educators (Okware et al., 2001). Their programs in local communities and schools allow UYAAS to directly and immediately affect the very real challenges facing the lives of individual youth.

The direct involvement of youth is particularly powerful as UYAAS facilitates peer education strategies that encourage youth to reach out and educate other youth (World Bank, 2002). UYAAS has also involved youth by taking advantage of mass media opportunities and facilitating the publication of critical educational materials, both of which align with and support their efforts.

The success of UYAAS represents an opportunity for other HIV/AIDS organizations to learn from UYAAS's experience and examine the extent to which they might be able to employ similar strategies. The driving strategic factors in UYAAS's success have been developing and communicating a clear and focused vision, building a broad national and international network, working at multiple levels simultaneously with an emphasis on decentralization, and directly involving youth. These effective strategies have made UYAAS a model organization that has proven over 14 years—and is expected to continue—to be a positive force for change in improving adolescent health in Uganda and worldwide.

NOTES

1. A canteen is generally a small snack bar or cafeteria located either on or adjacent to a school campus.
2. Each carton contains 5,040 condoms distributed in packets of three condoms each.

REFERENCES

Bennell, P., Hyde, K., & Swainson, N. (2002). *The impact of the HIV/AIDS epidemic on the education sector in Sub-Saharan Africa.* Sussex, England: Centre for International Education, University of Sussex Institute of Education.

Blanc, A. K. (2000). *The relationship between sexual behavior and level of education in Developing countries.* Geneva, Switzerland: UNAIDS.

DiClemente, R. J. (1997). Looking forward: Future directions for prevention of HIV among adolescents. In L. Sherr (Ed.), *AIDS and adolescents.* Amsterdam, Netherlands: Hardwood Academics.

Elford, J., Bolding, G., Maguire, M., & Sheer, L. (2000, July). *Peer-led HIV prevention among gay men in London: Outcome evaluation in controlled trial.* Paper presented at the Poster Session at XIII International AIDS Conference, Durban, South Africa.

Hite, J. M., & Hesterly, W. S. (2001). The evolution of firm networks: From emergence to early growth of the firm. *Strategic Management Journal, 22*(3), 275–286.

Jacob, W. J., Smith, T. D., Hite, S. J., & Cheng, S. Y. (2004). Helping Uganda's street children: An analysis of the model for orphan resettlement and education (MORE). *Journal of Children and Poverty, 10*(1), 3–22.

Malinga, F. (2000). Uganda: Designing communication and education programs to combat HIV/AIDS. *ADEA Newsletter, 12*(4), 13–14.

Ministry of Health (MOH). (2001). *Primary school teacher's guide on STDs/HIV/AIDS prevention education.* Kampala, Uganda: STD/AIDS Control Programme, Ministry of Health.

Mirembe, R. (2002). AIDS and democratic education in Uganda. *Comparative Education, 38*(3), 291–302.

Murdock, P. O. H., Garbharran, H., Edwards, M. J., Smith, M. A., Lutchmiah, J., & Mkhize, M. (2003). Peer-led HIV/AIDS prevention for women in South African informal settlements. *Health Care for Women International, 24*, 502–512.

Obbo, C. (1995). Gender, age, and class: Discourses on HIV transmission and control in Uganda. In H. T. Brummelhuis & G. Herdt (Eds.), *Culture and sexual risk: Anthropological perspectives on AIDS* (pp. 79–95). Amsterdam, SA: Gordon & Breach.

Okware, S., Opio, A. A., Musinguzi, J., & Waibale, P. (2001). Fighting HIV/AIDS: Is success possible? *Bulletin of the World Health Organization, 79*(12), 1113–1120.

Olson, T. D., & Wilkins, R. G. (2001). *The family, youth and AIDS: A neglected area of prevention.* Paper presented at the International AIDS Conference, Tunis, Tunisia.

Parker, R. G., Barbosa, R., & Aggleton, P. (2000). Framing the sexual subject. In R. G. Parker, R. Barbosa, & P. Aggleton (Eds.), *Framing the sexual subject: The politics of gender, sexuality and power.* Los Angeles: University of California Press.

Piot, P. (2001, November). *Speech.* Paper presented at the National AIDS/STD Conference, Beijing, China.

Population Council. (2001). On the socioeconomic impact of the HIV/AIDS epidemic. *Population and Development Review, 27*(3), 619–624.

Stoneburner, R. L., & Low-Beer, D. (2004). Population-level HIV declines and behavioral risk avoidance in Uganda. *Science, 304*(5671), 714–718.

UNAIDS. (1995). *A measure of success in Uganda.* Geneva, Switzerland: Joint United Nations Programme on HIV/AIDS (UNAID).

UNAIDS/UNICEF/USAID. (2004). *Children on the brink 2004.* Geneva, Switzerland: UNICEF.

UNAIDS/WHO. (2004). *Uganda epidemiological fact sheets on HIV/AIDS and sexually transmitted infections: 2004 Update.* Geneva, Switzerland: Authors

United Nations. (2001). *Declaration of commitment on HIV/AIDS.* New York: United Nations General Assembly Special Session on HIV/AIDS.

World Bank. (2002). *Education and HIV/AIDS: A window of hope.* Washington, DC: Author.

CHAPTER 10

MAXIMIZING HIV/AIDS PREVENTION THROUGH THE MEDIA

AN ANALYSIS OF THE STRAIGHT TALK FOUNDATION

Catharine Watson, Betty Kagoro, and Beatrice Bainomugisha

The mass media has been identified as a powerful tool for teaching young people about the consequences of sexual activity. The HIV-prevention media campaigns in Uganda were instrumental in reducing HIV prevalence among young women in the 1990s (Keller, 1997). Several major mass media campaigns throughout the country are thought to have (1) produced an increase in monogamy, (2) significantly increased condom use in risky sexual relationships, and (3) postponed the age of women's sexual debut. According to an October 1996 report from the Ugandan Health Ministry's STD/AIDS Control Program (STD/ACP) on HIV prevalence among pregnant women (research was completed at six hospitals between 1991 and 1995), HIV infection has been declining in parts of the country, and Ugandans have significantly changed their sexual behavior

Overcoming AIDS: Lessons Learned from Uganda, 189–208
Copyright © 2006 by Information Age Publishing
                                                                    189

to avoid infection ("Ray of Hope in Uganda in War against HIV," 1997). A 5-year study by the Medical Research Council (MRC) and the Uganda Virus Research Institute, which covered 15 villages and approximately 5,200 people over the age of 13 in the Masaka District of Uganda, indicates that the prevalence of HIV in men ages 20–24 has declined by 80%, from 11.8%–2.6%. Among girls ages 13–19 and women ages 20– 24, the decline was 62% and 34%, respectively. In the general population, the decline was from 8.2%–7.6%. Reasons for the decline are attributed to increased socializing influences and social values placed on sexual experience. Sources of social influence include parents, social functions, nature, peers, their paternal aunts and uncles,[1] school curriculum, and various media. Additional sources include church leaders, political leaders, and teachers, who often play important roles in this endeavor (Kinsman, Nyanzi, & Pool, 2000).

Stoneburner and Low-Beer (2004) provide excellent empirical documentation of how Uganda has responded to the AIDS epidemic, noting that a population with a risk-avoidance agenda can be easily mobilized through mass media approaches. Despite limited resources, Uganda has shown a 70% decline in HIV prevalence since the early 1990s, a reduction linked to a 60% reduction in casual sex. The response in Uganda appears to be distinctively associated with communication about AIDS through social networks. Despite substantial condom use and promotion of biomedical approaches, other African countries have shown neither similar behavioral responses nor HIV prevalence declines of the same scale. The Ugandan success is equivalent to a vaccine of 80% effectiveness, and its replication will require changes in global HIV/AIDS intervention policies and their evaluation.

Much of Uganda's significant reduction in HIV prevalence over the past decade is attributed to an explicit national policy known as "A, B, C": Abstinence, Be faithful, and Condoms. This strategy has garnered attention throughout the world (Green, 2003). Most programs anchor their prevention programs on the concept of abstinence, encouraging individuals to delay their sexual debut until a later stage of life, preferably at matrimony. However, not all adolescents are sexually naïve, and consideration must be given to the sexually active adolescent who responds more favorably to other prevention modalities, such as being faithful and using condoms. Although "be faithful" literally implies monogamy, it also includes reduction in casual sex and multiple sexual partnerships (and related issues of partner selection) that would reduce higher risk sex. While most of the often polarized discussion surrounding AIDS prevention has focused on promoting abstinence or the use of condoms, partner reduction has been the neglected middle child of the ABC approach.

THE EPIDEMIOLOGICAL RATIONALE
FOR PARTNER REDUCTION

It seems obvious, but there would be no global AIDS pandemic were it not for multiple sexual partnerships. The rate of change of sexual partners—especially concurrent partners—is a crucial determinant in the spread of sexually transmitted infections, including HIV (Garnett, 1995). Moreover, HIV's viral load, and therefore infectiousness, is dramatically higher during the early (acute) stage of HIV infection (Pilcher et al., 2004), so transmission would be particularly heightened by partner change among newly infected people. Transmission of HIV is also facilitated by the presence of other sexually transmitted infections, especially ulcerative ones. Consequently, increased risk of other sexually transmitted infections from multiple partnerships further magnifies the spread of HIV.

PARTNER REDUCTION EFFORTS

Partner reduction seems to have been pivotal to the success in two countries heralded for reversing their HIV epidemics, Thailand and Uganda. Thailand's "100% condom" approach in brothels is widely credited with reversing its more concentrated epidemic. This intervention was also followed by a striking reduction (about a twofold decline between 1990 and 1993) in the number of men who reported engaging in commercial and other casual sex (Bessinger, Akwara, & Halperin, 2003; Low-Beer & Stoneburner, 2003; Mills, Benjarattanaporn, Bennett, Pattalug, Sundhagul, & Trongsawad, 1997).

In Uganda, where the estimated prevalence of HIV in adults has fallen from about 15–18% to 5–7% during the past decade, each component of the ABC approach probably has played an important role. However, the least recognized element, partner reduction, was perhaps the key.

It is difficult to reconstruct the events that occurred during the late 1980s and early 1990s, when the rate of new infections was falling in Uganda (Bessinger et al., 2003; Hogle, Green, Nantulya, Stoneburner, & Stover, 2002; Low-Beer & Stoneburner, 2003). With respect to abstinence, demographic and health surveys between 1989 and 1995 show that the average age at sexual debut increased by less than one year during this time (Bessinger et al., 2003), and the proportion of single women aged 15 –24 who reported having sex during the previous year fell by about a third. Such changes were clearly important, but these changes alone probably cannot account for the large national decline in HIV infection across all age groups.

In the same surveys, use of condoms increased from 1%–6% for women, and by 1995 it had reached 16% among men (Hogle et al., 2002). The 1989 and 1995 surveys conducted by the World Health Organization's (WHO) Global Program on AIDS—which sampled a more urban population—reported ever use of condoms was substantially higher, increasing from 7%–20% in women and from 15%–30% in men (Bessinger, 2003). Especially in such a generalized epidemic, however, these levels of condom use are still relatively modest, and ever use encompasses much more than the correct and consistent use of condoms required to prevent HIV infection (Ahmed et al., 2001; Hearst & Chen 2003). Therefore, although condom use probably contributed to the decline in HIV infection rates, it seems unlikely that it could account for such a dramatic fall in HIV incidence in the late 1980s and early 1990s. By 2000, Uganda had one of the highest levels of reported condom use for nonregular partners in Africa (Bessinger et al., 2003), which probably supported the continuing stabilization of the epidemic in the later 1990s.

But evidently even more important changes in sexual behavior had occurred in Uganda. In the face of the pervasive national campaign at that time to encourage sticking to regular partners ("zero grazing"), reported multiple partner behavior dropped noticeably. The Global Program on AIDS surveys found that the proportion of men with one or more casual partners in the previous year fell from 35% in 1989 to 15% in 1995, and the proportion of women from 16%–6% (Bessinger et al., 2003; Hogle et al., 2002; Low-Beer & Stoneburner, 2003). Notably, the proportion of men reporting three or more nonregular partners fell from 15%–3% (Bessinger et al., 2003).

Because people with large numbers of sex partners are most likely to spread sexually transmitted diseases, such changes are profound. Indeed, modeling of HIV interventions in rural Uganda suggests that such degrees of partner reduction could have had a substantial effect on the incidence of infection (Robinson, Mulder, Auvert, & Hayes, 1995). Although a direct causal link cannot be definitively established between the campaign to promote monogamy and partner reduction and the concomitant fall in the incidence of HIV infection, it seems likely that it was critical to the success in Uganda (Bessinger et al., 2003; Hogle et al., 2002; Low-Beer & Stoneburner, 2003).

Other data provide more direct evidence of such behavioral change. Surveys from Cambodia, where prevention efforts seem to have reduced HIV infection (Rotello, 1997), indicate that the proportion of men who reported paying for sex has fallen greatly (Cambodia Ministry of Health, 2004). In Zambia, the prevalence of HIV reportedly fell among young

urban women during the 1990s (Bessinger et al., 2003, Fylkesnes, Musonda, Sichone, Ndhlovu, Tembo, & Monze, 2001; UNAIDS, 2002). At
about that time there was a large reduction in casual and multiple-partner
sex (Agha, 2002; Bessinger et al., 2003) in the wake of faith-based and
other grassroots efforts to promote a delay of sexual debut among young
people and to promote monogamy for those who were sexually active.
More recently, HIV prevalence has declined in Addis Ababa, Ethiopia,
where large reductions in commercial and other casual sexual encounters
have been reported among male factory workers (Mekonnen et al., 2003).
And in the Dominican Republic, where HIV also seems to have abated
(Green & Conde, 2000; UNAIDS, 2002), men have reported partner
reduction in addition to increased condom use with sex workers.

IMPLICATIONS FOR BEHAVIOR CHANGE PROGRAMS

Analysis of the importance of partner reduction and monogamy rests
largely on ecological and other observational evidence, including self-
reported behavioral findings. Nevertheless, the overall patterns and associations seem consistent and logical and suggest that partner reduction
could be a major factor in reducing the incidence of HIV infection. Yet it
is still given little attention in most HIV prevention programs, despite its
epidemiological importance and apparent behavioral "acceptability." We
believe it is imperative to begin including (and rigorously evaluating)
messages about mutual fidelity and partner reduction in the ongoing
activities to change sexual behavior. Formative research should identify
which changes are feasible for each audience, and programs should then
build on behavior changes that people already seem to be willing to make.

Moreover, it seems important and feasible to promote monogamy and
partner reduction alongside abstinence and the use of condoms. People
seem generally able to grasp that the root problem with HIV transmission
is risky sex and to adopt the behavior that best fits their circumstances. We
have a public health responsibility to help people understand the
strengths and limitations of each of the ABC components and not to promote one component to the detriment of another. For example, although
abstinence may be a viable option for many young people, for others it
may be an unrealistic expectation. Likewise, even though prospective
studies have shown that condoms reduce risk by about 80–90% when used
correctly and consistently (Hearst & Chen, 2003), in real life they are
often used incorrectly or inconsistently (Ahmed et al., 2001; Hearst &
Chen, 2003); therefore, condoms should not be advertised in ways that
lead to overconfidence or risky behavior.

Importantly, evidence from both Thailand and Uganda indicates that not only was individual behavior changed to promote partner reduction, but group behavioral norms were also altered (Hogle et al., 2002; Low-Beer & Stoneburner, 2003; Van Landingham & Trujillo, 2002). In Uganda, a combination of presidential pronouncements and the engagement of faith-based organizations, the governmental apparatus, the military, the health system, and community-based and mass communications—all in the context of the stark reality of people dying from AIDS—seem to have achieved a "tipping point" so that avoiding risky sex increasingly became the community norm, although it was not eliminated altogether. This experience supports the need to reinforce messages from multiple sources. In addition, most of the approaches that involve behavior change originated within Uganda (and similarly within Thailand) (Green, 2003; Hogle et al., 2002; Low-Beer & Stoneburner, 2003), suggesting external assistance should reinforce such locally developed approaches.

Of course, HIV prevention must extend beyond the ABC approach. Other behavior changes, such as avoiding the particularly risky practice of unprotected anal intercourse, are important (Halperin, Padian, Palefsy, & Shiboski, 2002), as are efforts to reduce risk from intravenous drug use, promote safe injection practices in health-care settings, expand access to voluntary counseling and testing, and treat other sexually transmitted infections, especially in high-risk populations. In addition, it is imperative to continue efforts to develop an effective AIDS vaccine, develop safe microbicides so that women can directly lower their risk, explore increased availability of male circumcision (Bailey, Plummer, & Moses, 2001), and remain open to other new tools in the fight against the pandemic. The method through which all these components are optimally promoted and deployed depends on many factors, including the stage and nature of a given epidemic and the particular subpopulations at risk. Additional research is also necessary to maximize the impact of partner reduction and other interventions. Rather than arguing over the merits of abstinence versus condoms, it is time for the international community to unite around a balanced, evidence-based ABC approach.

REACHING THE MASSES THROUGH THE MEDIA

The following sections describe the national media-based program in Kampala, Uganda, which has revolutionized national HIV/AIDS programs and has had a major impact on the prevention of HIV/AIDS in Sub-Saharan Africa. The Straight Talk Foundation (STF) originated out of the *Straight Talk* newspaper, which was first published in 1993 and funded by UNICEF. Today, STF is a health communication nongovernmental organization (NGO) that produces behavior change communication (BCC) materials for adolescents. The broad objective of the foundation is to contribute to the improved mental, social, and physical development of Ugandan adolescents (ages 10 through 19) and young adults (ages 20 through 24). The program also aims to keep its audience—mostly adolescents but increasingly also adults—safe from HIV/STD infection and early pregnancy.

More specifically, STF aims to increase understanding of adolescence, sexuality, and reproductive health and to promote the adoption of safer sex practices through its communications projects. The foundation also strives to help adolescents acquire necessary life skills and get a good grasp on child and human rights so that they can make the passage through adolescence safely.

Communication Through Straight Talk Clubs

Because of the popularity of STF's programs, Straight Talk Clubs have been formed in secondary schools and communities. These clubs are venues for open discussion about adolescent issues. Since 1994, over 400 Straight Talk Clubs have been independently formed. The clubs are initiated by the adolescents themselves to discuss the message of safer sex with their peers.

These clubs are affiliated with but are not controlled by STF. They are led by elected school leaders who work as a team in a committee. STF supports the clubs by training club leaders and by providing support visits from a development worker and a health worker. In addition, the clubs receive copies of the *Straight Talk* newspaper and other behavior change communication materials.

Straight Talk Radio—A Wake-up Call

It is six o'clock in the morning. I'm rolling in my bed. I switch on my small radio to catch the early morning news. Instead, my ears are tuned to a sound of the famous "Kangabaijje" drum. That was way back in the 1980s, when AIDS was spreading like a wildfire.

In traditional Africa, such drumming was done in times of danger. It alerted people to get their spears and shields and prepare to attack an enemy who had invaded their community. But this time around, the enemy was nothing human; it was the invisible Human Immunodeficiency Virus (HIV). It had claimed millions of lives in Uganda and other parts of the world. Many Ugandans—rich, poor, young, old—had been affected by the virus in one way or another. Yet nothing was in place to avert the situation. Something had to be done to alert the population about the scourge and what could be done to prevent it.

Using the drum on the national radio was one of the most successful media approaches adopted by the government. The sound of the drum was a constant reminder to people that AIDS is with us, AIDS is a killer, AIDS is an enemy. Radio was an ideal medium because it is more accessible than print, it is rich in content, it provokes emotion, and it appeals to all categories of people. But with time, the drum alone was not enough.

Combating HIV/AIDS became everybody's concern in the early 1990s, but it required a concerted effort from all sectors of society to realize positive results. Different approaches both in the media and other sectors had to be adopted by different stakeholders, both private and public, in order to reduce the impact of the scourge.

STF was organized out of the need to provide accurate, age-appropriate HIV-prevention information to young people. At the time, many young people were in high-risk situations, yet there were no specific interventions that targeted them. All the existing interventions neglected the fact that adolescents are a special group of people with unique concerns that need special attention. Someone had to do it, and Straight Talk chose to be the one.

STF is the first mass media source of adolescent health information, education, and communication organization in Uganda. Today, it boasts 11 years of successful communication for better adolescent health. Its major media interventions include the production and distribution of newspapers for in- and out-of-school youth in English and six Ugandan languages and the production and airing of radio shows in English and eight Ugandan languages.

In 2003, STF produced and distributed over 7 million copies of *Straight Talk* and *Young Talk* newspapers and broadcast over 2,100 radio shows. The organization has other outreach programs for youth and teachers that support STF's mass media interventions.

REACHING THE MASSES THROUGH PRINT

STF newspapers are adolescent driven and age appropriate. They are inserted in the major daily newspaper, *The New Vision,* and are posted to approximately 2,800 addresses, including schools, other institutions of learning, community-based organizations (CBOs), NGOs, churches, mosques, health centers, prisons, and police posts.

Straight Talk Newspaper

The *Straight Talk* newspaper started in 1993, when HIV infection was at its peak in many parts of the country. It targets in-school adolescents ages 15–19. At the time the newspaper began, all age groups in the country were at risk, but there were no special government interventions targeting adolescents (see Figure 10.1).

Young people constitute almost 50% of the population of Uganda. They have special needs with regard to information on how to handle the challenges of growing up, such as body changes, sexual feelings, and relationships, challenges that they encounter during the transition from childhood to adulthood. Because this group needs special attention, STF opted to address their needs through provision of accurate, age-appropriate, and culturally sensitive information.

Each month, the *Straight Talk* newspaper is posted to about 2,800 secondary schools throughout the country. A total of 260,000 copies are

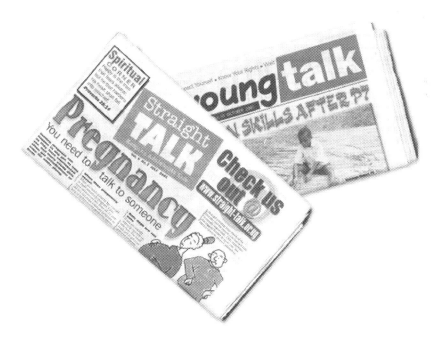

Figure 10.1.   Pictures of STF's *Straight Talk* and *Young Talk* Newspapers.

printed, and each school gets 30 copies free of charge. Key messages in *Straight Talk* relate to body changes, relationships and love, delaying sex or always using condoms, preventing HIV/STDs, and testing for HIV.

Young Talk

After successfully establishing a good relationship with older adolescents in secondary schools, STF realized there was a need to communicate to younger adolescents in upper primary schools. Research conducted by the African Medical and Research Foundation (AMREF), another NGO, showed that some adolescents aged 10–14 were engaging in sex and were therefore equally at risk.

Furthermore, because puberty begins as early as age 8 in some girls and age 10 in some boys, there was a need to give information to young people early enough so that they would know how to deal with sexual maturation as it unfolded and stay safe. STF thought it was important to start *Young Talk* to reach young people early so that when they enter secondary school, the information they received in primary school is reinforced by the messages they find in *Straight Talk*. Alternatively, if they do not gain a postprimary education, they will have had access to some sex education in primary school.

Each month, STF produces 430,000 copies of *Young Talk* newspapers that are sent to about 13,000 primary schools. Key messages include delaying sex, knowing your rights, avoiding early pregnancy or marriage, staying in school, and preventing HIV/STDs.

It is vital to note that messages in both *Straight Talk* and *Young Talk* emphasize abstinence as the number one way of preventing HIV/STDs. Abstinence is inexpensive, has no side effects, and is available to everyone. However, STF believes that emphasizing abstinence alone would eliminate a considerable portion of its target audience, namely, adolescents who are already sexually active.

There are many adolescents who are already engaged in premarital sex; they need information on how to best protect themselves. They need support to either abstain again or practice safer sex. At the same time, those who choose abstinence also need access to facts about condom use so that in the future, if they choose to engage in high-risk sexual relationships, they will be better prepared to protect themselves from HIV infection. A high-risk sexual relationship involves having sex with a person whose HIV status is not known to his or her partner.

Teacher Talk

In June 2002, STF introduced *Teacher Talk*, a newspaper targeting primary school teachers (see Figure 10.2). Its major goal is to foster a

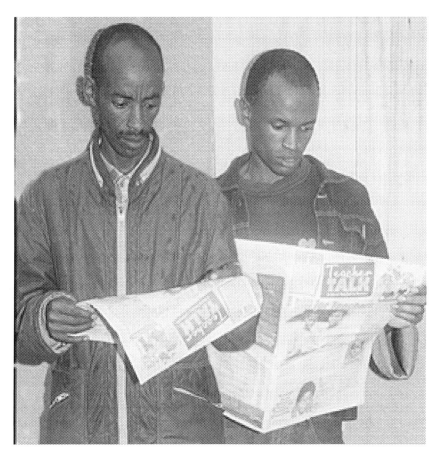

Figure 10.2.   Two primary school teachers reading *Teacher Talk*.

supportive environment at school for adolescent sexual and reproductive health (ASRH) development. Teachers spend about three quarters of the year with students, so it is important to empower teachers with ASRH information and skills so that they can ably discuss this information with their students. Teachers need to counsel, guide, and teach students skills relating to how to deal with ASRH challenges and how to support peer-to-peer activities in their schools. *Teacher Talk* also aims to support universal primary education and therefore increase teacher influence in school.

Many teachers are appreciative of STF activities in their schools as observed in the following letters:

Young Talk has helped me a lot in answering children's questions on issues like menstruation and sexually transmitted diseases. It also answers my own questions. For example, I didn't know why menstruation occurs twice in a month. (Teacher, Gulu Public School, Gulu District)

I love *Straight Talk* papers because now I do less talking about sexuality and growing up. (Headmaster, Bukedea Secondary School, Kumi District)

Parent Talk

Parent Talk, a newspaper for adults like *Teacher Talk*, was launched in 2004 with the goal of fostering a supportive environment at home for adolescent sexual development. Research conducted by STF in 2003 shows that parents still have a greater influence on their adolescent children than any other person. It further shows that adolescents who first hear about sex from their parents or teachers are more likely to delay sex than adolescents who first hear about sex from their peers.

There are many parents who do not talk about sex to their adolescent children for fear that such conversations will encourage children to become sexually active. This fear is misplaced. Other parents feel uncomfortable because they are not very knowledgeable about reproductive health and lack the skills to talk to their children about such sensitive issues. On the other hand, many more parents are willing to talk to their children about sex, but they lack the time to do so, since they spend much of their time working to provide for the family.

Parent Talk helps parents feel comfortable discussing ASRH issues with their children and allowing their adolescent children to express themselves freely. Parents should also allow and encourage emergence of life skills and complement the teachers' role in educating their kids about ASRH issues.

Ugandan-Language Newspapers

School dropout rates in Uganda mean that many adolescents remain illiterate and therefore cannot access much information that is in English; roughly one-third of all children who complete primary school go on to postprimary education. Consequently, STF recognized the need to address out-of-school adolescents who are equally at risk. Ugandan-language newspapers with low-literacy content in six local languages are today being produced and distributed in their respective regions. The major message for adolescents in this category is to stay safe through abstinence, use of condoms, faithfulness, regular access to contraceptives,

STD treatment, and increased access to antenatal testing services and voluntary counseling and testing (VCT) services.

RADIO SHOW PROGRAMS

A half-hour entertainment-education radio show is presented weekly on 18 FM radio stations strategically located countrywide, the English *Straight Talk* radio show targets in-school adolescents aged 15–19. It first went on the air in 1999 in English. Eight Ugandan-language radio shows target out-of-school adolescents with age-appropriate reproductive health messages: their audience appears to be mostly male. In 2004, a total of 2,132 Straight Talk radio shows were broadcast.

Straight Talk radio shows are meant to (1) reinforce the *Straight Talk* newspaper messages, (2) reach adolescents who have no access to *Straight Talk* newspapers, and (3) reach adolescents who cannot read or understand English. Like the *Straight Talk* newspaper, the show is created for and by young people, spiced up by weekly quizzes and music that appeal to them. Once every month a doctor program features listeners' questions answered by doctors, counselors, or other qualified health providers.

FEEDBACK FROM READERS AND LISTENERS

STF has always logged letters according to age, gender, topic, and district, and letters from adolescents have always driven the content of their publications. Producing materials in such large volumes brings responsibility. The materials must be accurate, attractive, and compelling to adolescents. They must remain relevant and on the cutting edge, and they must change as adolescents change. In 2004, STF received almost 30,000 letters from adolescents. Since 1993, these letters have provided a window into the thoughts and lives of 10–19-year-olds. Some letters include unsolicited questions and opinions, while others are solicited specifically for use in the magazines.

Examples of correspondences STF receives on a daily basis include letters from readers of the various STF newspapers and listeners of the weekly radio show programs. A secondary student from Tororo District said in a recent letter, "Since I started reading *Straight Talk*, I have stopped having sex. Had I began reading it much earlier, I would not have lost my virginity at such an early age." Another student lamented the cultural barriers that exist when discussing sexual matters in the home, "Here in Acholi, parents do not talk to us about sex. I thank the Straight Talk Foundation for talking to us about it." These examples highlight the

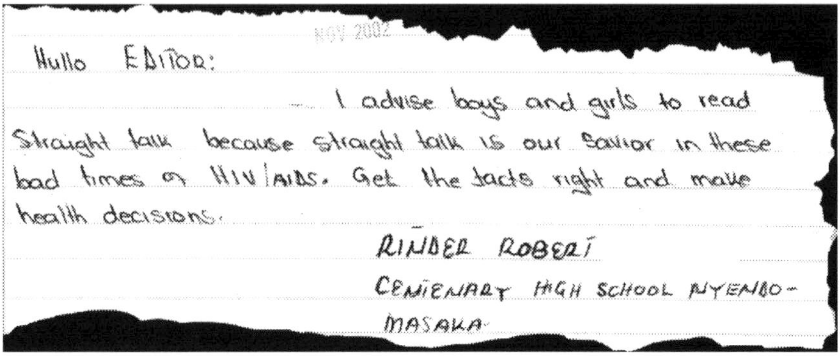

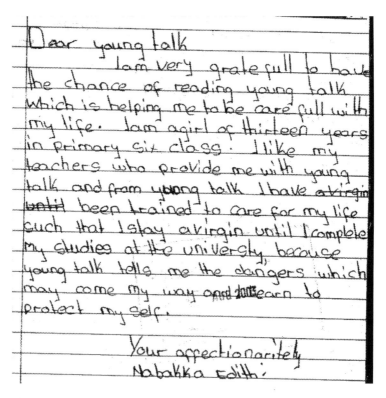

Hullo EDITOR:
            I advise boys and girls to read
Straight talk because straight talk is our Savior in these
bad times of HIV/AIDS. Get the facts right and make
health decisions.
                    RINDER ROBERT
                    CENTENARY HIGH SCHOOL NYENDO-
                    MASAKA

Figure 10.3.   Male student correspondence, secondary school in Masaka District.

Dear young talk
          I am very gratefull to have
the chance of reading young talk
which is helping me to be carefull with
my life. I am a girl of thirteen years
in primary six class. I like my
teachers who provide me with young
talk and from young talk I have a virgin
until been trained to care for my life
such that I stay a virgin until I complete
my studies at the university, because
young talk tells me the dangers which
may come my way and I learn to
protect my self.

                    Your affectionaritely
                    Nabakka Edith:

Figure 10.4.   Female student correspondence, primary school in Kampala District.

desire adolescents have to learn about sexual relationships, HIV/AIDS and other STD prevention methods, and the best ways to discuss these issues with their peers. The letters also emphasize that the mass media is often the only medium adolescents can turn to for facts about these culturally sensitive issues.

The majority of *Straight Talk* readers sending letters sought advice on general issues about sex (42.3%) and staying safe. Other issues readers were interested in include boy-girl relationships (26.5%), body changes (9.8%), condoms (5.1%), general health issues (4.8%), virginity (2.9%), pregnancy (2.5%), STDs (2.0%), and masturbation (1.0%). *Young Talk* readers tended to ask questions regarding body changes at puberty (48.6%). Questions regarding boy-girl relationships (16.7%) came in as the second most frequently asked about subject, followed by questions on pregnancy (14.5%), forced marriage (4.0%), child abuse (2.3%), and emotional changes (1.7%).

OTHER SUPPORT PROGRAMS

School Environment Program

The School Environment Program (SEP) is the face-to-face arm of the Straight Talk Foundation (STF) that complements the print and radio interventions. It aims to create a supportive environment for discussions about adolescent sexual and reproductive health in school settings. Teams of STF doctors, nurses, and counselors work with pupils, students, teachers, and parents on adolescent sexual and reproductive health issues.

School environment programs include secondary school workshops, primary school teacher training seminars, and support for Straight Talk and Young Talk Clubs. According to the Education Data Survey 2001, there are approximately 127,000 primary school teachers and 30,000 secondary school teachers in Uganda. Until recently, teachers have not been trained to teach pupils about reproductive health or life skills. In 2002, the President of Uganda instructed primary schools to address HIV/AIDS issues and answer students' questions about sex. Many teachers felt unprepared to teach this subject, and some head teachers disagreed that children in primary schools should learn about sexual and reproductive health. Through sensitization workshops, STF promotes discussion about sexual and reproductive health issues between pupils and teachers, counseling and guidance about sexuality and body changes, and life-skills education. STF training also encourages teachers to support peer-to-peer activities, such as drama and debates. This led to the development of the Presidential Initiative on AIDS Strategy for Communication to Youth

(PIASCY). Since 2004, PIASCY has led to much greater levels of sex education in primary schools.

Online Counseling

STF also undertakes online counseling for in-school adolescents to complement the other interventions. A number of schools have access to the Internet under the World Bank-funded *School Net* project in conjunction with STF. Through the arrangement, students send in their questions with an identification code instead of their names to ensure confidentiality.

Using the Internet to answer young people's concerns creates a multiplier effect, since the response is sent to all readers. The system is more active during holidays when students cannot easily access *Straight Talk* newspapers. Although this program is still being tested, the response has been positive.

Monitoring and Evaluation

STF's Monitoring and Evaluations Department keeps track of the foundation's activities but also seeks to answer larger question like "What impact does STF have on the behavior of adolescents?" A list of indicators and means of measuring them on a routine basis was developed to answer this question. The monitoring and evaluation system involves selecting sentinel communities, schools, and health facilities in a few districts at a time.

Data collection is done through periodic community surveys, interviews with adolescents in primary and secondary schools, reviews of health facility and school records, and reviews of club minutes. Also, the Monitoring and Evaluations Department continuously monitors and evaluates posttraining evaluations and the letters received from readers and listeners. In addition, a system for monitoring radio broadcasts and receiving feedback from schools, the district education offices, and post offices about the distribution of the publications was developed. Findings from the aforementioned research studies constitute the content of the newspaper and radio messages, which makes all STF programs adolescent and learner guided. This has kept STF focused on the needs of the target audience throughout its first decade of existence.

Collaboration With Local CBOs, NGOs, and Faith Groups

In a bid to link information to services, STF networks with over 3,000 NGOs, CBOs, mosques, churches, and health units involved in ASRH activities. STF specializes in BCC interventions. Its messages—like "seek STD treatment," "use condoms," and "go for voluntary counseling and testing"—create a demand among the target audience for STF to network with organizations involved in service provision.

STF publications are the main source of adolescent sexual mass media information in Uganda, so many organizations use the newspaper messages for counseling and for attracting young people to utilize their services, since they can easily identify with reading a newspaper or listening to a radio program. Collaborating organizations also serve as a significant distribution medium of STF newspapers to adolescents nationwide.

IMPACT ON THE BEHAVIOR OF ADOLESCENTS

Since *Straight Talk* was first published in 1993, there have been many notable behavioral changes in the lives of adolescents. For example, the average age of sexual debut among adolescents has risen. According to the Uganda Bureau of Statistics (UBOS) *Demographic and Health Survey 2000/2001*, the age of first sexual experience among girls has risen from 16.1 years in 1995 to 16.7 years in 2001. For boys, the change has been even greater—from 17.5 years in 1995 to 18.8 years in 2001 (UBOS, 2001).

Research has further found that when today's adolescents do become sexually active, they are likely to have fewer partners and are much more likely to use condoms than were their counterparts in the early 1990s. Condom use among unmarried females has also risen from "negligible" in 1995 to 24% in 2001. At the same time, the proportion of unmarried sexually active females who said they had had more than one sexual partner in the past year fell from 10% in 1995 to 4% in 2001 (UBOS, 2002).

One indication of this changed behavior is a decreased rate of HIV prevalence in the adult population. Prevalence among 15–19-year-old females in antenatal clinics in Kampala has fallen from over 30% in 1992 to 4–9% in 2002 (Ministry of Health (MOH), 2002). Another indication of sexual behavior change is fewer teenage pregnancies. The percentage of girls aged 15–19 who are pregnant or have ever delivered fell from 43% in 1995 to 31% in 2001 (UBOS, 2002). In addition, more young people are seeking information about VCT and actually taking advantage of these services where available. These and several others are some of the achievements to which STF has contributed. No other population group in Uganda has witnessed as much sexual behavior change in the past decade as adolescents.

While STF has helped in Uganda's battle to overcome HIV and AIDS, many challenges remain. More effort needs to be made to advocate proper utilization of print and radio materials. Print and radio messages would have greater impact in HIV/AIDS prevention if teachers, parents, and adolescents made better use of them. A careful analysis of STF's best practices and research findings would help disseminate prevention methods to a wider audience. Ideally, this analysis process should be ongoing, but it has not been fully developed at this point. Perhaps STF's primary strength is the power it holds in networking and partnering with the government, CBOs, NGOs, and faith groups. STF materials create or increase demand for services like VCT and STD treatment, among others. However the services currently offered in Uganda are frequently inadequate, and where they do exist, they are often not adolescent friendly.

NOTE

1. In Uganda, sexual learning was traditionally provided by the paternal aunt and uncle of adolescents. This sexual education network has shifted in recent years to include school senior teachers (both male and female) and mass media outlets such as *Straight Talk* and *Youth Talk*. See for instance, Lawrence Birken (1988) *Consuming Desire: Sexual Science and the Emergence of a Culture of Abundance 1871–1914* (Ithaca, NY: Cornell University Press).

REFERENCES

Agha S. (2002). Declines in casual sex in Lusaka, Zambia: 1996–1999. *AIDS*, 16, 291–293.

Ahmed, S., Lutalo, T., Wawer, M., Serwadda, D., Sewanlambo, N. K., Nalugoda, F., et al. (2001). HIV incidence and sexually transmitted disease prevalence associated with condom use: A population study in Rakai, Uganda. *AIDS*, *15*(16), 2171–2179.

Bailey, R. C., Plummer, F. A., & Moses, S. (2001). Male circumcision and HIV prevention: Current knowledge and future research directions. *Lancet Infectious Diseases*, *1*(4), 223–231.

Bessinger, R., Akwara, P., & Halperin, D. T. (2003). *Sexual behavior, HIV and fertility trends: A comparative analysis of six countries; phase I of the ABC study.* Chapel Hill, NC: Measure Evaluation.

Birken, L. (1988). *Consuming desire: Sexual science and the emergence of a culture of abundance 1871–1914.* Ithaca, NY: Cornell University Press.

Cambodia Ministry of Health. (2004). *Report on HIV sentinel surveillance in Cambo-dia, 2002.* Phnom Penh: National Center for HIV/AIDS, Dermatology and STDs.

Fylkesnes, K., Musonda, R. M., Sichone, M., Ndhlovu, Z., Tembo, F., & Monze, M. (2001). Declining HIV prevalence and risk behaviors in Zambia: Evidence from surveillance and population-based surveys. *AIDS, 15*(7), 907–916.

Garnett, G. P. (1998). The basic reproductive rate of infection and the course of HIV epidemics. *AIDS Patient Care and STDs, 12*(6), 435–449.

Green, E. C. (2003, March 1). The new AIDS fight: A plan as simple as ABC. *New York Times,* p. A19.

Green, E. C., & Conde, A. (2000). Sexual partner reduction and HIV infection. *Sexually Transmitted Infections, 76,* 145.

Halperin, D. T., Padian, N. S., Palefsy, J., & Shiboski, S. C. (2002). *High level of HIV-1 infection associated with anal intercourse: A neglected risk factor in heterosex-ual AIDS prevention.* Paper presented at the XIV International AIDS Conference, Barcelona, Spain.

Hearst, N., & Chen, S. (2003). *Condoms for AIDS prevention in the developing world: A review of the scientific literature.* Geneva, Switzerland: UNAIDS.

Hogle, J., Green, E. C., Nantulya, V., Stoneburner, R., & Stover, J. (2002). *What happened in Uganda? Declining HIV prevalence, behavior change, and the national response.* Washington, DC: USAID.

Keller, S. (1997). Media can contribute to better health. *Network, 17*(3), 29–31.

Kinsman, J., Nyanzi, S., & Pool, R. (2000). Socializing influences and the value of sex: The experience of adolescent school girls in rural Masaka, Uganda. *Culture, Health, and Sexuality, 2*(2), 151–166.

Low-Beer, D., & Stoneburner, R. L. (2003). Behaviour and communication change in reducing HIV: Is Uganda unique? *African Journal of AIDS Research, 2*(1), 9–21.

Mekonnen, Y., Sanders, E., Aklilu, M., Tsegaye, A., RinkedeWit, T. F., Sharp, A., et al. (2003). Evidence of changes in sexual behaviors among male factory work-ers in Ethiopia. *AIDS, 17*(2), 223–231.

Mills, S., Benjarattanaporn, P., Bennett, A., Pattalug, R. N., Sundhagul, D., & Trongsawad, P. (1997). HIV Risk Behavioral Surveillance in Bangkok, Thai-land: Sexual Behavior Trends Among Eight Population Groups. *AIDS, 11*(Supp 1), S43-S51.

Ministry of Health (MOH). (2002). *HIV/AIDS surveillance report, June 2002.* Kam-pala, Uganda: Author.

Pilcher, C. D., Tien, H. C., Eron, J. J., Vernazza, P. L., Leu, S. Y., Stewart, P. M., et al. (2004). Brief but efficient: Acute HIV infection and the sexual transmis-sion of HIV. *The Journal of Infectious Diseases, 189*(10), 1785–1792.

Ray of Hope in Uganda in War Against HIV. (1997, March). *AIDS Weekly Plus,* pp. 19–21.

Robinson, R., Mulder, D. W., Auvert, B., & Hayes, R. J. (1995). Modelling the impact of alternative HIV intervention strategies in rural Uganda. *AIDS, 9*(11), 1263–1270.

Rotello, G. (1997). *Sexual ecology: AIDS and the destiny of gay men.* New York: Dut-ton.

Stoneburner, R. L., & Low-Beer, D. (2004). Population-level HIV declines and behavioral risk avoidance in Uganda. *Science, 304*(5671), 714–718.

Uganda Bureau of Statistics (UBOS) & ORC Macro. (2001). *Uganda demographic and health survey 2000/2001*. Calverton, MD: Authors.

UNAIDS. (2002). *Report on the global HIV/AIDS epidemic 2002*. Geneva, Switzerland: Author.

Van Landingham, M., & Trujillo, L. (2002). Recent changes in heterosexual attitudes, norms and behaviors among unmarried Thai men: A qualitative analysis. *International Family Planning Perspectives, 28*(1), 6–15.

CHAPTER 11

THE ROLE OF RELIGION IN EDUCATING UGANDAN YOUTH ABOUT HIV/AIDS

Jeremy Liebowitz and Stephen Noll

Uganda has attracted considerable attention for its extraordinary success in combating HIV/AIDS, reducing its HIV prevalence rate from 15%–5% over a 10-year period (Hogle, Green, Nantulya, Stoneburner, & Stover, 2002). Attention to Uganda's success has led to debate as to what internal and external factors were responsible for the rapid decline in prevalence. Disagreements over which prevention strategies were most effective in the "Ugandan miracle" and what lessons can be learned for other countries in similar situations continue, showing few signs of resolution. One of the areas that has generated the most controversy has been the role of religion in campaigns to combat HIV/AIDS.

The impact of faith-based organizations (FBOs) in educating the Ugandan public about HIV/AIDS and carrying out programs of HIV/AIDS prevention, care and support has been considerable. Many FBOs have carried out formal programs or informal activities that have raised awareness and increased knowledge. They have also visited homes, supported orphans, counseled those infected and affected, and provided other kinds of care and support. FBOs have often targeted youth as those

Overcoming AIDS: Lessons Learned from Uganda, 209–224
Copyright © 2006 by Information Age Publishing
All rights of reproduction in any form reserved.

in greatest need of information, care and support. FBO programs for youth include paying school fees for orphans and vulnerable children, conducting education programs, and providing counseling and other support. Their education programs have been particularly effective, reaching large numbers of youth and using creative and participatory techniques to ensure that the programs are meaningful and have an impact. Nevertheless, the youth programs of FBOs have also displayed certain weaknesses, which include delivering inappropriate messages, functioning with limited resources and skills, failing to use peer communication effectively, and producing an unclear impact on behavior change.

RELIGIOUS ORGANIZATIONS IN UGANDAN HISTORY

Uganda was evangelized by Protestant Anglicans (1877) and Roman Catholics (1879), and both continue to play a significant role in Ugandan society. Religious affiliation is distributed as follows: Of the current population of approximately 26 million, almost 90% are Christian (42% Roman Catholics, 39% Anglicans), and 5% are Muslim (Barrett, 2001, p. 76).[1] A significant number of Catholics and Anglicans are nominal, but the total church-going population is significantly higher than in Europe. It may be true that the traditional churches have a stronger base among the older segment of the population and in the rural areas.

The other factor affecting religion and youth in Uganda is the history of revival movements. The "East African Revival," beginning in 1935 in Rwanda and Western Uganda, spread across the country and into Kenya and Tanzania. Though the passionate activity of this revival may have abated over the years, a tradition of evangelistic preaching and demand for moral purity continues, especially in the Protestant sphere. In the last 20 years Pentecostal churches have taken over much of the momentum of the revival, with a particular impact on urban youth.[2] Pentecostalism varies greatly in its social outreach. Some groups like the Miracle Center (Kampala) emphasize instant healing and prosperity. Others, most significantly Kampala Pentecostal Church, have entered into HIV/AIDS orphan work and youth choirs. The Catholic charismatic renewal has also provided some of the most motivated workers for church programs.

Uganda is also a hub for HIV/AIDS advocacy and ministry groups, with approximately 700 advocacy groups reported (Hogle, Green, Nantulya, Stoneburner, & Stover, 2002, p. 4), and for private Christian ministries, with over 1,000 resident missionaries.[3] It would be impossible to assess the total involvement of these various individuals and ministries in the training of Ugandan youth. It might be noted, however, that the vast majority of Christian ministries would be characterized as "evangelical," thus placing a strong emphasis on behavioral factors in preventing HIV/AIDS.

Islam, which predated Christianity in Uganda by more than 30 years, constitutes a smaller community; however this denomination does have more than one million members, and Muslims exercise a visible role in Ugandan politics and civil society. In this paper Islamic efforts receive less attention due to their smaller population, but their work has been considerable, as is evident in the section on the Madarasa project.

RELIGIOUS ORGANIZATIONS AND HIV/AIDS IN UGANDA

As people look to Uganda for lessons in preventing and mitigating HIV/AIDS, one of the areas that has generated considerable debate is the role of faith-based organizations (FBOs) and other religious responses to the epidemic (Green, 2003; Uganda AIDS Commission, UAC/UNICEF, 2003). In studies of religious responses to HIV in Africa, few disagree that FBOs possess significant advantages in certain kinds of HIV/AIDS prevention, care and support activities. FBOs often have extensive networks of people, institutions, and infrastructure, especially in rural areas where few other such institutions exist. In many cases, members of FBOs demonstrate more commitment to their FBOs than to other political, social and economic institutions. FBOs often have a direct impact on social institutions, such as schools, which socialize people and change values over time. In addition, their jurisdiction often includes a number of areas closely connected to HIV/AIDS, such as morality, beliefs about the spiritual bases of disease, and rules of family life and sexual activity (Baylies et al., 1999; Bond & Vincent, 1991; Kagimu, Marum, & Serwadda, 1995; Kagimu, Marum, Wabwire-Mangen, Nakyanjo, Walakira, & Hogle, 1998; Negerie, 1994; Liebowitz, 2002).

Given the complex nature of FBOs, however, this argument needs a number of qualifications. First of all, the level of strength of an FBO in a given community will affect its ability to promote meaningful change. Second, each FBO has different strengths and weaknesses in the areas of institutional structure, religious practices, systems of belief, and international connections. These strengths and weaknesses can determine to what extent an FBO is willing and able to deliver successful interventions in the area of HIV/AIDS. Third, within each FBO internal dynamics between clergy and laity or between youth groups and older church members can either undermine or support efforts in disease prevention and mitigation. Finally, it is clear that FBO programs that do not consider the community pressures on youth sexuality and behavior will not be successful (Awusabo-Asare, 1999a; Garner, 2000; Gregson, Zhuwau, Anderson, & Chandwana, 1999; Liebowitz, 2002; Preston-Whyte, 1999; Varga, 1999).

The impact of FBO activities has generated particular controversy in the areas of prevention and stigma. On the side of prevention, some observers argue that FBOs' emphasis on abstinence and faithfulness, perhaps rather than condom use, has weakened the overall response to the epidemic by discouraging one possible source of prevention (Amuyunzu-Nyamongo et al., 1999; Anane, 1999; Awusabo-Asare, 1999b; Mitchell, Nakamanya, Kamali, & Whitworth, 2002; Spira et al., 2000). Some argue that abstinence has not been a particularly widespread response among many demographic groups, including youth and widows (UAC/UNICEF, 2003). On the other hand, some studies claim that abstinence and faithfulness are the most appropriate and effective methods of prevention, and that FBOs' initiatives in promoting abstinence and fidelity have led to delay of sexual debut, fewer partners, and higher rates of abstinence (Green, 2003).

In the area of stigma, although most FBOs have emphasized the importance of loving and caring for the infected and affected, the inability of some FBO leaders to discuss HIV/AIDS publicly, along with its perceived connection with sinful behavior, may have helped to perpetuate the discrimination practiced against people living with HIV/AIDS (PWA) (Byamugisha, 1998a; Byamugisha, 1998b; Garner, 2000; Gregson et al., 1999).

In Uganda, FBOs have been extremely active in HIV/AIDS prevention and mitigation. A number of their programs have targeted youth. These programs have been effective at raising awareness among and providing education to youth. Despite FBOs' considerable success in such programs, a number of significant challenges remain. First, the types of messages delivered in education programs may not resonate well with youth, and may therefore be ineffective. Second, few FBO programs have achieved demonstrable behavior change among youth. Third, many religious education programs have been informal and inconsistent, not being regularly integrated into the school curriculum, which makes their sustainability and reach unclear. Finally, many programs have not involved youth sufficiently in the development of curriculum and the implementation of activities, developing a top-down approach that identifies youth as "beneficiaries" rather than implementers. This approach has made many programs less participatory and efficient than they might have been if youth had been involved.

RELIGIOUS PROGRAMS FOR PRIMARY AND SECONDARY EDUCATION

Religious organizations founded many of Uganda's historically prestigious schools, and many of these schools continue to be Uganda's top educational institutions today. Schools founded by Anglican and Catholic missionaries have held out a high standard of education over time and have groomed many of Uganda's leaders. Over time, some faiths (especially Anglicans) have lost significant forms of control over schools, as government has assumed an increasing role. At the same time, the number of educational institutions has increased dramatically, including both secular and religious schools. A massive increase in school attendance among primary and secondary age youth has made schools an attractive arena for youth education on HIV/AIDS. However, many attempts at religious education of youth on HIV/AIDS have taken place in other forums where FBOs can capture the attention of youth, since despite increased attendance many youth still do not attend school. According to one statistic, only 14% of boys and 9% of girls attend secondary school in Uganda; therefore, effective programs need to target out-of-school youth as well.

Support for Orphans and Vulnerable Children

Support for orphans and vulnerable children (OVC) is a common way that FBOs respond to congregations' needs. Over half of all religious bodies carry out an OVC support program of some kind (Muhangi, 2004). According to one study, providing school fees is one of the most common ways of supporting orphans and vulnerable children. Paying tuition for orphans provides an excellent way to ensure that those affected by HIV/AIDS develop skills and hope that they can support themselves constructively despite their challenges. Many congregations and faith communities at the local level provide such support, as in the case of the Church of Uganda in Iganga, where a parish supports 158 orphans to study at its local primary school.

Some programs to support OVCs integrate components of training into their programs. An initiative in Wakiso District, near Kampala, integrates a vocational skills training program for orphans with a component of AIDS education and prevention. This faith-based program established a school teaching vocational skills and provides the fees for its students. It also, however, includes a "life skills" component that encourages students to learn more about HIV/AIDS and develop life skills that they can use to keep themselves healthy or live positively. This program is a brainchild of Canon Gideon Byamugisha, an Anglican priest living with HIV/AIDS, who has carried out exceptional work in HIV/AIDS prevention, care and support for youth and other vulnerable groups as a trainer at Namirembe Diocese and as an activist throughout Uganda and Africa. His approach emphasizes the importance of combining peer education and training about HIV/AIDS with other life skills and employment skills to build a community that can sustain itself economically, spiritually, and socially to be better equipped to combat AIDS within the community. Such programs build on the strength of religious leaders to promote hope, faith, and behavior change among an affected community. They also realize the importance of developing activities that can generate resources that can be deployed to fight HIV/AIDS in a sustainable fashion.

The Mildmay Center, an interdenominational FBO based near Kampala, also carries out extensive programs for over 1,600 children living with HIV/AIDS, combing treatment, care and support with educational activities. The Jajja's Home program, for example, combines education and vocational training activities with care for children residing at its various homes. Mildmay also promotes Jajja's Home Clubs, which combine physical, spiritual, emotional, and social support and care through activities like singing and prayer, as well as peer education and age-specific sex education. The combination of high quality medical care with spiritual, emotional, social, and financial support makes for a uniquely effective popular program for youth.

Watoto Children's Ministries, based in Kampala Pentecostal Church, is another model program that combines education with support for OVCs. It has set up "Children's Villages" that provide housing, family care, and education to orphans. These villages house over 800 children in small family units under the care of "house mothers." These villages have facilities to support children, including a medical clinic, available water, a community hall, and a school. Watoto also supports the care of children in their extended families by providing food, clothing, and education. These activities are partially supported by the Watoto Children's Choir, an initiative to raise funds and provide a positive activity for children, while spreading the message of the ministries. The choir has toured all over the world and has generated valuable resources and publicity for the ministries. Similar to the Mildmay Center, Watoto has also integrated a component of HIV/AIDS education in their programs. These programs target educating children so that they are trained academically and spiritually with the goal of equipping them with fundamental life skills and moral values. The integration of care and support for OVCs with education provides an excellent opportunity for Watoto to impart values that can help children to avoid HIV/AIDS in the future.

Education and Awareness Programs for Youth

Although HIV/AIDS education is seldom integrated in the curriculum of secular or parochial schools, a number of FBOs have developed programs that provide education for youth in schools and other informal settings. These programs can be quite effective at communicating ideas to youth in a context that is comfortable for learning that can lead to behavior change. For example, Madarasa, an AIDS education program for youth sponsored by the Islamic Medical Association of Uganda (IMAU) and UNICEF, supports the integration of AIDS education curriculum into the religious teachings of Madarasa schools. The Ugandan Ministry of Health developed a curriculum in conjunction with UNICEF to educate youth about HIV/AIDS transmission, prevention and control. The program has used sheikhs, imams, imams' assistants, volunteers, and youth peers to reach a broad range of youth. In addition to discussing the importance of using sterile instruments and protecting oneself while washing the dead, program implementers decided to include a section on condoms in the curriculum during the program's second year. Since the program's inception in 1995, it has reached more than 36,000 children in 350 schools with messages of HIV/AIDS prevention (Islamic Medical Association of Uganda, 1998).

Youth Alive, a Catholic NGO founded in 1993, is another of the most successful initiatives in FBO youth programs. Initiated by the Kampala-based Kamwokya Christian Caring Community, Youth Alive works with youth through peer education programs that engage them in constructive activity and encourage them to change their behavior. Youth Alive also carries out creative programming for youth education through drama, music, and other activities. Youth Alive's programs have even discussed use of condoms (although only in explanation of why not to use them). The awareness of important subjects for discussion is a sign that peer education programs may be able to identify subjects in need of discussion to a greater extent than other less peer-centered programs. Youth Alive educated 40,000 youth directly during its first 2 years of activity; now over 80,000 youth in 72 clubs nationwide participate in Youth Alive's activities. Youth Alive claims that of its participants 88% of females and 67% of males have adopted "a more wholesome lifestyle" (Scottish Catholic International Aid Fund, 1996, p. 3). The Youth Alive model is being replicated in Tanzania and Zambia, based on its success in generating a peer response to HIV/AIDS and in involving youth in activities that increase their motivation to ensure positive behavior change despite peer pressure.

In other areas, youth programs have collaborated with FBOs to ensure effective efforts in prevention and mitigation. The African Youth Alliance has entered in collaboration with the Inter-Religious Council of Uganda and other faith-based groups to provide more youth-friendly medical services in medical facilities sponsored by faith communities. At the same time, these groups have worked on education programs in collaboration with faith groups to "increase knowledge, life skills and positive attitudes" that can help youth resist the dangers of HIV/AIDS. AYA's partners have included two dioceses of the Anglican Church of Uganda. These partners have worked to improve youth-friendly health services and outreach programs to youth who are at high risk or who lack other educational opportunities.

At a congregational or community level, similar programs provide support, counseling and awareness for youth on HIV/AIDS. In Namirembe Diocese of the Church of Uganda, post-test clubs provide support for HIV positive youth and allow them to take leadership roles in educating and counseling others about the disease (Diocese of Namirembe, 1999). The Naguru Youth Center, an FBO in Kampala, has used its center as a focal point for youth interaction, along with sustained support and counseling over time. The Church of Uganda's Balikyewunia health program in Luuka, Iganga uses peer education to raise awareness among the youth, encourage behavior change, and distribute condoms.

Such youth programs contrast with most youth education programs that exist in churches. Programs such as Youth Alive are participatory and creative; they involve youth not just as recipients of the message but as the developers and deliverers of communication about HIV/AIDS. These organizations attempt to address youth behavior on a sustained basis, with messages to youth in ways that are meaningful in addressing concerns. Youth education in FBOs may ignore youth concerns or neglect to involve youth in developing and designing programs. Many youth criticize their FBOs for failing to discuss condoms and deliver knowledge that includes condoms in its approach to prevention (Byamugisha, 1998a). Participants at a youth workshop in Mbale argued that leaders should not confuse technical issues with spiritual ones, and that condoms should be a subject of education programs. Attendees at a youth workshop in a rural area of Iganga District, in Eastern Uganda, suggested that messages from FBO leaders discouraging condom use either were simply ignored or were subverted by youth who disagreed but felt either unwilling or powerless to change their behavior.

Youth also resist programs that do not involve them in program design and implementation. For example, FBOs that do not make use of peer education in delivering awareness on HIV/AIDS find youth less likely to take an active role in programs and messages more likely to be disconnected from the reality of youth life.

HIGHER EDUCATION

Although not classified as FBOs, universities influence the mindset of students in a high-risk age bracket. They also prepare the country's leadership cadre, whose example and influence will have a ripple effect on the wider society, especially children. It is clearly important for universities to engage in HIV/AIDS education, as noted in the current Strategic Plan for Higher Education. So it is significant to know how the old and new universities are addressing the HIV/AIDS crisis. In particular, it is useful to assess how the religious groups, whether at the overtly religious institutions or through the chaplaincies at secular institutions, are dealing with this issue.[4]

Until recently, Uganda was a "one university country," dominated by Makerere University (founded 1922). Under British rule, Makerere was an elite institution admitting only a few hundred students a year from East Africa. After the failed experiment with the University of East Africa (1962–1970) and the devastation of the Amin and Obote II years (1971–1987), Makerere has begun to grow, both in numbers and in facilities, with over 35,000 students enrolled in 2004.

Education in Uganda is big business. Even before the baby boom caused by Universal Primary Education arrives at university, demand for higher education has been increasing exponentially. Foreseeing this eventuality in its 1992 *White Paper*, the government has encouraged the growth of higher education in both public and private sectors (Kasozi, 2003). Three public universities have joined the ranks: Mbarara University of Science and Technology (1989), Kyambogo University (2004); and Gulu University (2003). Given the history of church activity in Uganda, it is not surprising that many of the emerging private universities are church founded or affiliated: Uganda Martyrs University at Nkozi (Roman Catholic, 1993), Uganda Christian University at Mukono (Anglican, 1997), Bugema University (Seventh-Day Adventist, 1997), Busoga University (Anglican, 1998) and Ndejje University (1999).

It is sobering to report that while all institutions have given attention in one way or another to the global AIDS crisis, few have attempted to bring together the religious dimension of prevention with the "secular" medical and social science research.

The public and nonsectarian universities, for instance, appear to separate academic research, both medical and social science, from religious perspectives. Makerere University, for instance, has received multiple grants for the establishment of an Infectious Disease Institute for HIV/AIDS Care, Training, Research and Prevention. Likewise, the Makerere Institute for Social Research has produced reports on HIV/AIDS. There is no indication that religious leaders or religious perspectives have been included in this research.

This is not to say that religious leaders are not active on the Makerere campus. One chaplain commented, "Makerere does not have a policy. That is one reason the chaplaincies got involved." Roman Catholics, Anglicans, and Pentecostals at Makerere have active campus ministries that include preaching, teaching, and administering programs directed to sexual behavior.[5] The Catholic chapel participates in the Youth Alive movement by visiting and speaking to secondary schools. All three main religious groups put a primary emphasis on the "A" and "B" of Uganda's policy: "Abstinence" and "Be Faithful."

Among all universities, public and private, Nkumba University alone has developed a comprehensive HIV/AIDS policy (Nkumba University, 2002). Although the policy includes a section on prevention, which includes "condom education" and "skills on abstinence and general moral education," there seems to be no visible role for religion in this education, and indeed the university is unusual in not having a chaplaincy and in channeling behavioral guidance through the dean of students (p. 31).

The attitude of the Roman Catholic and Anglican universities to instruction is important because of the strength of their constituencies. The Roman Catholic university at UMU Nkozi has no HIV/AIDS policy as such; it relies on general orientation at the beginning of each year. The Vice Chancellor says, "We treat [students] as adults and [expect them] to behave accordingly." It should be noted that this university pioneered 'Ethics and Development Studies' as its main degree. Undoubtedly the Catholic moral tradition is communicated to students through required courses in ethics.

The main Anglican university, UCU Mukono, has been slow to develop official policies. However, since 2002 the chaplaincy at UCU has offered annual retreats at which students have been urged to commit themselves to abstinence before marriage, using the "True Love Waits" response cards. Like its Roman Catholic counterpart, UCU requires a basic course in "Ethics from a Christian Perspective," which explains and commends monogamy and has specific study questions regarding HIV/AIDS. In addition, the senate has approved a required "Personal and Community Health" course to include instruction on HIV/AIDS in the context of an overall wholesome and godly lifestyle. Finally, UCU has proposed to several donors the idea of an "AIDS Officer Training Corps": students who would be trained to offer leadership in their various professions and regions.

Bugema University, as part of the International Seventh Day Adventist Church, describes itself as "an implementing agency of the World Wide Church HIV/AIDS policy." This policy includes both an affirmation of the biblical principle to shun premarital "fornication" and also the commitment to persons living with AIDS "in a non-judgmental way." The university implements this policy through its Counseling Department, its chaplaincies, and its student code, which emphasizes that "there are boundaries beyond which individual male and female students should not pass."

General responses to the role of religion in responding to the HIV/AIDS crisis by most university administrators and faculty members are that it has a role to play in shaping moral character and behavior, but they have not attempted to integrate religion fully in with other medical and social dimensions of the problem. This should not be surprising, since most staff in Uganda are practicing Christians or Muslims, and they hold a generally positive attitude toward religious involvement in university life, as opposed to the "politically correct" hostility to religion found in some Western settings. The following comment from the dean of students at Mbarara University of Science and Technology may be taken as representative:

> I think religion has a positive impact on students' attitudes and behavior with regard to HIV/AIDS. It is difficult to single out a particular religion in our set-up, in terms of effectiveness in helping youth avoid and cope with HIV/AIDS. They all pass on the same message.

CONCLUSION: RELIGIOUS YOUTH PROGRAMS IN CONTEXT

FBO youth programs in Uganda form only one part of a broader multi-sectoral strategy that has made Uganda so successful in the fight against HIV/AIDS (Hogle et al., 2002). Within the education sector, FBOs have been effective in certain areas, but have also demonstrated weaknesses. First of all, given the lessening grip of certain FBOs on their educational institutions, some FBOs may not be as effective at implementing such programs in schools. For example, the low influence of the COU in some of the schools it founded has meant that COU programs in those schools may be ineffective. In fact, the most powerful actor within the primary and secondary education sector has been *Straight Talk*, a newspaper on health issues for youth, which has used creative media techniques to achieve impressive results in youth education.

Secondly, FBOs have delivered messages that have not always been relevant or appropriate. Many youth members of FBOs publicly or privately admit that abstinence is a strategy that is not realistic, even if such messages have led to others delaying sex until marriage (Byamugisha, 1998a). In the case of the Madarasa project, however, leaders made the eventual decision to allow for discussion of responsible use of condoms during activities. In some cases like Youth Alive, where peer education is used most effectively, the message can be based on a discussion between youth and for youth, rather than on lectures from elders about how youth should behave. The vast majority of educational efforts by FBOs on HIV/ AIDS, however, often generate messages that may be less relevant to youth.

Third, FBOs have limited capacities in a number of areas. Although peer education is an effective and inexpensive way to build knowledge and skills among participants, more specialized activities such as counseling and care require increased resources or technical skills that FBOs may lack. Even in areas like peer education, training and other skills needed to be effective peer educators and counselors may be insufficient among many FBOs. Respondents to a study in rural Iganga suggested that lack of trained counselors was a major barrier to effective use of counseling as a tool. Those who had partners who could provide training and technical assistance, however, were able to overcome these limitations to provide effective services. To the extent that FBOs can work together or in collaboration with NGOs to develop capacities for education of youth, they will be able to produce more impressive and creative results than in areas where FBOs are working alone or without such collaboration.

Fourth, most FBOs remain resource-poor and thus require small grants or other nonformal sources of funding to make their HIV/AIDs activities viable on a larger scale. Programs that have worked on a broader scale have usually drawn on international resources, whether they are from FBOs or other government bodies. Youth Alive, for example, has benefited from significant external resources to build their programs. UNICEF funded the Madarasa AIDS Education program of IMAU, which has reached youth in 350 schools. Many FBOs can carry out effective education programs in schools with limited resources, but can also benefit from targeted small grants that boost strategic areas.

Fifth, the quality of the awareness and education that FBOs deliver to youth depends on the FBO's ability to work closely with other stakeholders to ensure that information is up to date, accurate and useful. In many cases FBOs lack the technical knowledge of HIV/AIDS and reproductive health to pass on such material to youth in an effective and relevant manner. Information on availability of ARVs, stigma and technical aspects of the disease usually comes from public health or government officials. To this end, FBOs can strengthen their youth education programs by contracting technical assistance and engaging in such work in collaboration with public health, government and the NGO community.

Finally, it is still unclear or too early to tell to what extent FBOs have been responsible for generating real behavior change in prevention and support among youth. The few evaluations that exist on FBOs' HIV/AIDS programming generate unrealistic numbers on abstinence and faithfulness, but there is evidence to show that age of sexual debut has gone up, and at least some Ugandans are limiting their number of sexual partners or choosing abstinence (Green, 2003; Hogle et al., 2002). To what extent FBOs can be credited for these areas of behavior change needs further study. It is clear that FBOs have made a contribution to HIV/AIDS awareness, in that some people have changed behavior as a result of their efforts. However, continuing to evaluate and monitor how effective FBO programs are in educating youth on prevention and support will establish how this contribution can be expanded.

NOTES

1. The 2002 Census reports 22.7 million, but recent reports in 2004 suggest the population has hit 26 million. The U.S. Department of State (2004) estimates that as of September 15, 2004, approximately 75% of the population is Christian, 15% Muslim, and a variety of other religions, including traditional indigenous religions, Hinduism, and Judaism constitute the remaining 10%.

2. David Barrett (2001) estimates 5 million Pentecostals/Charismatics as of the year 2000, many of whom are baptized Catholics or Anglicans (see p. 162).

3. Missionary numbers are based on report obtained from the U.S. Embassy in Kampala.

4. Much of the data below is derived from a questionnaire submitted to vice chancellors of all public and licenced private universities in April 2004. Responses were received from Mbarara University of Science and Technology, Kyambogo University, Uganda Martryrs University (Nkozi), Uganda Christian University (Mukono), Nkumba University, Bugema University, Busoga University, and Aga Khan University. The following questions were asked: (1) Does your institution have an HIV/AIDS policy? What role does religion play in that policy? (Please include policy if possible.) (2) Do your dean of students, chaplain, or other officers give religious advice to students about sexual behavior and its relationship with HIV/AIDS? What impact do official persons have on student attitudes? (3) On balance, do you think religion has a positive, a negative, or a neutral impact on students' attitudes and behavior with regard to HIV/AIDS. Do you think one particular religion or tradition (Anglican, Catholic, Pentecostal, Muslim, Hindu, other) is most effective in helping youth avoid and cope with HIV/AIDS? How so?

5. Data was gathered from the Rev. Dr. Lawrence Kanyike of St. Augustine's Chapel (RC) and the Rev. Stephen Galenga of St. Francis Chapel (Anglican). The Rev. Martin Sempa, Pastor of Makerere Community Church, is also known as a strong advocate of abstinence to Makerere students.

REFERENCES

Amuyunzu-Nyamongo, M., Tendo-Wambua, L., Babishangire, B., Nyagero, J., Yit-barek, N., Mataha, M., et al. (1999). Barriers to behaviour change as a response to STD including HIV/AIDS: The East African experience. In J. Caldwell, P., Caldwell, J., Anarfi, K., Awusabo-Asare, J., Ntozi, I. Orubuloye, J., Marck, W., Cosford, R. Colombo, & E. Hollings. (Eds.), *Resistances to behavioral change to reduce HIV/AIDS infection in predominantly heterosexual epidemics in Third World countries* (pp. 1–11). Canberra, Australia: Health Transition Centre: National Centre for Epidemiology and Populations Health, Australian National University.

Anane, M. (1999). The soul is willing: Religion, men and HIV/AIDS in Ghana. In M. Foreman (Ed.), *AIDS and men: Taking risks of taking responsibility?* London: Zed Books.

Awusabo-Asare, K. (1999a). All die be die: Obstacles to change in the face of HIV infection. In J. Caldwell, P. Caldwell, J. Anarfi, K. Awusabo-Asare, J. Ntozi, I. Orubuloye, J. Marck, W. Cosford, R. Colombo, & E. Hollings (Eds.), *Resistance to behavioral change to reduce HIV/AIDS infection in predominantly heterosexual epidemics in Third World Countries* (pp. 125–132). Canberra, Australia: Health Transition Centre: National Centre for Epidemiology and Populations Health, Australian National University.

Awusabo-Asare, K. (1999b). Obstacles and challenges to sexual behavior change. In J. Caldwell, P. Caldwell, J. Anarfi, K. Awusabo-Asare, J. Ntozi, I. Orubuloye, J. Marck, W. Cosford, R. Colombo, & E. Hollings (Eds.), *Resistances to behavioral change to reduce HIV/AIDS infection in predominantly heterosexual epidemics in Third World Countries* (pp. 235–240). Canberra, Australia: Health Transition Centre: National Centre for Epidemiology and Populations Health, Australian National University.

Barrett, D. (2001). *World Christian encyclopedia: A comparative survey of churches and religions in the modern world* (2nd ed., Vol. 1). Oxford, England: Oxford University Press.

Baylies, C., Burja, J., Chabala, T., Kaihula, N., Liatto-Katundu, B., Lutimba, J., et al. (1999). Rebels at risk: Young women and the shadow of AIDS in Africa. In C. Becker, J.-P. Dozon, C. Obbo, & M. Toure (Eds.), *Experiencing and understanding AIDS in Africa* (pp. 319–341). Paris: Codesria, IRD, Karthala.

Bond, G., & Vincent, J. (1991). Living on the edge: Changing social structures in the context of AIDS. In H. B. Hansen & M. Twaddle (Eds.), *Changing Uganda* (pp. 113–129). Athens, OH: Ohio University Press.

Byamugisha, R. G. (1998a). AIDS, the condom and the church. In ecumenical association of Third World Theologians-Uganda Chapter (Ed.), *The theological and pastoral implications of AIDS to Uganda series*. Kampala, Uganda: Tricolour Designers and Printers.

Byamugisha, R. G. (Ed). (1998b). Am I my brother's keeper? Reflections on Genesis 4:9. In *Ecumenical association of Third World Theologians-Uganda: The theological and pastoral implications of AIDS to Uganda series* (Vol. 2). Kampala, Uganda: Tricolour Designers and Printers.

Diocese of Namirembe. (1999). The caring church: Integrating reproductive health, HIV/AIDS and general health care concerns into community worship, liturgy and spirituality. Kampala, Uganda: Author.

Garner, R. C. (2000). Safe sects? Dynamic religion and AIDS in South Africa. *The Journal of Modern African Studies, 38*(1), 41–69.

Green, E. (2003). *Faith-based organizations: Contributions to HIV prevention.* Washington, DC: USAID.

Gregson, S., Zhuwau, T., Anderson, R. M., & Chandwana, S. K. (1999). Apostles and Zionists: The influence of religion on demographic change in rural Zimbabwe. *Population Studies, 53*(2), 179–193.

Hogle, J., Green, E. C., Nantulya, V., Stoneburner, R., & Stover, J. (2002). *What happened in Uganda? Declining HIV prevalence, behavior change, and the national response.* Washington, DC: USAID.

Islamic Medical Association of Uganda. (1998). *AIDS education through imams: A spiritually motivated community effort in Uganda.* Geneva, Switzerland: UNAIDS.

Kagimu, M., Marum, E., & Serwadda, D. (1995). Planning and evaluating strategies for AIDS health education interventions in the Muslim community in Uganda. *AIDS Education and Prevention, 7,* 10–21.

Kagimu, M., Marum, E., Wabwire-Mangen, F., Nakyanjo, N., Walakira, Y., & Hogle, J. (1998). Evaluation of the effectiveness of AIDS health education interventions in the Muslim community in Uganda. *AIDS Education and Prevention, 10*(3), 215–228.

Kasozi, A. B. K. (2003). *University education in Uganda: Challenges and opportunities for reform.* Kampala, Uganda: Fountain.

Liebowitz, J. (2002). *The impact of faith-based organizations on HIV/AIDS prevention and mitigation in Africa.* Paper presented at the Health Economics and HIV/AIDS Research Division, University of KwaZulu-Natal.

Mitchell, K., Nakamanya, S., Kamali, A., & Whitworth, J. (2002). Exploring the community response to a randomized controlled HIV/AIDS intervention trial in rural Uganda. *AIDS Education and Prevention, 14*(3), 207–216.

Muhangi, D. (2004). *Documentation study of the responses by religious organizations to orphans and vulnerable children: Uganda country study report.* Kampala, Uganda: UNICEF/World Conference on Religious for Peace, Inter-Religious Council of Uganda.

Negerie, M. (1994). *The association of religious beliefs with AIDS risk behavior among Kenyan males.* Unpublished doctoral dissertation, Loma Linda University, Loma Linda, California.

Nkumba University. (2002). *Nkumba university HIV/AIDS Policy.* Kampala, Uganda: Author.

Preston-Whyte, E. (1999). Reproductive health and the condom dilemma: Identifying situational barriers to HIV protection in South Africa. In J. Caldwell, P. Caldwell, J. Anarfi, K. Awusabo-Asare, J. Ntozi, I. Orubuloye, J. Marck, W. Cosford, R. Colombo, & E. Hollings (Eds.), *Resistance to behavioral change to reduce HIV/AIDS infection in predominantly heterosexual epidemics in Third World countries* (pp. 139–155). Canberra, Australia: Health Transition Centre: National Centre for Epidemiology and Populations Health, Australian National University.

Scottish Catholic International Aid Fund. (1996). *Project Uganda: The Project-Kam-woyka/Youth Alive*. Glasgow: Scottish Catholic International Aid Fund.

Spira, R., Lagarde, E., Bouyer, J., Seck, K., Enel, C., Kane, N. T., Piau, J.-P., Ndoye, I., Mboup, S., & Pison, G. (2000). Preventive attitudes towards the threat of AIDS: Process and determinants in Senegal. *AIDS Education and Prevention, 12*(6), 544–556.

Uganda AIDS Commission/UNICEF. (2003). *The district response initiative on HIV/ AIDS action research: A synthesis report*. Kampala, Uganda: UNICEF.

U.S. Department of State. (2004). *Uganda: International religious freedom report 2004*. Washington, DC: Bureau of Democracy, Human Rights, and Labor.

Varga, C. (1999). South African young people's sexual dynamics: Implications for behavioral responses to HIV/AIDS. In J. Caldwell, P. Caldwell, J. Anarfi, K. Awusabo-Asare, J. Ntozi, I. Orubuloye, J. Marck, W. Cosford, R. Colombo, & E. Hollings (Eds.), *Resistance to behavioral change to reduce HIV/AIDS infection in predominantly heterosexual epidemics in Third World countries* (pp. 13–34). Canberra, Australia: Health Transition Centre: National Centre for Epidemiology and Populations Health, Australian National University.

CHAPTER 12

THE FAMILY, YOUTH, AND AIDS

Hope and Heartbreak for Africa[1]

Terrance D. Olson and Richard G. Wilkins

INTRODUCTION

A recent cover story in *Time Magazine* on AIDS in Africa asserted that
nothing less than changing the sexual practices of the entire continent
would avert disaster (McGeary, 2001). Unfortunately the collective
efforts of the international community generally have not been effective in making widespread alterations in sexual behavior. The reasons
for this failure are many. But perhaps the most neglected avenue of
intervention is the system of values and beliefs underlying current sexual practices. Without addressing (and changing) the beliefs and values,
there may be little hope indeed for averting disaster—not only in
Africa—but around the world.

The direct causes of AIDS can be reduced to five factors: sexual practices, illegal drug use, childbirth, nursing by infected mothers, and certain medical treatments gone awry (such as blood transfusions using HIV-
infected blood). The two overwhelmingly predominant factors in the

Overcoming AIDS: Lesson Learned from Uganda, 225–248
Copyright © 2006 by Information Age Publishing

spread of the infection—sexual practices and illegal drug use—are the result of voluntary behavior. And no physical consequences from voluntary behavior are more deadly than those related to AIDS.

IDEOLOGY IN PREVENTION

Long before AIDS became an issue of international concern and the hallmark of personal suffering for so many, Kurt Back, of Duke University, observed that prevention efforts that target problems related to human sexuality are essentially based on ideology. As a result, prevention efforts are not merely objective or scientific responses to a problem—they are ideological responses. Back was addressing adolescent pregnancy prevention in the United States, but his conclusion is valid for prevention efforts generally:

> The problem we are dealing with is the result of two components: increased sexual activity and insufficient contraception. Each of these factors can be analyzed in more detail, for instance, what is "insufficient," and from whose point of view? But keeping only these major factors in mind we are struck by the preponderance of research and application on the second factor—the use of contraceptives, to the virtual exclusion of the first, the increase of teenage, non-marital intercourse. Basic to this choice is [the adoption of] an underlying model of human nature. (Back, 1983, p. 2)

Accordingly, social responses are based, first on an ideology about human nature which then dictates the approaches that are considered realistic and practical. Back's observations were contemporary with a new direction in prevention efforts inaugurated by the U.S. Congress, grounded in a philosophy of sexual abstinence for the unmarried (Adolescent Family Life Act, Title XX, 1981).

Regarding AIDS and sexual behavior, the generally accepted ideology is that sexual involvement with multiple partners is inevitable, so the most legitimate prevention efforts are those which seek to change the conditions under which sexual involvement takes place. This response generally excludes as unrealistic attempts to reduce promiscuous sexual involvement, promote fidelity in marriage, or encourage abstinence in the young, unmarried generation. Ironically, the fidelity-abstinence approaches are often criticized as unrealistic precisely because they are ideological (rather than scientific), while the interventions that are promoted (such as mandatory condom use or "education") are falsely assumed to be free of ideology. In fact, there is no ideology-free intervention.

Cultural Ideologies

We propose that the reason attempts to combat AIDS are almost universally failing is that few programs address the values, beliefs, and philosophies that surround sexual practices. It is unclear whether philosophies that facilitate the spread of AIDS can be altered, yet it is imperative that risky AIDS-promoting human behavior must change. But changing behavior requires a fundamental change in values and beliefs—not mere distribution of knowledge. Why? Because belief systems—especially cultural belief systems—are the most robust predictor of actual behavior. Studies show that belief systems are more accurate predictors of behavior than knowledge—and this is particularly true regarding sexual behavior.

For example, in a sample of 10,000 15-year-old females in the United States, Hanson, Myers, and Ginsburg (1987), found that knowledge of human sexuality and birth control practices had "no effect on the chances that a black or White female will experience an out-of-wedlock birth as a teenager. However, when adolescents and their parents hold values that stress responsibility, the adolescents' chances of experiencing an out-of-wedlock childbirth are significantly reduced" (p. 241). In a demographic review of adolescent sexual behavior, Santelli, Lowry, Brener, and Robin (2000) speculate that "factors that are relatively pervasive in the culture may have more influence on adolescent sexual behaviors" (p. 1586) than socioeconomic status (SES) or other background factors. However, family structure—notably, reported residence in a two-parent family (among Whites)—was associated with significantly lower levels of sexual involvement. Although more than 73% of males and females in this sample were from two parent families, the percent of adolescents reporting ever having sexual intercourse was 45% for males and 41% for females. To go deeper than family structure to determine the interior life of adolescents in families would help tease out more specific family-related predictors of adolescent sexual behavior. A more sophisticated study should include assessments of individual values and beliefs and the content of parent-child conversations about sexuality. At the least, unless knowledge and information regarding sexual behaviors are linked to beliefs and values—to a philosophy relevant to the knowledge—providing knowledge and information alone is a very weak intervention tool. Moreover, instead of using intervention efforts which typically cut adolescents off from parental influence and consider parents intruders on the "autonomy" of a child, that very kind of parental influence should be encouraged. Discussions of values and beliefs do seem to enhance student responsiveness to prevention efforts, be they focused on abstinence or on condom use.

Abstinence programs vary in quality and effect, as do condom-use programs. For an example of the latter approach, Miller and Olson (1998) found increased condom use by adolescent females who reported they had discussed condom use with their mothers. However, as is typically the case in studies seeking to increase condom use, success never includes 100% of the sample using condoms 100% of the time. In terms of practical significance, and when AIDS (as well as a host of STDs) is the possible consequence, the statistical significance is not necessarily heartwarming. Abstinence programs do not reach 100% of the target audience either. Nevertheless, addressing cultural factors, including family structure and quality of interaction, and specific cultural or familial or peer group beliefs is a promising intervention possibility, especially given some data from Africa. (For studies that address beliefs as related to, or as an intervention strategy, see Hanson et al., 1987; Miller & Olson, 1988; Olson Wallace, & Miller, 1984).

Being Realistic

Some research in the United States suggests that the most effective interventions regarding sexual behavior are those typically defined as comprehensive sex education, where instruction in disease prevention and birth control techniques are linked with information on abstinence (Kirby, 2001). Currently, some professionals and some parents seem divided over whether to "mix the messages" of abstinence with that of condom use, since the philosophical starting points of the two strategies are in conflict. To promote condoms as a pragmatic response to the reality of adolescent sexual involvement seems legitimate, given what is at stake regarding the future health and social-emotional well-being of adolescents. Whatever the relative impact of a given abstinence program or a specific comprehensive sex education intervention, the sobering reality is that no intervention is successful with everyone. Even in studies that show a statistical increase in condom use, for example, the impact on STDs is not as great as hoped. (See DiClemente et al., 2004). Pedlow and Carey (2003), in a critique of HIV sexual risk-reduction programs, note numerous methodological flaws in studies, with the most practical problem being a lack of sustained findings over time.

An example of this problem is the admirable AIDS prevention program from Stanton, Ricardo, Galbraith, Feigelman, and Kaljee (1996). African American youth in the United Stages (ages 9–15) were randomly assigned to experimental and control groups. At baseline, 36% of the total sample was sexually experienced. At the 12 month follow-up, 49% of the sample was sexually active. The study showed an increase in condom use by the experimental group versus the control group (85%–57%) at the 6 month follow-up. However, by the 12 month follow-up, among sexually active youth in both groups, there was no significant difference in condom use. Moreover, in a practice that would be devastating in Africa, assume that the experimental group, at the height of the success period of the intervention, reported using condoms 60% of the time, while the control group reported such use only 40% of the time. How successful are we going to be in Africa if we simply settle for people being at risk for AIDS 4 of 10 times instead of 6 of 10 times? Stanton et al. do not report what percentage of experimental or control group youth initiated sexual intercourse in the course of the study. They do make this general observation summarizing a common problem in AIDS intervention in the United States:

> Among other populations there is accumulating evidence that, in the absence of sustained intervention (or boosters), newly acquired protective behaviors may rapidly revert to baseline. Therefore, once they have demonstrated that under certain conditions behavioral interventions can alter certain high risk practices, researchers must begin to assess the sustainability of intervention effect. (p. 363)

This problem could be due to the preference for interventions that focus on changing a single aspect of sexual behavior (such as condom use) without addressing or confronting beliefs and values that foster, promote or, at the least, permit approaches to human sexual behavior that assist and support youth in deciding whether to engage in sexual activities in the first place. Numerous intervention studies, moreover, are single-minded in the assumption that condom use is the only measurable and realistic goal, and the option to attend to or take seriously the abstinence option is foreign to the philosophical and theoretical design of the studies themselves.

The results of various studies reveal a wide range of effectiveness, variables measured, and degree of success. For example, in a controlled trial similar to that of the Stanton group, DiClemente et al. (2004) found consistent condom use and even a slight reduction in number of sexual partners in a randomized sample of African American youth in the United States, even at the 12 month follow-up measure. The prime focus of the study was on reducing HIV risk-taking *behaviors*. Quite importantly, however, in spite of the success of increased condom use, actual rates of infection of HIV or various STDs evidently were not statistically significant between the treatment and control groups.

In these experimental designs the decision regarding what to measure often does not include serious consideration of the ultimate objective animating the interventions themselves: a statistically and practically significant reduction in actual pregnancy and disease rates, with the virtual extermination of AIDS being a prime goal. Also, measurement issues and the perceived need for practical intervention strategies may explain why many randomized trials neither take abstinence seriously nor parental involvement as necessary or possible. Consideration of abstinence and parental involvement interventions are called for by the National Coalition to Prevent Teen Pregnancy (Kirby, 2001), but not all researchers in the health field have picked up that challenge. Parental influence seems to be a positive factor whenever it is included in a well-designed study (Hanson, Myers, & Ginsburg, 1987; Jacard & Dittis, 1991; Stanton et al., 2004). In any event, thus far, it seems that short-term behavioral programs seem to produce only short-term results and that the long-term results necessary to affect the AIDS pandemic may require long-term programs.

Practical experience, as well as documented research, shows the inadequacy of sexual education and condom distribution programs to halt the AIDS crisis. Even if "graphic demonstrations" of condom use are given, studies have shown that the pregnancy and sexual activity rates among youth continue to increase (Kirby, Waszak, & Ziegler, 1989 as quoted in Hartigan, 1997). As a result, efforts to reduce AIDS infection rates through intensive counseling and condom use have proved almost uniformly unsuccessful, even when the persons being counseled are adult females who are very strongly motivated to avoid pregnancy. In one study, 404 uninfected adult European women with HIV positive partners received intensive counseling. But despite the training—and the high motivation to use condoms to avoid infection from their partners—only 49 of these women used condoms all or most of the time. And of these 49, 6 still became infected (see summary in Hartigan, 1997). Moreover, during AIDS projects in Thailand, studies of young men showed 1.04 new cases of HIV per 100 people not visiting sex workers, and 3.47 cases per 100 people among those visiting sex workers—even though the men visiting sex workers *always* used condoms (UNAIDS/WHO, 2000). This outcome sustains the argument from, among others, Richins, Imrie, and Weiss (2003) that structural or contextual factors must be addressed (not just information regarding condoms) which can affect sexual behavior in ways that actually reduce infection rates. Accordingly, the epidemic of AIDS in Africa presents a moral—not just an educational or an informational—crisis. It is a crisis related to citizenship and responsibility and to living by philosophies and beliefs regarding human sexuality that are nondestructive to present and future generations.

This point is conclusively illustrated by a well-designed study in the United States by Polit and Kahn (1985) which placed disadvantaged pregnant teens in two separate groups. One group was nurtured in contraceptive practices, the other was not. When participants were interviewed 12 months into the program, the repeat pregnancy rate of the contraceptive-educated group was significantly lower than that of the comparison group (14 pregnancies compared to 22). But at 24 months, 1 year after the end of the educational program, the repeat pregnancy rate of the contraceptive educated group had regressed to that of the comparison group, and rates of contraceptive use by the two groups was virtually the same (p. 152). Unfortunately, results of numerous condom advocacy programs show, generally, not only that greater numbers of adolescents participate sexually when such programs are in place in U.S. schools, but that virtually no population of the sexually active adolescents in those programs use condoms 100% of the time (see Kirby et al., 1989, 1991 as quoted in Hartigan).

The African Condition

The social and contextual factors related to sexual relationships in Africa are formidable. If, as has been noted by many, Africa's unique explosion of AIDS among generally innocent women and children is due to cultural and social practices, a quick and ready solution to the problem seems unlikely. When one studies the means of infection in African nations, a recurring theme is the vulnerability of women to the advances of men. These vulnerabilities include young girls being subject to the intimidations and invitations of teachers (McGeary, 2001; U.S. Congressional Research Service, 2000). The vulnerability of women is also increased by sexually promiscuous husbands, who also refuse to use condoms for various reasons related to cultural attitudes, habits and practices. If these practices continue to be as unresponsive to education or behavioral programs as they have been so far, the future for the next generation in Africa is grim indeed.

Caldwell (2000), in describing factors in Africa related to the general failure to curb the spread of AIDS, echoes the view that merely providing knowledge will not stem the crisis when the real issue is changing behavior. Caldwell notes that cultural beliefs about sexual practices are so pervasive that behavioral approaches, such as encouraging condom use, have failed. These cultural beliefs include attitudes against the use of condoms, expectation of sexual promiscuity by men, emphasis on fertility as a defense against a high mortality rate, prevalence of polygyny, employment of husbands in distant locations, and beliefs about predestination and death. Thus cultural beliefs—and the practices which spring from them—seem to be more fundamental than behavioral approaches which seek to change behavior based on knowledge alone. Caldwell even notes that educational programs, though "successful" in providing knowledge, fail because the cultural beliefs about sexuality undermine the "facts" presented.

Generally, beliefs—cultural and personal—are the greatest help or the greatest hindrance to solving social problems, even those as devastating as the spread of AIDS. Studies have shown that behavioral approaches that are not closely tied to stable and deeply held belief systems have little chance of success. For example, in a study from Thailand, Hanenberg, Rojanapithayakorn, Kunasol, and Sokal (1994, as cited in Caldwell, 2000) noted that, when commercial sexual establishments were forced by the government to require condom use, levels of STDs "fell steeply among prostitutes, and HIV prevalence among army recruits declined by two-thirds" (p. 119). But this success depended on close governmental monitoring. According to the UNAIDS/WHO *Epidemiological Fact Sheet–2000 Update* for Thailand, the percentage of AIDS infection for sex workers from 1991–1997 was, consecutively, 7.4%, 17.82%, 8.59%, 13%, 9.61%, 6.89%, 13.02%. This is a disheartening fluctuation. It indicates that a program that was supposedly successful with a relatively small target group was successful only temporarily. Furthermore, the current data demonstrate that the study's limited "success" is not likely to reach the total population, even if the government could successfully expand the aggressive monitoring procedures it applied to visible and targeted sexual establishments.

These conclusions are sustained by Richens, Imrie, and Copas (2000), who point out that condom distribution is often related to an *increase* in nonmarital sexual behavior and, thus, to a greater percentage of the population being at risk when condoms fail or are not used. This prediction, of course, does not include the spread of less lethal STDs that are not restrained by condom use.

In the African context we do not have the luxury of reducing sexual promiscuity a little bit, or increasing condom use 10–20% points. True, any improvement in those factors is better than nothing. But when the whole population is at risk, and when orphans are multiplying as parents are dying, solutions must be bold and multifaceted, and new (or revisited old) philosophies of intervention must be given a place. This includes direct challenges of beliefs and values that sustain sexual practices that are destructive of the participants, and ultimately, of the next generation. The approach of Uganda is unique and challenged by many, but seems to be an approach worth consideration. There may be cultural and contextual reasons for hope.

TRANSFORMING IDEOLOGIES IN CULTURES AND INTERVENTION EFFORTS

The above studies may be prototypical of what happens when the AIDS epidemic is addressed only by behavioral programs. We will not change at-risk practices by knowledge alone. And we will not reach a substantial portion of the most at-risk populations if the targeted changes in behavioral practices are not linked to a transformation of the fundamental beliefs and values related to sexual behavior. Moreover, the striking success of AIDS prevention efforts in Uganda invites a rethinking of the "received view" of what our starting points for prevention really could be (Green, 2003a, 2003b; Stoneburner & Low-Beer, 2004).

The unprecedented and unique decrease of HIV/AIDS in Uganda is likely due to a multiplicity of factors that address—directly and boldly—the idea that behavior change is linked to philosophical and cultural values. The program fostered by President and Mrs. Museveni of Uganda has been labeled the ABC approach. The sequence of the letters is deliberate and is proving to be consequential. *Abstinence* is the first message—presented unequivocally. *Be faithful*, the second component of the program, appears to be the source of a dramatic decrease in number of those engaging in sex with multiple partners. The third and apparently the least significant contributing factor in Uganda to the decrease in HIV/AIDS is *condom* use (Green, 2003b, Stoneburner & Low-Beer, 2004). According to Stoneburner & Low-Beer's research, between 1989 and 1995 in Uganda, there was a 60% reduction in persons reporting casual sexual partnerships in both rural and urban populations. Declines in casual sex among those 15–24 years of age were unique to Uganda, as compared to the neighboring countries of Malawi, Zambia and Kenya. In urban Kampala, Uganda, "HIV declined most in younger age groups, . . . with declines of 75% in 15 to 19 year olds and 60% in 20 to 24 year olds" (p. 715). The authors note that condom use was roughly the same in Uganda as in neighboring countries that did not experience a decline in infections during the same period. They note:

> Only sexual abstinence in males distinguishes Uganda from comparison countries. These findings suggest that reduction in sexual partners and abstinence among unmarried sexually inexperienced youth (particularly in urban areas and in males), rather than condom use, are the relevant factors in reducing HIV incidence. A reduction of casual sex across the whole population, not in a particular segment or age group or only in those exposed to a specific intervention, reduced the size of high-risk sexual networks and the efficiency of HIV transmission. (p. 715)

This population-wide increase in risk-avoidance behavior is extraordinary. How has Uganda achieved such an outcome? It is likely that intervention programs that stress abstinence and fidelity as the *primary* approaches to prevention are not operating in a cultural vacuum. A country-wide network of communication discusses how deadly AIDS is, converses about the behaviors that increase risks, and stresses the importance of abandoning promiscuity (by adopting a practice described as "zero grazing"—the goat stays tethered close to home). These efforts, with the support of the President and First Lady of Uganda, have achieved what had seemed impossible in previous AIDS prevention efforts. In the opinion of Ugandan President Yoweri Museveni, these efforts are also consistent with long-standing cultural taboos against premarital sex and sex out of wedlock that began eroding in the 1940s in Uganda. He notes that AIDS is not merely a biological disease, but progresses in a social contexts which either promote or retard the behaviors that place people at risk. President Museveni notes,

> The sexual opportunities available to an individual and the type of partners deemed appropriate will vary from one social group to another. It is in view of this background that I have been emphasizing a return to our time-tested cultural practices which emphasised fidelity and condemned premarital and extramarital sex. I believe that the best response to the threat of AIDS and other STDs is to reaffirm publicly and forthrightly the respect and responsibility every person owes to his or her neighbour. Just as we were offered the "magic bullet" in the early 1940s, we are now being offered the condom for "safe sex." . . . I feel that condoms have a role to play as a means of protection, especially in couples who are HIV-positive, but they cannot become the main means of stemming the tide of AIDS. (Museveni, 1992, pp. 273–274)

What makes the abstinence efforts in Uganda of practical significance may be the sociological context in which the abstinence message is presented. When the voices at the top are making abstinence the first priority (The A in the ABC approach), and being faithful the second priority, the legitimacy of the idea is affirmed by powerful cultural forces and becomes a central feature of the AIDS prevention dialogue. When, on the other hand, the idea of abstinence is seen as a contextual afterthought, and is not treated as a genuine possibility by commentators and experts alike, there is little reason for the general population to consider abstinence a realistic possibility. When we assume that premarital and promiscuous sexual involvement is inevitable or unavoidable, then condom use becomes the prevention strategy of choice, and abstinence philosophies are merely an add-on for that miniscule portion of the population willing to so live. The call to action made by Back (1983) 25 years ago (which involved both reducing sexual involvement and increasing contraception) seems finally to have been addressed in one culture in the continent that is most at risk for AIDS. That a systematic, culture-wide philosophy is taking hold suggests both that abstinence and fidelity efforts are empirically defensible and that individual prevention programs must be philosophically supported in the wider culture if they are to be taken seriously. Jim Shelton, in commenting on the success in Uganda, notes,

> What happened in Uganda . . . is that a lot of forces at one time were promoting more responsible sexual behavior, so you get to a social norm, a tipping point kind of thing. At some point all these messages, plus seeing people dying, get people to change their sexual behavior . . . . And I guess this has reinforced and awakened us to the virtue of emphasizing more the A and B in the ABC strategy. (Allen, 2002, pp. 14–15)

The foregoing conclusion is grounded in an often-overlooked reality: (1) the cultural values and beliefs that contribute to the spread of AIDS are fundamental components of the AIDS crisis itself, and (2) behavioral monitoring programs, in the long term, cannot counter the influence of those cultural values and beliefs. As a result, when a problem has become culture wide, and when cultural beliefs accelerate rather than inhibit the problem, no solution is likely. Accordingly, interventions based on merely changing behavior or requiring government coercion will inevitably fail. In short, the common ideologies of purportedly "scientific" interventions—which limit their focus to providing knowledge and offering behavioral interventions and government control or monitoring—are inadequate for the comprehensive prevention philosophies and practices needed. To continue in a path of intervention that ignores cultural values and beliefs will be like trying to overtake a cheetah in the bush with an elephant. The next generation will be lost, in large part, because by focusing our intervention efforts on knowledge or behavioral change alone we will have failed to take seriously (or be realistic about) the fact that beliefs predict (and govern) behavior better than either knowledge or external behavioral controls. The success in Uganda seems to be grounded in cultural change encouraged "from the top" and into which abstinence and fidelity programs naturally work to enhance results.

It is time, therefore, for the world community to consider more seriously an alternative intervention ideology—just as empirically valid as the so-far minimally successful behavioral approaches. This intervention ideology would emphasize sexual chastity prior to marriage and sexual fidelity within marriage. In making this proposal, we are not so naive as to believe that such an approach will halt the AIDS crisis overnight. But such an approach offers hope for certain target populations who are most likely to adopt beliefs which protect the rising generation. To succeed with *some* populations is essential for the economic and cultural survival of the infected countries of Africa (and the world).

Incidentally, typical responses to any call for abstinence education as a potentially effective weapon in the war on AIDS and STDs argue that such an approach is unrealistic (humans are sexual beings and will participate), it is ideological (and thus is imposing values), and positive research results are scanty (Green, 2003b; Kirby, 2001; Kristof, 2003; SIECUS, 1999). These points are typically invoked to indicate that, while AIDS prevention efforts should include the abstinence option, it must be only one tool in the content of the curriculum, since many youth and adults are not going to abide by the abstinence doctrine. These responses neglect the reality that *all* AIDS prevention efforts are falling short (Kirby, 1985) and thus are as unrealistic as current portrayals of abstinence efforts. Within the philosophical position that to address values is to impose them, *all* AIDS education efforts are ideological and are "imposing values." It is imposing values to suggest that a man not be coercive with a woman. It is imposing values to suggest that people should care about the consequences of their sexual behavior for both themselves and others. It is imposing a philosophy of sexuality to assume that "everyone is going to have sex" irrespective of age, context, or marital status. What should be fundamental to all AIDS prevention efforts is a stark, open admission that such efforts will fail without a change in the values that currently promote those behaviors that place participants at high risk for AIDS. It is not enough to make progress. It is not enough to achieve a percentage change in a behavioral measure, such as condom use, that has no established track record over time in reducing HIV transmission rates. Regarding AIDS, STDs, and so forth, one instance of risky behavior is enough to change an abstract risk into a deadly and miserable reality.

One of the first scientists to document the extensive success of the ABC approach in Uganda was concerned that the "received view" of the success was often touted in the AIDS-prevention scientific community as being increased condom use. The data, however, show no difference in condom use between Ugandans and residents of neighboring countries that have not come close to the success in Uganda. Importantly, the studies do show dramatic increases in the percentage of those reporting abstinence (especially in younger age groups) and strong decreases in reported casual sex. It is also important to note that the significant declines in HIV/AIDS in Uganda began before condoms were widely available (Green, 2003b). In his discussion, Green calls the ABC approach to AIDS prevention atypical both in philosophy and in success rates. Green declares:

> One would expect that those involved in international AIDS prevention would become very interested in . . . the Uganda model of how to promote

this [the emphasis on abstinence and fidelity]. Yet this has not happened, at least prior to 2003. For one thing, there has been little acceptance of the version of events as I have laid them out. The dominant view, at least until recently, is that condoms deserve the credit. (p. 216)

How can the neglect of the empirical reality of the Uganda model be explained? Perhaps because typical prevention efforts are guided by a presumption that precedes the development and implementation of sex education and AIDS prevention programs. This presumption is philosophical, and rarely made explicit; it is at least logically linked to the typical efforts of the current prevention industry. If, for example, it is presumed that sexual access, from a young age through adulthood, is not only inevitable, but practically and morally legitimate—not tied to contexts of commitment, permanence and fidelity—then it is understandable that efforts that promote the context of abstinence prior to marriage and fidelity afterwards are seen as unrealistic. It may look as if the United States has also embraced the ABC approach so successful in Uganda. But the U.S. model is probably more like C, then perhaps B and occasionally A. That is, instead of making abstinence the prime call of the culture, the United States seems to have deferred to the "practical reality" that teenagers are going to have sex. Hence, we must start with the C. In Africa, sexual participation and extensive promiscuity *is* the reality and in Uganda, at least, the abstinent message seems to be realistic. Perhaps this message has been effective, in part, because the leaders of the country have been unequivocal in presenting, promoting and teaching the program.

Some opponents of "abstinence only" programs have dismissed them as fostering "guilt and shame" (Haffner, 1997; Whitehead, 1994). Although some curricula may make the pedagogical and moral mistake of demeaning young sexual participants, it is neither typical nor necessary to do so. Programs that recommend abstinence should (and usually do) deliver their message with as much compassion, understanding and encouragement as claimed by those programs that earnestly plead with youth to use condoms. The issues of guilt and shame are not necessary, inevitable nor endemic to abstinence programs.

Nevertheless, to many the proposal regarding premarital abstinence and marital fidelity may seem like Don Quixote tilting at a windmill. To be truly effective, such efforts require not only a shift in individual beliefs about human sexuality, but often a transformation of the beliefs of an entire culture. Given that behavioral approaches have failed, given that providing knowledge and even practice in contraceptive use has proven less effective than desired (and sometimes claimed), and given the life or death stakes confronting anyone serious about preserving the health and well-being of the next generation, being bold and direct about transforming philosophies and beliefs that promote destructive consequences to those that prevent those consequences is necessary to succeed in the battle against AIDS. It is absolutely essential that the context of beliefs regarding human sexuality be transformed in Africa.

Moreover, even if the starting points we propose are unrealistic or ineffective, then in the absence of some medical breakthrough, everyone should be honest enough to admit, regardless of ideology and in spite of possibly divergent views of the available social science, that there may not be any practical, realistic solution to the HIV/AIDS problem when it is as extensive and destructive as it is in portions of Africa. We can not continue to reduce prevention efforts to political battles which are merely conflicts of ideologies, while the people we wish to help, including the next generation, are sick and dying.

The legitimacy of a values-based intervention program is based in the research which shows the powerful link between people's beliefs, values, and commitments—and their behavior. This research shows that, although behavioral approaches rarely change underlying beliefs, a change in values and beliefs *can and does* change behavior. We recognize that, while it may be unlikely that a whole culture will respond to abstinence and fidelity efforts, it is also less than likely that a whole culture will respond to government coercion promoting condom use. President and Mrs. Museveni were willing to be bold about the fundamentals governing the survival of their culture. Those who *do* respond and who *do* change their beliefs are likely to be those who will preserve the culture and give the next generation—or the generation after that—the chance to be free of AIDS.

The two major causes for the spread of AIDS—sexual practices and drug use—involve voluntary behaviors. We must, therefore, transform cultural beliefs regarding these voluntary behaviors, and the invited transformations must be grounded in love and compassion, not in coercion, lest the results be temporary. Also, the restored values must include a commitment to the well-being of the young. Cultures that last are built on values and belief systems that foster and protect children—especially from sexual or drug-related predation.

STUMBLING BLOCKS TO SUCCESS

The least likely populations to respond to the efforts we propose are those who are self-centered and narcissistic and who, though knowledgeable, ignore the risk to which their behavior places themselves and others, especially those they claim to love. The invitation to transform values and beliefs in order to preserve others will, of course, include offering knowledge. But the knowledge offered will be exact and pointed: All those who are at risk for AIDS, educated and uneducated, will be offered a moral call to act on behalf of the next generation. In brief, we are suggesting that a beginning, low level but recurring message of AIDS obliteration efforts be "If you choose not to be sexually faithful for yourself, do it for them." A higher level philosophy is "Choose to live in support of your own and others' *best* interests—not your self-interests."

These are admittedly moral messages, because they focus on the quality of life people set in motion by their own choices. But the moral content of this approach does not, as some may claim, distinguish it from (presently) more widely promoted behavioral methods. Those who have accepted the philosophical belief that behavioral practice (not sexual access) is the problem are also fostering their moral version of "best interests," with the focus generally being the best interests of the individual. Our proposal focuses on moral obligations (grounded on the impact of individual conduct) in promoting—or harming—the best interests of *relationships*, both in the present and across generations.

Such a moral call must address the specific values and beliefs that fuel the ongoing AIDS crisis. The moral call, for example, must point out with great clarity that sexual promiscuity places women at great risk. Sexual promiscuity is bad citizenship. It undermines cohesion in families and, therefore, in society. Most grievously, it winks at the misuse of women and children. In a typical example, in Kisumu, Kenya, in 1997/1998, 23% of 15–19-year-old women in the general population were already infected with HIV, compared with just 3.5% of boys of the same age" (UNAIDS/WHO, 2004, p 2). Such a disparity in infection rates is just one indicator that women may be unable to escape sexual coercion in cultures where sexual promiscuity has become a prominent feature of cultural life. Commitment to the well-being or value of other persons is a starting point to abandoning self-centered, mutually destructive behaviors. We cannot continue to condone sexual promiscuity if we expect to offer a solution to AIDS.

THE FAMILIAL DIMENSION: A MORAL CALL

How would such an idea as startling as what we propose be implemented? It would involve many avenues of pursuit, but the first would be to restore or renew the idea of the generational family. It would foster the idea that husbands and wives, at their best, act on behalf of the next generation by, among other things, not placing children and the women who bear them at risk (through no fault of their own) of infection, disease and death. By appealing to beliefs about family, we address preservation of a culture. We address, in effective and realistic terms, the need to improve the status of women, who must be recognized as unique and valuable persons rather than mere objects for pleasure, subject to destructive practices and risks.

Women as persons of value are persons worthy of being treated with sexual fidelity. We may not be able to halt the spread of AIDS if society continues to consider women as secondary to the cohesion and strength of a community and society. Also, children infected at birth become painful evidence that the destructive consequences of some parental acts can not be easily contained. Infected children are the ultimate evidence that the heart of solving the AIDS epidemic lies in believing and living by relational ethics, where the consequences of our acts are seen as having familial and cultural outcomes.

One prevention program that is showing promise in Kenya and Uganda, which makes abstinence and fidelity central to the content of the curriculum, involves parents in discussions with children. The curriculum teaches consequential thinking, through which children are shown the relationship between actions and outcomes. The philosophical myths and cultural beliefs that actually spread AIDS and STDs are challenged directly, and correct information is delivered. This all takes place in a curriculum that extols and demonstrates the value and possibility of individual responsibility and generational commitments (Sheffield, Cox, Panos, & Panos, 2004).

More recently, Janet Museveni explained the philosophy of her country's ABC prevention efforts, indicating the priorities of a quality response to the problem:

> The message was simple, and it was this: That AIDS is transmitted mainly through heterosexual contact (in the Ugandan context); that it has no cure and leads to death; that young people should stick only to their marriage partners and be faithful, and those who have risky lifestyles should use the condom to reduce the likelihood of infection or re-infection in the case of the already infected. (Museveni, 2004, p. 2)

Museveni also acknowledges the practical reality of condom use—although her pragmatism applies to those groups already "set in their ways"—and proposes reasons for the "C" in the ABC approach that do not match those typically advocated by Western experts:

> Condom use, as a preferred method of prevention or reduction of infection, is definitely not in the interest of Ugandans. Our people are still poor and the majority of them still live in remote villages in rural areas. Even if they had money to buy condoms regularly, they would find it a problem to access them. When condoms are not used consistently, they are even less effective.

Therefore, it is wiser to show our people that there is a surer way to stay safe and alive; because the truth is that there is no "safe sex" outside of the situation of faithfulness to a partner. (Museveni, 2004, p. 3)

Make no mistake: our proposal sounds a moral call. But, quite importantly, the proposal is not simply "religious." We advocate promotion of those practices which place the next generation at the least possible risk. This message, of course, is often a component of religious belief, perhaps because the welfare of future generations is central to the theology of so many of the world's established religions. *The Qur'an* states that "Allah has made for you mates from yourselves and made for you out of them, children and grandchildren" (Sura 16:72). *The Holy Bible* reflects the same truth: "And the Lord God said, It is not good that the man should be alone" (Genesis 2:18). The profound importance of the family unit established by Adam, Eve, and their children is recognized in *The Torah* (Bereishis 2:18) and explained in the *Catechism of the Roman Catholic Church*, ¶ 2207 (1994). The fundamental truth that the natural family is the basic unit of society, furthermore, extends beyond the great monotheistic religions of Christianity, Islam, and Judaism. The classic Taoist text, *The Chuang Tzu*, explains that familial ties are the basis of a stable society because "[w]hen people are brought together by Heaven, . . . when troubles come, they hold together" (Palmer & Breuilly, trans., 1996). The inherent value of future generations, however, is not inherently or necessarily a religious concept. And, given that many religious groups seem to be able to dramatically reduce AIDS-risk behaviors in their congregations, including their young people (Garner, 2000), we are mystified that many who hope to reduce the spread of AIDS spurn and even ridicule such efforts. It is another sign that ideology is embedded in our current "received views" of how to attack the spread of the disease.

But despite the embedded ideology that education regarding sexual "facts" and condom distribution are the only methods for attacking the AIDS epidemic, there is proof that values-based programs *do* work. The Report of the Secretary General to the Special Session on HIV/AIDS notes "well documented evidence of successes . . . particularly among young people" (United Nations, 2001, p. 11). This success comes from values-based programs in Zambia, Uganda, and Tanzania that encourage chastity and sexual abstinence. According to the report of the Secretary General, these programs have "resulted in less premarital sex, increased male sexual abstinence, and less frequent casual sex" (p. 11). Nevertheless, the ultimate determinants of success are not the results demonstrated by individual programs. The potential success of any intervention effort is vastly multiplied when the powerful agenda setters in a country support cultural beliefs that are compatible with responsible sexual behavior that protects present and intergenerational relationships. That, at least, seems to be the ménage of Uganda's experience.

The Secretary General's report demonstrates that changing beliefs can change sexual behavior in ways that halt the spread of the crisis. Therefore, if the beliefs of a group reduce the likelihood that their members will take sexual risks, why not sustain and support their efforts? The world community should strengthen, for example, the efforts of communities that encourage their populations in abstaining from AIDS-risk lifestyles. The Report of the Secretary General notes that the predominantly Islamic nations of North Africa and the Middle East "have so far been the least affected by the epidemic" (p. 11). Why not strengthen, rather than deride, cultural norms that halt or avoid the crisis? If sexual promiscuity is bad citizenship, and if drug use places individual well-being at risk, society must call upon people to be good citizens, and responsible family members, by not placing themselves, others, and their own culture at risk.

In his testimony before a U.S. House Subcommittee, Edward C. Green, Senior Research Scientist at the Harvard Center for Population and Development Studies, summarized Ugandan efforts in the ABC programs this way:

> The AIDS message was not soft-pedaled. People were made to fear HIV infection, but not to fear people with AIDS. People were also told clearly what to do to avoid infection. The main lessons from Uganda are that: (1) sexual behavior can change; (2) a comprehensive program of promoting abstinence, faithfulness and condom use for nonregular partners can be implemented and this may lead to higher levels of all three outcomes; (3) AIDS prevention programs benefit greatly from top-level political commitment and involvement; (4) condoms do play a role in risk reduction, but focus exclusively on condom use is not a panacea for HIV prevention, especially in high prevalence, generalized epidemics as we find in Africa. (Green, 2003a, p. 46)

The success of any call for abstinence and fidelity may not be significant if only behavioral changes are emphasized. But if there is a change in philosophy, commitments and beliefs about how to treat each other, about how to behave on behalf of the members of one's family and for the next generation, many more individuals are more likely to forgo risky behaviors. Indeed, it is within the smallest unit of society, the generational family, where face-to-face daily interaction is available, that the battle against AIDS is won or lost. Parents at their best teach and live beliefs and philosophies that preserve the next generation. On the other hand, when parental beliefs or example invite destructive lifestyles, the risk to the next generation is extreme.

Thus we believe families must be the hub of prevention efforts regarding beliefs and values because parents are the most likely adults to be committed to the long-term well-being of their children. After government policies have been installed, after educational programs have been delivered, after medical treatments have been obtained, it is parents who are involved with the lives of their children for the long term. Families continue after programs and policies have faded. Parents are the ones who transmit values and beliefs (Dittus, Jacard, & Gordon, 1999; Hanson et al., 1987; Lees & Tinsley, 2000). Families deserve to be supported in examining how to transform a culture—or more properly, restore a culture—to the beliefs and practices which are family, child and next-generation friendly.

RESTORING FAMILIAL-FRIENDLY STARTING POINTS

What cultural and familial beliefs are relevant to reducing the risk of exposure to AIDS? The transformation of beliefs on behalf of the next generation might include the following:

1. Restoring the idea that abstinence prior to marriage and fidelity afterward— even in polygynous societies—is evidence that marriage, family and sexual matters are neither casual nor inconsequential.
2. Rejecting the idea that men have the right or the need to pursue sex wherever it is available. This also suggests that men are something other than mere animals.
3. Granting women their deserved status as persons of worth, who must not be sexually or economically exploited as things.
4. Protecting children from exploitation by those in authority, and making sexual access to children an absolute cultural taboo.
5. Revising business and economic practices which require men to be employed in cities or countries where it is not possible to locate their families.
6. Protecting refugees from predatory sexual behavior and seeking ways to restore them to homes and homelands.
7. Seeking economic support for infrastructures which minimize the need for migration.

The choice in intervention efforts is not between merely giving facts or addressing cultural beliefs. In fact, it is philosophically and practically impossible to present facts which do not express a philosophy. It also is not a question of "whose values we are going to *impose*." This invokes an assumption that humans are mere receptacles into which values and beliefs are poured—which then either enhance or ruin their lives. While it is possible for humans to be victimized by destructive cultural beliefs, humans are not mere victims of cultural practices. It is also possible for people to be exposed to, understand and then respond to those beliefs that are in their best interests. The question concerning values is what we are willing to *expose* cultures, families, and individuals to, rather than what we are going to *impose* on them. The former approach grants the value of education *and* the reality that individuals have the ability to choose whether or not to act in their own and others' best interests. The latter approach seems to deny a place for a human moral sense regarding those best interests. Any intervention must acknowledge the capacity that humans possess to live true or false to the knowledge they have. This aspect of the human condition—the ability to respond to facts and knowledge by living by them or by ignoring-rejecting them—is the Achilles heel of all prevention efforts.

Whether our efforts are grounded in a philosophy that knowledge and facts are enough or in the philosophy of our proposal to also confront cultural beliefs, the reality remains that humans frequently do not live by what they know. This is a sobering reality that reflects why so many prevention efforts fail—no matter what philosophy they are grounded in. The reason for hope, however, regarding the success of efforts to reduce HIV/AIDS is that most behavior that produces the disease is voluntary, and the possibility to change consequences by changing behavior is always available. Since values and beliefs are strong predictors of actual behaviors, when education and knowledge do include the support of AIDS-preventive cultural, familial, and personal beliefs, the chances of success are multiplied.

If a society places philosophy and beliefs that nourish, encourage, and reward commitment to family and to the next generation at the heart of its culture, it has a base from which to attack a disease that is spread primarily through voluntary behavior and ignorance. If, as we now know, providing knowledge is not enough, behavioral monitoring is insufficient, and cultural beliefs about sex, women, marriage, and family are major factors which contribute to the AIDS crisis, surely it is time to marshal beliefs which help one generation to preserve the next, and those of the next generation to preserve themselves. Such beliefs are most likely moral beliefs which sustain familial, generational commitments.

Africa generally has a history of family-centered cultural beliefs. Practices from those cultures may not all be beneficial; as the family culture has eroded, the AIDS crisis has accelerated. To seek a restoration of a family culture—of the idea that one generation is committed to the well-being of the next and ought to step forward to act in behalf of that generation—is a worthwhile tool in the life or death AIDS battle. To take the family factor seriously may be one of our greatest allies in the fight against AIDS. Those who undermine family commitments invoke an ideology which threatens the greatest resource available for scientists, governments, the medical profession, and religious groups to use in acting in behalf of the next generation: the family (Fagan, 1999, 2001). Those voluntary organizations, including religious ones, that teach abstinence and family commitment, should be encouraged, not criticized. Then our attempts in Africa to preserve the young, to protect refugees, to reduce the necessity of migration, to keep families together by strengthening local economies, to treat women as persons of value—all are more likely to succeed. Cultural beliefs and values operate for or against the next generation. Values and beliefs that invite the preservation of the next generation are legitimate and central to our prevention efforts. They become the hope, rather than the heartbreak, of preserving the next generations in Africa.

NOTE

1.   This chapter is an adaptation of a paper accepted by the Organization of African Unity, September, 2001.

REFERENCES

Adolescent Family Life Act, Title XX, U.S. Congress. (1981)

Allen, A. (2002, May). Uganda v. condoms. *The New Republic*, 226(20),14–15.

Back, K. W. (1983). Teenage pregnancy: Science and ideology in applied social psychology. In R. F. Kidd & M. J. Saks (Eds.), *Advances in applied social psychology* (pp. 1–17). Hillsdale, NJ: Erlbaum.

Caldwell, J. C. (2000). Rethinking the African AIDS epidemic. *Population Development Review*, 26(1), 117–135.

DiClemente, R. J., Wingood, G. M., Harrington, K. F., Lang, D. L., Davies, S. L., Hook, E. W., Oh, M. K., Crosby, R. A., Hertzberg, V. S., Gordon, A. B., Hardin, J. W., Parker, S., & Robillard, A. (2004). Efficacy of an HIV prevention intervention for African American adolescent girls: A randomized controlled trial. *Journal of the American Medical Association*, 292(2), 171–179.

Dittus, P. J., Jacard, J., & Gordon, V. V. (1999). Direct and nondirect communication of maternal beliefs to adolescents: Adolescent motivations for premarital sexual activity. *Journal of Applied Social Psychology*, 29(9), 1927–1963.

Fagan, P. (1999, June). How broken families rob children of their chances for future prosperity. *The Heritage Foundation: Backgrounder* No. 1283.

Fagan, P. (2001, February). How U.N. conventions on women's and children's rights undermine family, religion and sovereignty. *The Heritage Foundation: Backgrounder* No. 1407.

Garner, R. C. (2000). Safe sects? Dynamic religion and AIDS in South Africa. *The Journal of Modern African Studies, 38*(1), 41–69.

Green, E. C. (2003a). *HIV/AIDS, TB, and Malaria: Combating a global pandemic.* The Committee on Energy and Commerce: Subcommittee on Health. Washington, DC: U.S. Government Printing Office.

Green, E. C. (2003b). *Rethinking AIDS prevention: Learning from successes in developing countries.* Westport, CT: Praeger.

Haffner, D. W. (1997). What's wrong with abstinence-only sexuality education programs? *SIECUS, 25*(4), 9–13.

Hanenberg, R. S., Rojanapithayakorn, W., Kunasol, P., & Sokal D. (1994). The impact of Thailand's HIV-centred programme as indicated by the decline of sexually transmitted diseases. *Lancet, 344*(8917), 243-245.

Hanson, S. L., Myers, D. E., & Ginsburg, A. L. (1987). The role of responsibility and knowledge in reducing teenage out-of-wedlock childbearing. *Journal of Marriage and the Family, 49*(2), 241–256.

Hartigan, J. D. (1997). *The disastrous results of condom distribution programs.* Washington, DC: Family Research Council.

Jacard, J., & Dittis, P. (1991). *Parent-teen communication: Toward the prevention of unintended pregnancies.* New York: Springer-Verlag.

Kirby, D. (1985). Sexuality education: A more realistic view of its effects. *Journal of School Health, 55*(10), 421–424.

Kirby, D., Waszak, C., & Ziegler, J. (1989). *An assessment of six school-based clinics: Services, impact and potential.* Washington, DC: Center for Population Options.

Kirby, D., Waszak, C., & Ziegler, J. (1991). An assessment of six school-based clinics: Their reproductive health services and impact upon sexual behaviors. *Family Planning Perspectives, 23*(1), 6–16.

Kirby, D. (2001). *Emerging answers: Research findings on programs to reduce teen pregnancy.* Washington, DC: The National Campaign to Prevent Teen Pregnancy.

Kristof, N. D. (2003, January 10). The secret war on condoms. *New York Times,* p. A23.

Lees, N. B., & Tinsley, B. J. (2000). Maternal socialization of children's preventive health behavior: The role of maternal affect and teaching strategies. *Merrill-Palmer Quarterly, 46*(4), 632–651.

McGeary, J. (2001, February). Death stalks a continent. *Time, 12,* 36–45.

Museveni, Y. G. (1992). *What is Africa's problem?* Kampala, Uganda: NRM.

Museveni, J. (2004, June). *Address.* Presented at the Common Ground: A Shared Vision for Health Conference, Medical Institute for Sexual Health. Washington, DC.

Miller, B. C., & Olson, T. D. (1988). Sexual attitudes and behavior of high school students in relation to background and contextual factors. *Journal of Sex Research, 24,* 194–200.

Miller, K. S., Levin, M. L., Whitaker, D. J., & Xu, X. H. (1998). Patterns of condom use among adolescents: The impact of mother-adolescent communication. *American Journal of Public Health, 88*(10), 1542–1544.

Olson, T. D., Wallace, C. M., & Miller, B. C. (1984). Primary prevention of adolescent pregnancy: Promoting family involvement through a school curriculum. *Journal of Primary Prevention, 5*(2), 75–91.

Palmer, M., & Breuilly, E. (1996). *The book of Chuang Tzu.* London: Arkana, Penguin.

Pedlow, C. T., & Carey, M. P. (2003). HIV sexual risk-reduction interventions for youth: A review and methodological critique of randomized controlled trials. *Behavior Modification, 27*(2), 135–190.

Polit, D. F., & Kahn, J. R. (1985). Project redirection: Evaluation of a comprehensive program for disadvantaged teenage mothers. *Family Planning Perspectives, 17*(4), 150–155.

Richens, J., Imrie, J., & Copas, A. (2000). Condoms and seat belts: The parallels and the lessons. *The Lancet, 355*, 400–403.

Richens, J., Imrie, J., & Weiss, H. (2003). Sex and death: Why does HIV continue to spread when so many people know about the risks? *Journal of the Statistical Society Association, 166*(2), 207-215.

Santelli, J. S., Lowry, R., Brener, N. D., & Robin, L. (2000). The association of sexual behaviors with socioeconomic status, family structure, and race/ethnicity among US adolescents. *American Journal of Public Health, 90*(10), 1582–1588.

Schaeffer, K. W., Nottebaum, L., Smith, P., Dech, K., & Krawczyk, J. (1999). Religiously-motivated sexual orientation change: A follow-up study. *Journal of Psychology and Theology, 27*(4), 329–337.

Sheffield, W. W., Cox, S. E., Panos, P. T., & Panos, A. (2004). Stay alive: *A Family Based Deterrent to the Spread of HIV/AIDS.* Manuscript submitted for publication.

SIECUS. (1999). *Developing guidelines for comprehensive sexuality education.* New York: Author.

Stanton, B. F., Li, X., Ricardo, I., Galbraith, J., Feigelman, S., & Kaljee, L. (1996). A randomized, controlled effectiveness trial of an AIDS prevention program for low-income African-American youths. *Archives of Pediatrics & Adolescent Medicine, 150*(4), 363–366.

Stanton, B., Cole, M., Galbraith, J., Li, X., Pendleton, S., Cottrel, L., Marshall, S., Wu, Y., & Kaljee, L. (2004). Randomized trial of a parent intervention. *Archives of Pediatrics & Adolescent Medicine, 158*(10), 947–955.

Stoneburner, R. L., & Low-Beer, D. (2004). Population-level HIV declines and behavioral risk avoidance in Uganda. *Science, 304*(5671), 714–718.

UNAIDS/WHO. (2000). HIV sentinel surveillance. Epidemiological fact sheet. *Thailand, 4,* 6.

UNAIDS/WHO. (2004). *Kenya epidemiological fact sheets on HIV/AIDS and sexually transmitted infections.* Geneva, Switzerland: Authors.

United Nations. (2001). *Report of the secretary general, special session of the general assembly on HIV/AIDS, A/55/779.* New York: Author.

U.S. Congressional Research Service. (2000). *AIDS in Africa.* April 19, 2000, pp. 1-18.

Whitehead, B. D. (1994, October). The failure of sex education. *The Atlantic Monthly, 274*(4), 55-80.

PART IV

DEALING WITH AIDS ORPHANS AND STREET CHILDREN

CHAPTER 13

POVERTY, AIDS, AND STREET CHILDREN IN UGANDA

Troy D. Smith and Acou Sam Ogojoi

Systemic poverty, significant HIV/AIDS prevalence, and 2 million orphaned children pose a threat to the future of Uganda. The number of street children in the country is expected to rise in the immediate future, impacting not only individual lives, but the larger society. In recent years Uganda has been heralded as a pattern of effective development in Sub-Saharan Africa (SSA). Specifically, a recent government program to help street children has been suggested as a model that other countries in the region can follow.

Less than 20 years ago, Uganda emerged from decades of chaos and a bloody civil war that decimated the country's rich natural resources, devastated its population, and left many of its people in turmoil. Since that time, the government has continued to battle rebel groups in Northern Uganda and the population has suffered immensely as one of the hardest hit by the HIV/AIDS epidemic sweeping through Africa. Approximately 1 million people have died as a result of HIV/AIDS, and another 1 million people are currently living with AIDS in the country. It is estimated that

Uganda has over two million orphan children, the majority of whom were orphaned by HIV/AIDS. This number is expected to increase over the next

Overcoming AIDS: Lessons Learned from Uganda, 251–273
Copyright © 2006 by Information Age Publishing
251

decade, increasing the risk of children becoming street children, beggars, thieves, or being a target for abuse and exploitation. (Ministry of Finance, Planning and Economic Development [MFPED], 2003, p. 152)

These millions of orphans represent current and future challenges to the stability and long term productivity of the country. Street children in Uganda are a growing subset of the 2 million orphan children in the country. Many eke out dangerous lives on the streets of large Ugandan cities. Their lives are characterized by violence, filth, drugs, crime, and loneliness. Their individual capacities and potentials are stunted through lack of opportunity. Street children often engage in several high-risk behaviors, making them especially vulnerable to Africa's ever-growing HIV/ AIDS epidemic. Because of the long latency period of the disease, many of these children will escape street life only to be cut down in their mid-twenties by the disease (English, 1991). Because they have little access to education, skills training, and other resources, street children further represent a future drain on the productive capacity of the country. According to Hecht (1998):

> Street children are a reminder ... just outside the five-star hotels where the development consultants stay, of the contradictions of contemporary social life: the opulence of the few amid the poverty of the majority, the plethora of resources amid the squandering of opportunities. They embody the failure of an unacknowledged social apartheid to keep the poor out of view. At home in the street, they are painful reminders of the dangerous and endangered world in which we live. (p. 214)

This chapter first chronicles the number of street children in Uganda and explores why children choose to live on the streets of urban cities. It then describes the life these children live in the streets and details the risk of HIV/AIDS for this vulnerable subpopulation. Finally, programs by governments and NGOs working to effectively deal with street children will be examined.

REPULSION AND ATTRACTION: WHY CHILDREN LIVE ON THE STREETS

Reasons that children leave their homes to pursue new lives on the streets of major urban areas have been well documented in the literature (see, for example, Hecht, 1998; Kilbride, Suda, & Njeru, 2000; UNESCO, 1995; Vélis, 1995). Despite wide geographic separation and cultural differences, the causes leading children to the streets are hauntingly similar through-

Table 13.1. Reasons Cited for Leaving Home by Street Children in Uganda

Causes	Frequency
Mistreatment	34.6
Orphaned	18.7
Poverty	10.0
Unemployment	96.0
Peer pressure	44.0
Rebel activity	1.3
Family conflict	0.9
Adventure	3.5
Witchcraft	0.4
Committed offences—on run/wanted	0.4

Source: Friends of Children Association (FOCA) (1999). Because of multiple responses per participant, percentages sum to more than 100.

out the world. War and political insecurity, abuse, neglect, poverty and orphanhood are some of the major "push" factors (see Table 13.1).

There is widespread agreement among international organizations, government officials, academics, and NGOs that poverty is the most prevalent factor driving children to the streets (Ministry of Gender, Labor, and Social Development [MGLSD], 1999, 2001; Munene & Nambi, 1996; UNESCO, 1995). Although poverty has been declining in recent years, 35% of Ugandans lived below the poverty line in 2000. This poverty line is roughly equivalent to the dollar-a-day measure often used by the World Bank (MFPED, 2003; Appleton, Emwanu, Kagugube, & Muwonge, 1999). Low returns from income-generating activities at the household level make many families unable to provide for the basic needs of their children. Sending children to school, for instance, is beyond the ability of many parents, even where universal primary education is offered, because the children's services are needed at home to help support the household. Also poverty is often the root of peripheral reasons why children leave home, including abuse, neglect, abandonment, child labor, domestic violence, boredom, and crime. It is the slums surrounding most major urban areas that are "the real breeding-grounds of street and working children" (UNESCO, 1995, p. 282). Too many homes with scarce food, few resources, and a lack of educational opportunities make life on the streets a "materially rational alternative for some children" (Hecht, 1998, p. 196). The sad reality for millions of poor children is that the conditions they face at home are no better than, and in some cases are actually worse than, those faced on the street.

Abuse and maltreatment are also major factors driving children to the streets. Step-parents are repeatedly implicated as perpetrators of abuse or neglect towards a spouse's previous children (Jacob, Smith, Hite, & Cheng, 2004; Williams, 2002). A lack of necessary skills to manage conflict at the household level aggravates domestic violence and has had a grave impact on the spiritual, emotional, physical, and sexual conditions and behaviors of children. Repeated abuse and rejection by adults leave many children emotionally empty. A search for acceptance and belonging may lead children to the streets where, as one child reports, "The street never rejects children, it is always proud of them and remains their best friend" (UNESCO, 1995, p. 41). Further situations that may lead to abuse are often fostered by social conditions in Uganda including poverty, large families, polygamy, and the increasing death rate from HIV/AIDS and other diseases. When parents cannot care for their own children because of death, illness, or poverty, the children are often farmed out to relatives for whom they are expected to work as domestic help in compensation for school fees, housing, and food. While this tradition of extended family involvement has been of great benefit to orphans throughout the country, in many cases it has facilitated abuse and marginalization of children, leading some to strike out on their own.

In conjunction with these "push" factors are several "pull" factors enticing children to relocate to the streets of large urban cities. Many children are attracted to big cities hoping to find employment, excitement, autonomy, and opportunity. Children already living on the streets often persuade friends or siblings to join them, with stories of freedom and fun. Especially in rural areas, false information about the glamour of city life is passed around, attracting both adults and children to migrate to urban slums. Many now recognize that charitable donations given by NGOs and private individuals, as well as petty employment opportunities, may be a further incentive to entice children to the streets (Wiehler, 2002; Malcomson, 2003). In guidelines established in 1999 for working with children by the government of Uganda, special attention is brought to this pull factor. The government recommends that all handouts "must be linked to learning or working experience, which contributes to the rehabilitation of the street child" (MGLSD, 1999, p. 22). While this is a rational policy, it is often very difficult to enforce, especially among members of the general population who feel cruel when they deny money or food to a homeless child. Many people find it easier to give petty handouts than to put forth the enormous effort needed to make the problem permanently disappear.

HIV/AIDS has had a devastating impact on Africa generally and Uganda specifically. All other factors that bring children to the streets are magnified by HIV/AIDS. Despite the fact that Uganda is one of only two countries in the world that have been able to reverse overall HIV adult prevalence rates, many extended families are already overburdened trying to care for children of relatives and friends left behind by the disease, and single-parent as well as child-headed households are becoming ever more common in the country. A recent draft of a report by the Ministry of Gender, Labor and Social Development (MGLSD) notes that 25% of Ugandan households include at least one orphan (Nandawula, 2002). Tragically, the number of orphans is expected to continue to increase for the next 10 to 15 years, as persons already infected succumb to AIDS and die, leaving behind children who have been within their care (UNICEF, 2002a, 2002c; USAID/UNICEF/UNAIDS, 2002; UNAIDS, 2002). Thus HIV/AIDS continues to be a leading cause of orphanhood and eventual street children status throughout much of SSA.

NUMBERS OF STREET CHILDREN

Although the number of street children worldwide is estimated to be 100 million (UNICEF, 2002b, p. 37), the exact figure is difficult to determine. Part of the ambiguity comes in the definition of a "street child." Generally children who participate in street life during the day and return home at night are termed "children on the street" or "part-time" street children, whereas those who live and sleep on the street are termed "children of the street" or "full-time" street children as portrayed in Table 13,2 (Kilbride et al., 2000, p. 2; MGLSD, 1999; Munene & Nambi, 1996). Numbers of street children are also hard to ascertain because of the high mobility of the population and because, due to frequent harassment by the police and other members of the public, street children have an incentive to become invisible whenever possible.

Although street children have always been present in modern Uganda, decades of war and violence put hundreds of orphans on the streets as early as the 1970s. These children, averaging between 8 and 10 years old, were called *bayaye*, the Luganda word for thieves (UNESCO, 1995, p. 177). Today some sources put the number of street children in Uganda as high as 10,000, with an estimated 2,500 in Kampala alone (Consortium for Street Children, 2002; Friends of Children Association [FOCA], 2002). Other sources argue for a more modest number. A MGLSD study in 1993 put the number at 3,827 (see Tables 13.2 and 13.3). A study published in 1996 of 10 of the largest cities in Uganda found 3,728 street children, of whom 924 were females (Munene & Nambi, 1996). In the capital city, Kampala, a government relocation campaign found nearly 1,000 children living on the streets

**Table 13.2.   Street Children by Time Spent on the Street in
Selected Urban Centers**

Town	Part-Time (%)	Full-Time (%)	Total
Jinja	82.5	17.5	200
Busia	93.75	6.25	1,120
Malaba	85	15	600
Mbale	90	10	200
Gulu	32.9	67.1	85
Arua	90	10	200
Masaka/Nyendo	50	50	120
Kampala central	65.7	34.3	405
Kampala surburb	97.7	2.3	742
Kabale	85.3	14.7	95
Mbarara	50	50	60
Total	85.6	14.4	3,827

Source: Munene and Nambi (1993).

between May 2002 and June 2003 (Kampiringisa National Rehabilitation Center, 2003). In the industrial city of Jinja, in 2003 there were estimated to be approximately 60 full-time street children (Malcomson, 2003). Although no systematic research has been done in recent years, most people who work with street children believe that the numbers have increased dramatically, as would be suggested by comparing recent estimates to those detailed in the 1993 and 1996 studies.

Most of the street children are from the Central Geographic Region of Uganda (67%), with the Northern Region reporting the smallest number (Figure 13.1). Proximity to the country's capital city, greater access to transportation, and violence in the Luwero Triangle have fueled rural-urban migration and may partly explain the high number of street children in the Central Region.

The general population of Africa is poor and young. Nearly half of the population is under the age of 16, and this continent includes many of the poorest countries in the world. The high birthrate coupled with poverty and the impact of HIV/AIDS indicates that the number of street children will continue to increase into the foreseeable future. This will further increase the competition among children for employment, food, and other resources (Jacob et al., 2004). Sustainable programs and policies must be enacted today to adequately prepare for increasing numbers of street children in the future.

Table 13.3.   Street Children by Sex and Age in Selected Towns

Town	Gender (%)		Age Group	No.	%
	Girls	Boys			
Jinja & Mbale	35	65	5–9	44	11.0
			10–14	270	67.5
			15–19	86	21.5
Busia	41	59	4–7	134	12
			8–14	661	59
			15–18	325	29
Malaba	41	59	4–7	72	12
			8–14	366	61
			15–18	162	27
Masaka	0	100	8–13	60	50
			14–18	60	50
Mbarara	0	100	8–13	28	47
			14–18	32	53
Kampala	10	90	8–13	331	29
			14–18	816	71
Gulu	12	88	8–12	60	71
			13–15	25	29
Arua	8	93	8–13	22	11
			14–18	178	89
Kabale	8	92	14–18	95	100
Total	23	74		3,827	

Source: Munene and Nambi (1993).

LIFE ON THE STREETS

Street life is very difficult, and "immediate survival" dominates the lives of street youth (Luna, 1991, p. 512). One of the greatest pressures for street children is the daily task of finding food and other resources. Many, especially the younger ones, beg to get money or food from the public. For this reason many street children congregate around venues frequented by wealthy people, such as hotels, shopping centers, and local attractions. Street children often do odd jobs such as guarding parked cars, picking up garbage for recycling, and carrying items around the market to earn money for food and other necessities. Older street children are also likely to engage in petty crime and thievery (Hecht, 1998; Kilbride et al., 2000; UNESCO, 1995; Vélis, 1995). Trash heaps, which are prevalent through-

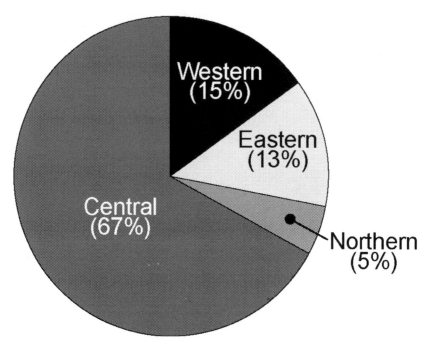

Figure 13.1.   Regional distribution of street children in Uganda, adapted from Genei (2000).

out urban areas in Uganda, provide warmth as well as food and other items which can be sold or traded (Munene & Nambi, 1996). Participation in this informal economy often leaves these children open to exploitation for labor or sex, as well as to harassment and abuse by law enforcement officers.

Most street children have had very little, if any, formal schooling. Drop-out rates of children, especially girls, are high across Africa. However, the cultural value placed on education in Africa is also very high, and most street children desire to return to school or to receive vocational training, although many of them are unable to articulate what specific training they need because they do not know about available options. UNESCO (1995) notes that

> there is a direct link between the lack of education prospects and the presence of children on the street . . . . In 1990, 75% of those who had completed their primary education [in Uganda] were unable to go on to a higher level. (pp. 188–189)

However, as challenging as it may be for street children to gain access to schooling, remaining in and finishing their schooling is even more problematic as many have never learned to function in a school environment and find the classroom very boring and monotonous compared to street life (Vélis, 1995). A child brought in off the street "will, potentially, be the poorest student that one can imagine" (UNESCO, 1995, p. 112). The difficulty of keeping street children in school is further compounded by the low quality of educational opportunity in Africa. According to a recent Oxfam report, Africa has 24 of the "world's worst-performing nations in providing educational opportunities for children" (Kilbride et al., 2000, p. 151). Programs successful at educating street children often focus on vocational education and nonformal teaching techniques. Given the self-reported high demand for schooling among street children, more effort must be invested in creating educational opportunities suited to their particular needs, desires, and constraints.

For economic as well as social and psychological reasons, many street children work in groups. As well as providing friendship, other members of the group can provide protection and access to resources as long as one is able to accept the authority of dominant members of the group. These groups or gangs of young people exhibit some characteristics of a family as well as characteristics of a business organization. In addition to providing emotional support, these groups may increase their resource base by having individual members specialize in certain activities and then share proceeds with the rest of the group (Kilbride et al., 2000; Vélis, 1995).

Drugs are a common feature of street life all over the world (Hecht, 1998; Kilbride et al, 2000; UNESCO, 1995; Vélis, 1995). Alcohol, marijuana, and petrol fumes are often used when they are available, but by far the drug of choice is glue, which is cheap and easy to obtain. Glue-sniffing is nearly universal among street children. Many children sniff glue to forget their problems; others claim that it keeps them warm, suppresses hunger, or gives them courage to beg or steal. Rather than being used for clothing or food, much of the money obtained from the public by begging or from working is spent to acquire glue and other drugs. Hecht (1998) found that among the street children he studied in Brazil, over half claimed to spend more on drugs than they did on food. Drugs and sex (often unprotected sex) are among the only "pleasures" available to street children.

Full-time street children often sleep out in the open, in abandoned buildings, or on verandas with other street children who are members of their group. A lack of shelter exposes them not only to dirt and disease, but also to violence from other street children, police, or the general public (Kilbride et al., 2000).

By virtue of their lives on the street, these children suffer from a number of health problems. Cuts, bruises, infectious diseases, and sexually transmitted diseases (STDs) are all common. Lack of health services often compounds these problems, as a small cut or laceration can lead to a life-threatening infection (Vélis, 1995).

Lack of family, mistrust of adults in general, and constant harassment and condemnation from the public lead to low self-esteem, loneliness, emotional problems, and hopelessness. Often born into poor families and slum areas, many street children have never been "exposed to mainstream society's cultural norms" (Munene & Nambi, 1996, p. 346). In a type of self-fulfilling prophecy, street children live up to the public's expectations of them. Caught in the vicious cycle of the streets, they are often unable to escape without outside intervention.

HIV/AIDS and Street Children

Because of their marginalized status, relatively little is known about HIV/AIDS prevalence among street children, and no systematic studies have been conducted on the issue in Uganda (Baligonzaki, 2002). However, given the findings of studies of similar populations in other areas of the world, along with the high-risk behaviors characteristic of street life, there is much cause for alarm. A 1988 study of street youth in New York found that 10.5% were HIV positive and that incidence of infection among them was increasing (Luna, 1991). Studies of Brazilian street children report HIV infection rates from as low as 1.0% to as high as 68.6% in some subpopulations (Luna, 1991; Raffaelli et al., 1993). Some people working with street children in Uganda estimate that as many as 3 in 10 street children could be victims of HIV/AIDS (Rukundo, 2004).

Globally, street children's behavior typically includes activities known to be high risk for contracting the HIV virus, such as various sexual encounters and injected drug use. A study of New York City runaways in 1988 found that 70% of the males and 59% of the females had been sexually active in the previous 3 months. The males averaged 2.7 partners and 9 sexual occasions, while the females averaged 1.3 sexual partners and 5.3 sexual experiences; 27% of the males and 47.2% of the females reported never using a condom (Rotheram-Borus & Koopman, 1991). A comprehensive study of Brazilian street youth is particularly alarming regarding the sexual behavior of street children. The study reports:

> Equal proportions of boys and girls reported that their friends were sexually active (71.5%), exchanged sex for money (32.3%), had sex under the influence of alcohol or drugs (42.9%), and had sexually transmitted diseases

(39.4%). Sixty-nine percent of the girls said their friends had been pregnant, and 43.4% that their friends had abortions. Forty-four percent of the boys said that their friends had impregnated a girl or woman. (Raffaelli et al., 1993, p. 663)

The study further reports that the age of first sexual experience among the street child population was 10.8 for boys and 12.4 for girls and that sexual initiation often occurred as a result of coercion, especially for girls (Raffaelli et al., 1993). While injected drug use is not a primary mode of HIV infection among street children in SSA and Uganda, sharing unsterilized razors or knives is a continuous threat.

A less formal study of 250 Ugandan street children found that 48% knew of a friend who had an STD, and 24% had a friend who was HIV positive. More than 70% knew of a girl of their same age who had been pregnant. For 31% of respondents sexual initiation was forced upon them, and 34% of those who had had sex thought it was wrong for a young woman to refuse sex. (This figure dropped to 14% among those who had not had sex.) An alarming 42% of the children said that they had never been shown how to use a condom by an adult, and only 22% said they had used one the last time they had sex. Over half (54%) had a boyfriend or girlfriend with whom they had sex, and 60% were having sex once a month or more. Regarding drug use, 36% reported "always" or "sometimes" taking drugs before having sex and 28% "always" or "sometimes" had sex in exchange for gifts or money. Overall, 15% responded "always" or "sometimes" when asked if they were forced into having sex, but the forcing was significantly more likely to happen to girls than to boys (Baligonzaki, 2002). Other studies have found that the mean age of first sexual experience among Ugandan youth (not limited to street youth) is 14 years for both boys and girls (Amuyunzu-Nyamongo et al., 1999).

Munene and Nambi (1996), in one of the only empirical studies of street children in Uganda report:

> There is also widespread understanding that these girls tend to be sexually abused both by street boys and other men. An indication this may be largely true is found in the street children's sexual language, used to refer to the sexes. The boys are referred to as Kawo or cowboys, while girls are called Busege or little wolves. The idea is that the cowboys hunt the wolves. When a street girl picks a boy friend among a gang of boys, it is not unknown nor is it uncommon that she may be forced to have sex with other boys in the gang. In general there is sexual delinquency among street children of both sexes particularly older ones. (pp. 346–347)

Because they lack food and other material resources, street youth engage often in "survival sex," selling sexual services for money, clothing,

262 T. D. SMITH and A. S. OGOJOI

or other gifts (Glasser, 1994; Kibride et al., 2000; Raffaelli et al., 1993). These sexual services may include anal, vaginal, or oral sex. Where other regions such as Latin America, North America, and Europe often involve homosexual experiences, sexual encounters among street children in SSA and Uganda largely occur within heterosexual relationships. The social networks from which street youth draw their sexual partners are also likely to increase their risk level of contracting HIV/AIDS (Rotheram-Borus & Koopman, 1991). Many customers refuse to use condoms with their partners. Having sex under the influence of drugs or alcohol is also a common element of street life. Alcohol is often used to give courage or to dull pain, especially during a first sexual experience. Sex with peers is often a part of street culture and socialization; and punishment and rape by other street youth is common. In addition to providing entertainment and comfort, street children engage in sex as a means of exerting power and establishing dominance. Sex with other street children can even be a form of protection as street girls ally themselves with strong street boys in order to avoid being taken advantage of by other street boys. Some street youth see "high-risk sexual activity as a different or exciting way to express or receive some semblance of affection" (Luna, 1991, p. 513).

Many street youth believe that they have no control over what happens in their lives. This may be enhanced by some cultural and religious beliefs that teach that the day of death is preordained by God and there is nothing that an individual can do to change this deterministic event (Amuyunzu-Nyamongo et al., 1999; Caldwell, Orubuloye, & Caldwell, 1999). High risk behaviors and a fatalistic attitude seem to suggest that "for some of the young people on the street, contracting HIV is, among other things, a function of time" (Anarfi, 1999, p. 88).

The pressing needs of day to day survival often outweigh the possible costs of the distant future. As one researcher noted, "If kids don't know where their next meal is coming from or where they will sleep tomorrow night, why should they worry about dying from AIDS 10 years from now?" (Heise, 1991).

A lack of self-esteem and a lack of respect for life in general often give street children a careless attitude about death, which may further prevent them from protecting themselves. Hecht (1998) reports asking a 14-year-old boy what he feels when one of his street friends dies. Without hesitation the boy replied, "Nothing. I don't feel anything. When I die, no one will cry" (p. 145). Luna (1991) quotes another street youth who typifies this attitude: "I live on the street, I don't really have anyone. I die every day. I'm not afraid of death, I'm afraid of life" (p. 513).

Special consideration must also be taken when deciding whether street children should be tested for HIV/AIDS. Without a social support system, a positive test result may lead to suicide, increased risk-taking behavior, or further segregation by society and alienation by a peer group. Benefits to testing may include a modification of behavior (for those testing negative as well as for those testing positive) and the possibility of obtaining early treatment (English, 1991; Konde-Lule, Musagara, & Musgrave, 1993). Since street children in Uganda are unlikely to have the necessary resources to obtain treatment for HIV/AIDS, a positive test result is more likely to bring depression and hopelessness than an extension of life. Along with the potential for obtaining treatment, organizations providing HIV/AIDS testing must take into account the relevant ethical and legal considerations. Specifically, issues of confidentiality and the question of whether a sexual partner should be informed of a positive diagnosis must be addressed (English, 1991). Further, some authors have cautioned that HIV testing programs should "not assume that knowledge of HIV status automatically enables individuals to take measures to reduce or eliminate HIV risk to others ... knowing one's HIV status may not be sufficient to achieve long-term consistent safe sexual behaviour" (Meursing, 1999, p. 38).

Cultural beliefs and attitudes can also present serious problems in controlling the spread of HIV/AIDS among street children. An early study in the Rakai District of Uganda found that condoms were not widely trusted by the population, as many believed that they were not effective barriers to the HIV virus and some believed that they could "get stuck in the female and lead to serious illness" or other problems (Konde-Lule et al., 1993, p. 681). Other beliefs have spread among street children that hospitals and medical treatment facilities shortened the lives of AIDS patients. Widespread myths and incorrect beliefs regarding HIV/AIDS transmission are perpetuated among street children groups and this lack of information is further complicated because of limited access to educative prevention information. Because of increasing fear of AIDS, adults are more likely to seek out sex partners among youth because young people are less likely to be infected, often turning to destitute street children (Amuyunzu-Nyamongo et al., 1999). In addition, cultural beliefs that having sex with a young person, especially a virgin, will rid one of the virus and that having sex with many people will decrease the potency of the virus in infected individuals lead to further victimization of young people, especially street children, who are particularly vulnerable.

While the government of Uganda has been very proactive in educating its citizens about the threat of HIV/AIDS, street children are less likely to have access to correct knowledge about HIV/AIDS than the population as a whole. Because of their low education and high illiteracy levels, many street children are unlikely to benefit from pamphlets and other printed AIDS education media. A 2001 study by the GOAL Project in Uganda among 250 street children found that knowledge about sex and pregnancy was low. For example, 31% of participants thought that if a boy does not have sex on a regular basis, his penis will stop functioning properly and get smaller. Although knowledge about HIV/AIDS was higher than about sex in general, "61% of respondents thought it was possible to tell whether someone had HIV or AIDS by looking at them" (Baligonzaki, 2002, p. 4). The study further found that "82% of children affiliated with NGOs and 85% of children on the street thought they were at risk of catching HIV/AIDS" (Baligonzaki, 2002, p. 5). Given their high risk behaviors, more efforts must be made to effectively educate street children about the dangers of HIV/AIDS. It is disturbing that some studies have found that high risk practices continue even when youth are aware of the potential risks (Amuyunzu-Nyamongo et al., 1999; Goulart & Madover, 1991; Luna, 1991).

Condoms are not widely used in Uganda, especially among the youth, many of whom feel invincible. Because HIV can take up to 10 or more years to manifest the symptoms of AIDS, many youth are not afraid of the disease because they have never known a young person who has died from it. Many youth are afraid that if they suggest using condoms their partners will think that they are promiscuous or that they are already infected with HIV/AIDS (Amuyunzu-Nyamongo et al., 1999; Konde-Lule et al., 1993). In addition, condoms are likely to be inaccessible to street children, who spend what limited resources they do have on food and drugs. Although condoms may be stored for distribution in local health clinics, several obstacles prevent street children from accessing these distribution centers. Two such obstacles include the shame of being perceived as promiscuous and the fear of having a parent, family member, or friend find out that he or she is using condoms (implying the notion of illicit sexual activity). Making condoms available to youth, including street children, is a controversial topic in Uganda today; many believe that this will only encourage immoral sexual habits ultimately leading to societal decay.

PROGRAMS TO HELP STREET CHILDREN

Despite its many challenges, Uganda is working to steadily improve the living standards of its people and become an example of success in SSA. Politically, the future holds the promise of transition from a dictatorship to a fledgling democracy. Economically, Uganda is trying to escape the title of "least developed" and push itself toward the level of "middle-income" countries. Socially, it is striving for high ideals such as gender equality, legal justice, and education for all.

As part of the efforts to improve social conditions in the country, NGOs and government agencies are working to improve the situation of street children. Despite implementing different development strategies, 17

NGOs working with street children in the Kampala area have been meeting together for the past few years to try to coordinate efforts and learn from each other (Williams, 2002). Along with this successful inter-NGO network in Kampala, the Jinja Network for the Marginalized Child and Youth was formed in 2002 to bring together NGOs and local government officials to help street children in Uganda's second largest city (Malcomson, Kulaba, & Obbo, 2003). Munene and Nambi (1996) characterize many effective NGO programs:

> Successful interventions employ four main strategies including befriending the children and building trust between them and the change agent; reclaiming them from the street by getting them interested in spending less and less of their wakeful and active hours on the street while gradually introducing them to alternative lifestyles; rehabilitating the children by providing them with resources to live like normal members of society; and finally, resettling them by assisting them to return to mainstream society without assistance from the change agent. (p. 348)

Specifically addressing the problem of HIV/AIDS among street children is a program by an international NGO called GOAL, which operates in conjunction with 12 local NGOs[1] in five districts of Uganda. This project, called Baaba, the first of its kind in Uganda, was initiated in 2001.[2] The project takes selected street youth and trains them in HIV/AIDS and sexual health issues, along with participatory teaching methods. To date, over 360 Baabas have been trained. The Baabas act as peer educators, teaching what they have learned to other street children and to the community at large (GOAL, 2004; Nyakake, 2004). Teaching is often done through roleplays, drama, song, dance, and poetry. Other activities include clubs, seminars, counseling, and condom distribution, as well as day and night outreaches. These efforts have been very successful because in Uganda stories, dramas, and roleplays are often viewed as culturally effective ways of communicating new ideas. Using drama festivals, the NGOs have taken HIV/AIDS prevention messages to the wider community and also helped disseminate positive publicity to participating street children. The program helps to provide self-esteem instead of dependency for street youth and gives them the confidence to succeed in other areas of life. The NGOs also work to bring together health service providers and others to improve street children's access to sexual health services as well as encourage further research into the sexual knowledge and behaviors of street children (GOAL, 2004; Nyakake, 2004).

In relation to street children, UNESCO (1995, p. 303) urges that "it is only by strong commitment from governments in identifying or combating the underlying causes, and in the implementation and financing of preventive and rehabilitation measures, that valid solutions will really be created." Anarfi (1999) further suggests that it is "absolutely necessary to get (them) [street children] out of the street if we are to effect any meaningful change in them" (p. 89). Taking this advice, the government of Uganda is striving to take an active role in the issue of street children. After months of deliberation, in May 2002 the Ministry of Gender, Labor, and Social Development (MGLSD), together with several local NGOs working with street children, embarked on an ambitious program to collect and resettle children living on the streets of the capital city Kampala. (For a more detailed discussion of this program, see Jacob et al, 2004.) Over a period of a few nights, children living on the streets of the city were collected by police and transported to a youth correction facility on Masaka road, called the Kampiringisa National Rehabilitation Center (hereafter Kampiringisa). Although the facility is generally used to house youth offenders, a wing of the facility has been set aside for the street children. It was found that 80% of the children did have some family, and plans were set up for resettlement of these children. The government also provided a resettlement package including a mattress, blanket, hoe, basin, and 100,000 Ugandan shillings (UGS).[3]

In the summer of 2003 several street children from Jinja, the second largest city in Uganda, were also taken to the facility. In the future, instead of housing children at Kampiringisa, the Jinja Network hopes to build its own secured facility to complement a small transit center that it currently operates (Malcomson et al., 2003).

After the first year of operation, 973 street children had been taken to Kampiringisa. Of these, 198 had been taken by their parents, 533 had been resettled with their families, 16 refused to go back to their families, and 177 had run away. Of those who ran away, 79 had been reinstigated into the program. As of June 2003, there were 53 street boys and 11 street girls at the facility. There were also 42 juvenile offenders at the facility (Kampiringisa, 2003).

Given the complexities governments face to effectively deal with the issue of street children, the proactive approach of the Ugandan government and its efforts to create partnerships among many organizations are admirable. One of the greatest accomplishments of the program was taking the children off the streets and giving them a chance to change their lives. The public in general also benefited from a decreased danger level on the streets of Kampala, as many street children are involved in theft and other public crimes. The program may further provide a disincentive for children to come to the streets in the future. The cooperation between government agencies and NGOs sets a positive precedent for future coordination in tackling other social problems (Jacob et al., 2004).

However, several NGOs condemned the use of coercion in trying to get the street children to change their lives. Many worry that the "criminalization of the child has been the traditional criterion of a round up mentality. The assumption is that every street child is so because of deviancy rather than being a victim of family dysfunction" (Malcomson, 2003, p. 5). Often the desire to change is a prerequisite for lasting change to occur. Street children need "mostly their own willpower" to instigate change in their own lives (Hecht, 1998, p. 186). Many argue that the government-led initiative is problematic by forcing street children to participate in the program (Jacob et al., 2004).

The use of a youth correction facility—particularly one with very negative associations among the population at large—to house the children together with youth offenders was also criticized by many people involved in the program. The facility itself was in poor condition, not adequately equipped to effectively help the hundreds of street children who were brought there (Jacob et al., 2004; Rukundo, 2002). This problem has since been addressed, and the facilities at Kampiringisa have been much improved. Kampala-based NGOs now have people on-site to provide counseling and other services to the children, and the World Food Program has stepped in to provide adequate meals. While the government still pays staff salaries, many local businesses as well as international organizations have participated in improving the facility (Rukundo, 2004).

Political commitment and government funding are vital to the continued success of the program. Recently the Ugandan Minister of Gender, Labor and Social Development, Zoe Bakoko Bakoru, pledged that the Ugandan government would spend U.S.$56 million to educate street children in the country (Uganda to Spend 56 Million Dollars to Educate Street Children, 2003).

Lasting change requires more than one government program or participation of many committed NGOs. Children will not stop coming to the streets until the root causes of their leaving home are addressed. Some NGO workers report that many (perhaps half) of the children resettled through the program have run away because the underlying issues of poverty that initially made them leave home have not been sufficiently addressed (Rukundo, 2004). According to the Independent Commission on International Humanitarian Issues (1986),

> It is one thing to prevent the occurrence of individual events, like accidents or lawbreaking, but another to prevent the emergence of a general condition. To prevent the marginalization of children, the marginalization of women and communities must also be prevented. Before the stresses of survival in slum conditions cause the breakdown of the family, problems must be tackled at their source ... street children are the end-product of a long chain of innumerable causes and effects, and can themselves be seen as a cause of further effects, such as delinquency and violence. The further one

goes back from the child himself, the more tenuous the causal link. (pp. 85–86)

To fully address the problems of street children, society as a whole must be reformed.

As the number of orphans and street children in Africa continues to escalate, due largely to the spread of the HIV/AIDS epidemic that is ravaging the continent, the problems that these children face will become ever more pressing. A generation of children raising themselves in Africa has stark implications, not only for the future of the continent but for the future of humanity. With a natural creativity, facility in trading and business, and rich natural resources, Africa has the potential for a bright future. However, this future will only be realized if policies and programs are enacted today to ensure opportunities for vulnerable children. Efforts must be made today to reclaim this lost generation.

NOTES

1. Organizations include Katwe Youth Development Association (KAYDA); Dwelling Places; Buddukiro Children's Agency; Tigers Club; An Open Door; Bambejja Project/Oasis; Kids in Need (KIN), Kisenyi; Kids in Need (KIN), Nansana; Adolescent Development Support Network (ADSN); Child Restoration Outreach (CRO), Jinja; Child Restoration Outreach (CRO), Mbale; and Child Restoration Outreach (CRO), Masaka.
2. In Luganda, a *Baaba* is an older sibling who counsels and gives advice.
3. In May 2002, UGS 1,750 equaled U.S.$1.

	Appendix:	Organizations Working With Street Children			
Organization Name	District	Contact Person	Phone*	Email	Road
Buyengo child and family project	Busia	Ojiambo James	077-420637		
Odongkara children's home	Gulu	Abitimo Odongkara	077-580687		Moroto Rd
Unity vocational training school	Gulu	Director	077-473524		5 Tank Rd
Adolescent development support network	Jinja	Mary Kafuko	077-642656		Spire Rd
Child restoration outreach-Jinja	Jinja	Harriet Obbo	043-121191	cro-jinja@source.co.ug	Oboja Rd
St. Mugagga boys home	Jinja	Wasswa Pual			Rubaga Rd
Africa evangelistic enterprises-Uganda	Kampala	Ephraim Gensi	041-250386	aee@imul.com	Berkely Rd
Africa foundation	Kampala		041-290528		P.O. Box 4100
An open door	Kampala	Diane Pardoe	041-272187	anodu@infocom.co.ug	Sentema Rd
Ambassadors of hope	Kampala	Lubwama Robinah	041-532225	ambhope@starcom.co.ug	Nanfumbambi Rd
British council voices of street children project	Kampala		041-234725	bc.kampala@bc-kampala.swiftuganda.com	P.O. Box 7070
Child welfare and adoption society	Kampala	Francis Mbayire	041-510224	babiea@utl.co.ug	Nsambya Church Rd
Companionship of work association (COWA)	Kampala		041-286932		P.O. Box 6785
Cornerstone Dev't Ltd	Kampala	Tim Kreutter	041-251911	cstone@imul.com	Acacia Avenue
FOCA	Kampala	Tumuheirwe Juliet M	041-236156	foca@infocom.co.ug	Old Kampala Rd
Give me a chance	Kampala	Kenneth Kamese	041-270122	achance@starcom.co.ug	Musajjalumbwa Rd
GOAL Uganda	Kampala	Mark Adams	041-266742	reception@goaluganda.com	P.O. Box 33140
Kampala city council	Kampala		041-231440		
Kamwokya Christian caring community	Kampala		041-532600		P.O. Box 25432
Katwe Youth development association	Kampala		041-230903		P.O. Box 10741

Organization	City	Contact person	Phone	Email	Address
Kids in need	Kampala	Christopher Wakiraza	041-271009	kin@infocom.co.ug	Rugaba Rd
Methel Kawempe children's center	Kampala	Lawrence Kalule	075-628195		Kawempe-Lugoba Rd
Ministry of gender, labor and social development (street children's desk)	Kampala	Sam Acou Ogojoi	041-258686		P.O. Box 7136
National council for children (NCC)	Kampala		041-232311		P.O. Box 21456
Rainbow house of hope Uganda	Kampala	Geoffery Tumusiime	077-489224	rhhumail@yahoo.com	Kabega Estate Rd
Rubaga youth development association	Kampala	Geoffrey Kyeyune	041-271129	ryda.org@infocom.co.ug	Kisingiri Rd
Tiger's club project	Kampala	Andy Williams	041-342220	tigers@starcom.co.ug	Mengo Hill Rd
Uganda youth anti-AIDS association	Kampala	Edward Baligonzaki	041-259397	uyaas@infocom.co.ug	Bombo Rd
Uganda youth development link	Kampala	Rogers Kasirye	041-530353	kasiryer@yahoo.com	Sir Apollo Kaggwa Rd
Voluntary workers organization	Kampala	Mark Mugerwa	041-273180	uoschool@yahoo.com	Butikiro Rd
Youth adults association	Kampala		041-530098		P.O. Box 24936
Buddukiro children agency	Masaka	Priyl Jones	077-519953		
Child restoration outreach-Masaka	Masaka		045-33382		P.O. Box 1610
UWESO Masindi branch	Masindi	Prossy Isingoma	077-660495		
Child care and family rehabilitation	Mbale		045-33160		Malukhu Rd
Child restoration outreach Uganda	Mbale	Christine Kamiti		cro_ug@infocom.co.ug	Biship Wasikye Rd
Elim Pentecostal temples of the Lord ministries	Mbale	James Kakonya	077-454676	mbalecitytemple@yahoo.com	Makukhu Rd
Watenga childcare center	Mbale	John Mukhwana	077-569073	cjgmukhwana@yahoo.com	Bududda Rd
Kagarama Entunguka women's club	Mbarara	P. Rutahwaire	077-571433		Kagarama Nyakitunda Rd
Simu family helper project	Sironko	Namunyali Nuhu	078-260070	ccf@ccf.or.ug	Buluganya Rd
Bweya children's home	Wakiso	John Kiwanuka	041-200239	homebwey@yahoo.com	Old Entebbe Rd
Voluntary workers organization	Wakiso	Hassan Kateera	075-445555	tawhidorphan@yahoo.com	Ndejje Rd

*For calls from outside of Uganda, dial 256 and drop the first zero of the given number.

REFERENCES

Amuyunzu-Nyamongo, M., Tendo-Wambua, L., Babishangire, B., Nyagero, J., Yit-barek, N., Mataha, M., & Omurwa, T. (1999). Barriers to behaviour change as a response to STD including HIV/AIDS: The East African experience. In J. Caldwell, P. Caldwell, J. Anarfi, K. Awusabo-Asare, J. Ntozi, I. Orubuloye, J. Marck, W. Cosford, R. Colombo, & E. Hollings. (Eds.), *Resistances to behavioral change to reduce HIV/AIDS infection in predominantly heterosexual epidemics in Third World countries*. Canberra: Health Transition Centre, National Centre for Epidemiology and Population Health, Australian National University.

Anarfi, J. K. (1999). Initiating behavioural change among street-involved youth: Findings from a youth clinic in Accra. In J. Caldwell, P. Caldwell, J. Anarfi, K. Awusabo-Asare, J. Ntozi, I. Orubuloye, J. Marck, W. Cosford, R. Colombo, & E. Hollings. (Eds.), *Resistances to behavioral change to reduce HIV/AIDS infection in predominantly heterosexual epidemics in Third World countries*, Canberra: Health Transition Centre National Centre for Epidemiology and Population Health, Australian National University.

Appleton, S., Emwanu, T., Kagugube, J., & Muwonge, J. (1999). *Changes in poverty in Uganda, 1992–1997: Paper series.* England: Centre for the Study of African Economies, University of Oxford.

Baligonzaki, E. M. (2002, February). *Street children/youth and HIV/AIDS in Uganda: A case of the Uganda Youth Anti-AIDS Association.* Paper presented at the East and Southern African Civil Society Forum on Promoting and Protecting the Rights of Street Children, Nairobi, Kenya.

Caldwell, J., Orubuloye, I. O., & Caldwell, P. (1999). Obstacles to behavioural change to lessen the risk of HIV infection in the African AIDS epidemic: Nigerian research. In J. Caldwell, P. Caldwell, J. Anarfi, K. Awusabo-Asare, J. Ntozi, I. Orubuloye, J. Marck, W. Cosford, R. Colombo, & E. Hollings. (Eds.), *Resistances to behavioral change to reduce HIV/AIDS infection in predominantly heterosexual epidemics in Third World countries.* Canberra: Health Transition Centre, National Centre for Epidemiology and Population Health, Australian National University.

Consortium for Street Children. (2002, February). *A civil society forum for East and Southern Africa on promoting and protecting the rights of street children.* Nairobi, Kenya: Author.

English, A. (1991). Runaway and street youth at risk for HIV infection: Legal and ethical issues in access to care. *Journal of Adolescent Health, 12*(7), 504–510.

Friends of Children Association (FOCA). (1999). *Baseline survey report on street children: Save the children.* Denmark: Red Barnet through DANIDA and the International Solidarity Foundation of Finland.

Friends of Children Association (FOCA). (2002). *Girls that live and work on the streets of Kampala.* Denmark: Koegel Local Committee of Denmark through Red Barnet.

Genei, E. K. (2000). *A situation analysis on street children in Uganda.* Unpublished manuscript.

Glasser, I. (1994). *Homelessness in a global perspective.* New York: G. K. Hall.

GOAL. (2004, August). *Giving a voice to children: The Baaba Project review of peer education activities.* Kampala, Uganda: Author.

Goulart, M., & Madover, S. (1991). An AIDS prevention program for homeless youth. *Journal of Adolescent Health, 12*(7), 573–575.

Hecht, T. (1998). *At home in the street: Street children of northeast Brazil.* New York: Cambridge University Press.

Heise, L. (1991, April 21). Killing the children of the Third World. In *Street children: A global disgrace: Hearing before the select committee on hunger.* Washington, DC: U.S. House of Representatives.

Independent Commission on International Humanitarian Issues. (1986). *Street children: A growing urban tragedy.* London: Weidenfeld and Nicolson.

Jacob, W. J., Smith, T. D., Hite, S. J., & Cheng, S. Y. (2004). Helping Uganda's street children: An analysis of the Model for Orphan Resettlement and Education (MORE). *Journal of Children and Poverty, 10*(1), 3–22.

Kampiringisa National Rehabilitation Centre. (2003). *Street children and Kampiringisa National Rehabilitation Centre children on order* [Bulletin]. Mpigi, Uganda: Author.

Kilbride, P., Suda, C., & Njeru, E. (2000). *Street children in Kenya: Voices of children in search of a childhood.* Westport, CT: Berlin and Garvey.

Konde-Lule, J.K., Musagara, M., & Musgrave, S. (1993). Focus group interviews about AIDS in Rakai District of Uganda. *Social Science and Medicine: An International Journal, 37*(5), 679–684.

Luna, G. C. (1991). Street youth: Adaptation and survival in the AIDS decade. *Journal of Adolescent Health, 12*(7), 551–514.

Malcomson, T. (2003). *Removal, rehabilitation and resettlement of full-time street children.* Paper presented for the Jinja network for the marginalized child and youth, Jinja, Uganda.

Malcomson, T., Kulaba, B., & Obbo, H. (2003). Interview by T. D. Smith, Jinja, Uganda, 20 June 2003. Malcomson is the Chairperson, Jinja Transit Centre for Full-time Street Children; Kulaba is the Assistant Town Clerk, Social Welfare—Jinja Municipal Council; and Obbo is the Project Manager, Child Restoration Outreach—Jinja.

Meursing, K. (1999). Barriers to sexual behaviour change after an HIV diagnosis in SSA. In J. Caldwell, P. Caldwell, J. Anarfi, K. Awusabo-Asare, J. Ntozi, I. Orubuloye, J. Marck, W. Cosford, R. Colombo, & E. Hollings (Eds.), *Resistances to behavioral change to reduce HIV/AIDS infection in predominantly heterosexual epidemics in Third World countries.* Canberra: Health Transition Centre, National Centre for Epidemiology and Population Health, Australian National University.

Ministry of Finance, Planning and Economic Development (MFPED). (2003). *Uganda poverty status report.* Kampala, Uganda: Author.

Ministry of Gender, Labour, and Social Development (MGLSD). (1999). *Practice guidelines for work with street children in Uganda.* Kampala, Uganda: Author.

MGLSD. (2001). *Training manual for practitioners working with street children in Uganda.* Kampala, Uganda: Author.

Munene, J. C., & Nambi, J. (1993). *Operational research on street chil*dren. Unpublished manuscript.

Munene, J. C., & Nambi, J. (1996). Understanding and helping street children in Uganda. *Community Development Journal: An International Forum, 31*(4), 343–350.

Nandawula, J. (2002, February 19). Orphan crisis in Uganda. *World Vision International.* Retrieved January 2, 2006, from http://www.wvi.org/wvi/archives/africa/uganda.htm

Nyakake, M. (2004). Personal communication with Troy D. Smith, Provo, Utah to Kampala, Uganda. Nyakake is a member of the Baaba Project Team for GOAL Uganda, Kampala, Uganda. Nyakake is a member of the Baaba Project Team for GOAL Uganda, Kampala, Uganda.

Raffaelli, M, Campos, R., Merritt, A. P., Siqueira, E., Antunes, C. M., Parker, R., Greco, M., Greco, D., Halsey, N., & The Street Youth Study Group. (1993). Sexual practices and attitudes of street youth in Belo Horizonte, Brazil. *Social Science and Medicine: An International Journal, 37*(5), 661–670.

Rotheram-Borus, M. J., & Koopman, C. (1991). Sexual risk behaviors, AIDS knowledge, and beliefs about AIDS among runaways. *American Journal of Public Health, 81*(5), 208–210.

Rukundo, C. (2002, July 12). Interview with T. D. Smith, Kampala, Uganda. Rukundo is the director of the Street Children Programme for Cornerstone Development, Kampala, Uganda. Rukundo is the director of the Street Children Programme for Cornerstone Development, Kampala, Uganda.

Rukundo, C. (2004, June 7). Personal correspondence with T. D. Smith, from Kampala, Uganda to Provo, Utah.

Uganda to spend 56 million dollars to educate street children. (2003, December 22). *Xinhua News Agency-CEIS.*

UNAIDS. (2002). *Young people and HIV/AIDS: Opportunity in crisis.* Geneva, Switzerland: Author.

UNESCO. (1995). *Working with street children: Selected case-studies from Africa, Asia and Latin America.* Paris: UNESCO/International Catholic Child Bureau.

UNICEF. (2002a). Orphans and other children affected by HIV/AIDS. New York: Author.

UNICEF. (2002b). *State of the world's children 2003.* New York: Author.

UNICEF. (2002c). *Young people and HIV/AIDS.* New York: Author.

USAID/UNICEF/UNAIDS. (2002). *Children on the brink 2002: A joint report on orphan estimates and program strategies.* Washington, DC: Author.

Vélis, J. P. (1995). *Blossoms in the dust: Street children in Africa.* Paris: UNESCO.

Wiehler, S. (2002). An examination of the "Pull Factors" affecting Kampala's street children and the shape of a comprehensive solution. In J. Lugalla & C. G. Kibassa (Eds.), *Poverty, AIDS, and street children in East Africa* (pp. 235–58). Lewiston, NY: Edwin Mellen Press.

Williams, A. (2002, August 26). Interview by T. D. Smith, Kampala, Uganda. Williams is the project director for the Tiger's Club Project, Kampala, Uganda.

CHAPTER 14

FROM RECOVERY TO CATASTROPHE

A Comparative Look at the Orphan Crises in Uganda and South Africa

Christopher B. Meek and W. Joshua Rew

INTRODUCTION

Whether it is conflict, poverty, or HIV/AIDS, the African continent has either experienced such a calamity or is currently experiencing a combination or a mutable form of it. The direct and indirect wreckage left behind from such calamities takes the form of shattered economies, severe poverty, racial and ethnic inequalities, and disintegrated and displaced families. While some individuals may live through such calamities unscathed, the unfortunate reality is that entire families seldom do. In such circumstances, families are torn apart as the father becomes a combatant, the mother dies from AIDS, and the children are left in a state of malnutrition and orphanhood. As calamities such as conflict and poverty are partial and confined to specific geographical regions within and between African countries, HIV/AIDS permeates all countries and affects

Overcoming AIDS: Lessons Learned from Uganda, 275–300
Copyright © 2006 by Information Age Publishing
All rights of reproduction in any form reserved.

every family. Moreover, the HIV/AIDS pandemic, alone or accompanied by additional calamities, magnifies the precarious impact already exerted on families. The direct consequence of HIV/AIDS on the family is the death of the parent, the caregiver, or the child; however, the indirect and perhaps more devastating consequence is orphanhood (Preble, 1990).

A substantial amount of literature has documented the devastating impact that HIV/AIDS has on orphanhood in Africa (Bicego, Rutstein, & Johnson, 2003; Hunter & Williamson, 2000; Meier, 2003; Preble, 1990; UNAIDS/UNICEF/USAID, 2004; UNICEF, 1999, 2003a, 2003b). Amongst this literature, many studies have examined orphanhood in countries where the orphan crisis is most acute such as the cases of Uganda and South Africa (Bennell, Hyde, & Swainson, 2002; Bradshaw, Hunter, 1990; Jacob, Smith, Hite, & Cheng, 2004; Johnson & Dorrington, 2001; Johnson, Schneider, Bourne, & Dorrington, 2002; Ntozi, 1997; Sengendo & Nambi, 1997). The orphan crises in Uganda and South Africa are not new phenomena. Orphanhood is pedestrian to Uganda and South Africa because of the nearly 30 years of civil war in Ugandan and the 46 years of apartheid in South Africa. What makes the current situation for each distinct from the past is the notion that the majority of children have become orphans due to HIV/AIDS as an alternative to conflict, poverty, or apartheid.

Although both Uganda and South Africa are considered to have acute orphan crises, it is argued in this chapter that the orphanhood trends for each country are headed in opposing directions. This chapter comparatively examines the orphanhood trends for Uganda and South Africa, and concludes that while both are considered crises, only orphanhood trends in Uganda appear to be improving. In addition, this chapter acknowledges that while orphanhood in Uganda has and is projected to substantially improve and orphanhood in South Africa appears to be worsening at catastrophic rates, the outcomes of orphanhood in each country are appalling and deserve discussion. Therefore, these outcomes are discussed, and in light of the orphanhood trends in each country, priority areas are outlined and recommendations are made as to reduce orphanhood in Uganda and South Africa and forestall its horrific outcomes.

BACKGROUND TO HIV/AIDS IN UGANDA AND SOUTH AFRICA

Uganda and South Africa present similar but distinct backgrounds with respect to HIV/AIDS. The first Ugandan and South African AIDS cases were recorded in 1982. However, the first AIDS cases in Uganda were identified among Black heterosexuals and the first AIDS cases in South

Africa were identified among White homosexuals. While HIV/AIDS in Uganda continues to be a heterosexual pandemic, HIV/AIDS in South Africa is now found throughout all segments of the population, especially in Black male and female heterosexual youths and adults. As both countries became centers of crisis regarding HIV/AIDS during the 1980s and 1990s, each initially responded in distinct manners which produced the polar extremes of recovery and catastrophe. These distinct manners along with the resulting outcomes are discussed below.

HIV/AIDS in Uganda: Recovery

The HIV/AIDS crisis in Uganda occurred as the civil war between the National Resistance Movement (NRM) and former regimes ended in 1986. With the end of the conflict and the establishment of the NRM government, 1986 marked the beginning of government intervention and response to the HIV/AIDS pandemic. By 1992, the Uganda AIDS Commission (UAC) was established to coordinate multi-sector efforts to address the disease (UAC, 2001). That same year, HIV prevalence peaked at 30% in urban areas and began to decline (UAC, 2001). Since the initial outbreak, Uganda has aggressively counteracted HIV/AIDS as can be seen in the reduction of HIV prevalence rates from 18.5% in 1995, to 8.3% in 1999, and to 4.1% in 2003 (Meier, 2003; UAC, 2001; UNAIDS/WHO, 2004). Uganda's actions to curb the spread of HIV/AIDS and recover from its devastation gained international attention and acclaim. These actions are attributable to the following: (1) the end of the civil war and the establishment of a stable government; (2) immediate government action to address and respond to HIV/AIDS; and (3) progressive action by top-level leadership including the President of Uganda, Yoweri K. Museveni.

HIV/AIDS in South Africa: Catastrophe

The HIV/AIDS crisis in South Africa occurred in the middle 1980s, a decade before apartheid ended. Although the outbreak led to a relatively quick response with the formation of an AIDS advisory group appointed by the government in 1985, the response was severely hindered by both the hostile relationship between the White-dominated government and the Black population as well as the government's very limited understanding of the nature of the disease and the causes of its transmission among affected populations. By 1990, South Africa had 48,818 HIV positive cases (Dorrington, Bradshaw, & Budlender, 2002). In 1992, the first official government response to HIV/AIDS was taken when Nelson Mandela addressed the newly-formed National AIDS Convention of South Africa (NACOSA). However, this official response represented little in terms of specific actions to be taken, and this was the state of affairs for several years to follow. In 1995, a year after apartheid ended, the number of HIV positive cases had substantially increased to 1,203,847, and by 2003, this number had increased to 7,027,931 HIV positive cases (Dorrington et al., 2002). According to Fredriksson and Kanabus (2004), it is estimated that as many as 600 people died daily in South Africa in 2003 due to HIV/AIDS. Fortunately but rather belated, the HIV/AIDS pandemic is projected to peak in South Africa by 2006 with an estimated 7.7 million HIV positive cases, and is projected to decline to 7.2 million HIV positive cases by 2010 (Dorrington et al., 2002). South Africa's inaction and unresponsiveness with respect to HIV/AIDS not only fueled the crisis but transformed a potential biological threat to a national catastrophe in 5 years. The factors that attributed to the inaction and unresponsiveness are the following: (1) the apartheid and postapartheid reconstruction environment; (2) government impassiveness and indolence; (3) the cultural and sexual attitudes, stigmas, and myths of the populace including that of rape, child sex abuse, and the extreme shame for publicly admitting HIV infection; and (4) the facetious, venal, and ignorant attitude and knowledge regarding HIV/AIDS, its causes, its transmission, and its resolution by top-level government leadership including but not limited to the President of South Africa, Thabo Mbeki.

Initially, the apparent outbreak of HIV/AIDS led to a relatively quick response with the formation of an AIDS Advisory Group appointed by the government in 1985. However, the potential for successful intervention by this group was sharply limited by the hostile relationship between the White-dominated government and the majority Black population as well as the government's very limited undertanding of the natue of the disease and the causes of its transmission among the most affected populations.

Antenatal testing in 1994 yielded nearly a doubling of prevalence rates at 7.6% compared to the 4.3% rate reported in 1993. Consequently, the Minister of Health officially adopted what was called the NACOSA strategy as the foundation for the government's AIDS intervention plan. However, many activists, public health experts, and politicians complained that the plan was disorganized and not rigorously thought through. This South African organization aimed at producing a number of media based public service announcements and television commercials to educate the population about a variety of health issues including HIV/AIDS and derivative health problems such as tuberculosis.

A brief but important boost, in concern with the HIV/AIDS problem, was created when South Africa hosted the 1996 International Conference for People Living with HIV and AIDS. This was the first time that the annual conference had been held anywhere in Africa. Then Deputy President, Thabo Mbeki, also finally acknowledged the seriousness of the HIV/AIDS epidemic in South Africa, however, it also became clear that he held the strange belief that no connection existed between HIV and AIDS. This viewpoint would ultimately become a very serious impediment to adoption of an urgent and effective treatment of HIV/AIDS and for protecting unborn fetuses from contracting HIV.

In 1996, the South African Ministry of Health also began to release statistics on the rapid spread of HIV/AIDS throughout the heterosexual population. The Ministry of Health estimated that some 850,000 people, approximately 2.1% of South Africa's population, were infected. It was also estimated that 8% of all pregnant women were becoming infected with this rate rapidly rising with no end in sight.

The prevalence rate rose to 17.0% in 1997 and 22.8% in 1998. At this point, the government finally decided to launch a new campaign called the Partnership against AIDS. At this time he also announced the alarming fact that 1,500 new HIV infections were being contracted daily. However, he also continued to stubbornly cling to his belief that HIV did not lead to AIDS, but, rather, AIDS is caused by widespread poverty and the resultant poor sanitation and nutrition it creates.

In 1998, a political pressure group, and eventually class-action lawsuit group, was formed called Treatment Action Campaign (TAC) (Fredriksson & Kanabus, 2004). In this year it also became apparent that rape and sexual assault were significantly contributing to the spread of HIV/AIDS with 49,280 incidents occurring in that year alone. Many rape and child sexual abuse cases were the result of myths and urban legends spread by South African traditional healers, called *nsangomas*, who claimed that men who had sexual intercourse with a virgin would be cured of their HIV/AIDS infection. In its most devastating form, the myth held that having sexual intercourse with 100 virgins would completely cure HIV/AIDS. This belief thus created an incentive for men to behave in ways that accelerated the spread of HIV and, therefore, also increasing the extent to which children would either die from AIDS or become orphans because of it. Sexual attacks on young females and even new born infants also began to increase due to these myths.

In 1999 the HIV/AIDS prevalence rate was 22.4%. However, the national government started to take the epidemic more seriously by distributing over 160 million free condoms and initiating a public relations and educational campaign called Lovelife. Lovelife involved the development and implementation of educational curricula dealing with sex and protecting oneself from HIV infections at the secondary level as well public service commercials on television, radio, and bill boards. As a result of this program the term condomize for safe sex became popularly known and used throughout South Africa.

In 2000 the prevalence rate rose to 24.5%. The International AIDS Conference was held in Durban, South Africa. Unfortunately, the newly elected President, Thabo Mbeki, was still openly arguing that AIDS is a disease that is caused by poverty and not by HIV. Because of this stance, Mbeki justified a policy of refusing to allow the treatment of AIDS patients with anti-retroviral drugs. Moreover, it was declared illegal for doctors to prescribe nevirapine to pregnant women in order to reduce the chances of them passing on the virus to their fetus.

In line with his anti-mainstream opinions, President Mbeki set up a group charged with solving the country's AIDS problems which included such "HIV dissidents" as Peter Duesberg, who dogmatically argued that anti-AIDS drugs, such as AZT, actually caused AIDS rather than treating the disease and reducing the debilitating symptoms. Duesberg, and other members of the committee, believed that lifestyle choices such as homo-sexuality and drug addiction were the cause of AIDS in spite of the large and growing number of HIV/AIDS-infected individuals who were strictly heterosexual and had never been illegal drug users much less addicts. The committee's work also resulted in the promulgation of laws and regu-lations that made it illegal for physicians to prescribe or give pregnant women nevirapine, and, if they were caught doing so, then they would lose their licenses and serve jail time.

In May of 2000 the government also completed a 5-year strategic plan for dealing with HIV/AIDS in South Africa (AIDS Helpline, 2000). The plan laid out a description of the progression of the disease between 1990 and 1999, discussed problems and limitations related to prior responses, and it created a plan involving a complex set of inter-locking committees and task forces ranging from the President and his cabinet all the way down to local and provincial leaders. The plan also produced a lengthy set of goals and objectives under specific dimensions called "Priority Areas" including promoting safe and healthy sexual behavior, improving the management and control of sexually transmitted diseases, reducing mother-to-child HIV transmission, research, monitoring and surveillance, and human rights (AIDS Helpline, 2000). Unfortunately, this elaborate strategic plan was severely limited by, firstly, the complex and elaborate system required to coordinate all of the many councils, committees and task forces created as well as a wide array of priority areas set to address and numerous goals and objectives laid out under each and, secondly, the government's adamant position against the use of any anti-retroviral and other drugs for treating or blocking the transmission of HIV/AIDS. Fur-thermore, all of the strategic plan's goals and activities focused solely on preventing the further spread of the disease and not the treatment of those individuals who had already contracted it. No part of the plan what-soever addressed the issue of HIV/AIDS orphans resulting from the disease which had already established an incredibly strong foothold in South Africa. Thus, here, two decades into the evolution and growth of the HIV/AIDS epidemic, no plan nor organization had been established to address the growing population of orphans being produced by the deadly disease, and the government was stuck in a stalemate between legislators and HIV/AIDS activists who believed anti-retroviral drugs should be made available immediately and the President and his committee who were blocking such actions.

Unfortunately, with so much attention having been devoted to creating new local governmental entities and jurisdictions, and the majority of educational programs, both governmental and private, being focused from the national level, or else carried out by very small NGOs in the provinces, then virtually no government planning or capacity building has been developed to this date on a national or local governmental level for dealing with the increasing numbers of orphans now being produced by the HIV/AIDS epidemic. Virtually all responses to providing resources and care for children who become paternal, maternal or double orphans as a result of their parents becoming incapacitated first, and then dying from AIDS has and is solely being addressed by small religiously-owned orphanages, residential schools, and resource centers focused on assisting street children.

By 2003 antenatal testing revealed that the HIV prevalence rate had grown to 27.9%. This was a highly eventful and unusual year; for TAC campaign members embarked upon a two-pronged strategy of civil disobedience through demonstrations and litigation against government officials for what TAC called criminal behavior. Demonstrations and civil disobedience were intended to publicly shame the government into finally acting responsibly in addressing the AIDS epidemic by aggressively making AIDS drugs available to all of the nation's victims for free or very low cost depending upon their ability to pay for medication. Litigation began in March of 2003 when TAC handed over a docket of charges to the police charging the Minister of Health, Mantombazana Edmie Tshabalala-Msimang and her colleague, Alexander Erwin, the Minister of Trade and Industry, with culpable homicide. The campaign was timed to coincide with the anniversary of the Sharpville Massacre that occurred on March 21, 1961, which is known worldwide as the International Day for the Elimination of Racism (Africa Action, 2003). The reasons for TAC's actions and nature of their strategy and tactics are outlined in a statement from TAC, which was issued on March 20, 2003.

Tradition and the Spread of HIV

The actions of TAC, through this lawsuit, finally moved the government into action with respect to finally addressing the HIV/AIDS epidemic on a national scale including the intervention of making antiretroviral medication in order to both lengthen the lives of people who had already contracted the disease as well as prevent the babies of AIDS mothers from contracting the disease in utero or from mothers' breast milk. However, comprehensive planning and active intervention to address the growing population of orphans has only recently come to take place, and this makes perfect sense because until the nature and causes of HIV/AIDS had been addressed the problem of the increasing number of orphans was simply ignored and not dealt with by government action in any way at all.

Tradition, among the members of South Africa's Black ethnic groups, also presents some serious barriers to significantly reducing the spread of HIV/AIDS. This is no more clearly apparent than among the members of the Zulu tribe, the primary ethnic group in the province of Kwa-Zulu Natal which is the region that has consistently had the highest HIV/AIDS prevalence rates.

For example, among the Zulu it is expected that a young man will have proven his virility by the time he reaches his early to mid-twenties then he is considered less than a "real man" or even a "man" at all. One's male virility, or the actuality of their manliness, for many Zulu families is ascertained by whether or not their sons have fathered several illegitimate children before they actually become married. A male who has refrained from sexual intercourse before marriage, or even if they have been sexually active but have failed to father any children with different women before officially becoming married, is considered weak and unmanly or an *isishimane* in Zulu terms. An individual who has conquered several women, and fathered at least one child by each, is considered a very manly individual having demonstrated his virility, and his status is recognized by referring to him as an *isoka* (Varga, 1997).

Obviously, in such a society trying to convince men to use condoms to prevent the spread of HIV is extremely difficult, and all the different educational programs thus far undertaken by the government and private organizations has had little if any impact on changing such attitudes. This is further complicated by the fact that most adult educational programs on HIV/AIDS seem to be generally held for women and not men. Such programs promise little if any long-term success if all the responsibility for safe sex or late sex rests solely on the shoulders of women. If a woman asks a male sexual partner to use a condom, or tries to use a female condom, then the male is likely to be very strongly opposed to the suggestion.

If a man feels his reputation can only be enhanced by producing another illegitimate child, he is certainly not going to be very supportive of this idea, and this is especially true of a young man who is out to establish his virility. This situation is further complicated by the fact that if a woman suggests the use of either type of condom the male partner typically assumes that it is the woman that has contracted HIV, and she is trying to avoid spreading the disease to him. In other words, the male assumes that the female has been unfaithful to him (a clear double standard here) and even worse she has been unfaithful with a known HIV/AIDS-infected male. Such a situation can only lead to the woman being chastised and often beaten up by her male lover. Indeed, it is often seen as perfectly reasonable for a man to beat up his woman if she denies him sex when he wants it, and the criticism and social sanction fall to the female and not the man (Varga, 1997).

COMPARING CONTINENTAL, NATIONAL, AND REGIONAL TRENDS

If it is the dramatic decrease in HIV prevalence in Uganda or the rapid increase in the numbers of HIV positive persons in South Africa, the quantity of AIDS orphans will continue to increase in both countries due to the substantial lag between HIV infection and death (UNICEF, 2003a). Due to conflict and poverty, Uganda has had substantial quantities of orphans. The civil war of the 1980s, the Tanzanian invasion, the insecurity in Northern Uganda, and the poverty resulting from these conflicts have contributed to the mass displacement and disintegration of families. From the late 1960s until the late 1980s (even until now with respect to Northern Uganda), men and women have died directly and indirectly due to these conflicts leaving many children without parents, caregivers, and income producers. Likewise, South Africa has had considerable amounts of orphans due to 46 years of apartheid and the resulting poverty that was produced as a by-product of social, political, and economic segregation and inequalities. From 1948 to 1994, military police enforcement of segregation, institutional discrimination, and racial inequality led to the death and/or imprisonment of men and women, leaving their respective families and children without fathers and mothers. Although Uganda and South Africa share similarities in terms of historically having quantities of orphans, to better understand orphanhood and to determine the state and direction of the current orphan crisis in Uganda and South Africa, it is imperative to compare the continental, national, and regional trends for each.

Comparing Continental Trends

In 2001, amongst a sample of 11 Sub-Saharan African countries (see Table 14.1 for more details), Uganda had the fourth largest quantity of total orphans and orphans due to AIDS with 1,731,000 and 884,000, while South Africa had the sixth largest quantity of total orphans and the seventh largest quantity of orphans due to AIDS with 1,528,000 and 662,000 respectively (UNICEF, 2003a). Nigeria, the Democratic Republic of Congo, and Kenya had larger quantities of orphans due to AIDS in 2001, while in that same year, Nigeria, the Democratic Republic of Congo, and Tanzania had larger quantities of total orphans. In 2003, Uganda's population of orphans due to AIDS slightly increased to 940,000 but its standing among the 11 other nations decreased to the fifth largest quantity of orphans due to AIDS behind Nigeria, South Africa, Tanzania, and Zimbabwe (UNAIDS/WHO, 2004). South Africa's population of orphans due to AIDS nearly doubled from 662,000 to 1,100,000, while its standing moved from seventh in 2001 to the second largest population of orphans due to AIDS. In 2010, Uganda is projected to have the sixth largest quantity of total orphans with 1,554,000, while South Africa will have the third largest quantity of total orphans behind Nigeria and the Democratic Republic of Congo with 2,303,000 (UNICEF, 2003a). Finally, Uganda is one of two countries projected to have a percent decrease in total orphans between 2001 and 2010 with a 10% decrease accompanied by Senegal with a 2% decrease. On the other hand, South Africa is the only country projected to have a percent increase in total orphans greater than 50%, while Botswana and Zimbabwe will have percent increases greater than 30% between 2000 and 2010.

That Uganda is projected to have a 10% decrease and South Africa is projected to have a 51% increase in total orphans by 2010 points to the distinct directions each country is headed with respect to the orphan crisis. Compared to other Sub-Saharan African countries, Uganda and South Africa not only represent regional leaders in recovery and catastrophe with respect to HIV/AIDS, but it appears that this could be the case regarding orphanhood too. It is plausible that each country's previous and respective response to HIV/AIDS is an indication of its response towards orphanhood. In fact, the response to orphanhood and the subsequent result mirrors that of HIV/AIDS for Uganda and South Africa. In Uganda, the action towards HIV/AIDS and the decline of HIV/AIDS is paralleled by the action taken towards orphanhood and the subsequent projected decline. This is the same for South Africa, the inaction taken towards HIV/AIDS and the following spread of HIV/AIDS is equivalent to the inaction taken towards orphanhood and the devastating projected increase in the number of orphans.

**Table 14.1.   Total Number of Orphans and
AIDS Orphans for Selected Sub-Saharan African Countries**

Country	AIDS Orphans 2001	AIDS Orphans 2003	% Change 2001- 2003	Total Orphans 2001	Total Orphans 2010 (Projected)	% Change 2001– 2010 (Projected)
D. R. Congo	927,000	770,000	-17	2,733,000	3,268,000	20
Kenya	892,000	650,000	-27	1,659,000	2,099,000	27
Rwanda	264,000	160,000	-39	613,000	687,000	12
Uganda	884,000	940,000	6	1,731,000	1,554,000	-10
Sudan	62,000	—	—	1,190,000	1,396,000	17
Tanzania	815,000	980,000	20	1,928,000	2,152,000	12
Nigeria	995,000	1,800,000	81	5,421,000	6,686,000	23
Senegal	15,000	17,000	13	402,000	395,000	-2
Botswana	69,000	120,000	74	98,000	136,000	39
South Africa	662,000	1,100,000	66	1,528,000	2,303,000	51
Zimbabwe	782,000	980,000	25	1,018,000	1,341,000	32

Sources: Adapted from UNIADS/WHO (2004) and UNICEF (2003a).

Comparing National Trends

From 1990 to 2000, Uganda experienced a gradual national increase in orphanhood. In 1990, orphans represented 10% of all children in Uganda (this percentage is the national orphan prevalence rate). By 1995, it had increased to 13%. In 2000, the national orphan prevalence rate increased two percentage points to 15%. The 2000 value marked the peak national orphan prevalence rate. From 2000 to 2003, the national orphan prevalence rate decreased one percentage point to 14%, and by 2010, it is projected to have decreased three additional percentage points to 11%. The 2010 value is one percentage point higher than the 1990 value. Presumably, the slight decline from 2000 to 2003 and the projected decline until 2010 in national orphan prevalence rates is a possible indication of successful interventions and a continued decline to natural levels of orphanhood not attributable to HIV/AIDS.

Similar to Uganda, South Africa experienced an increase in the national orphan prevalence rate. Although South Africa had the same percent of orphans as Uganda in 1990, the increase in the national orphan prevalence rate did not occur until 2003. From 1990 to 2000, South Africa maintained virtually the same rate (10%). In 2003, the national orphan prevalence rate increased to 13%, and by 2010, it is projected that 19% of all South African children will be orphans. From 1990 to 2010, South Africa's national orphan prevalence rate will increase nine percentage points, and based on the 2010 projection, it is showing no indication of declining. South Africa's rapid and abrupt increase in the national orphan prevalence rate from 2000 to 2010 is plausibly due to government inaction and poor leadership similar to what occurred concerning HIV/AIDS, while Uganda's slow and gradual decrease from 2000 to 2010 is due to government action and intervention.

While the Ugandan national orphan prevalence rate is in a projected decline, during the same time period, the percentage of maternal and double orphans due to AIDS is projected to increase from 29.1% in 1990, to 55.3% in 2000, and to 59.1% in 2010 (see Table 14.2). The increase from 29.1% to 59.1%, a difference of 30 percentage points, over a span of 20 years not only indicates an upward trend in AIDS orphans, but it is also considerable evidence that the source of orphanhood is shifting from historically influential sources such as conflict and poverty to contemporary and highly influential sources like HIV/AIDS. The government of Uganda, as it transitioned from despotism and economic nonexistence to single party democracy and economic growth during the 1990s, naturally addressed areas such as conflict and poverty, thus, reducing the national orphan prevalence rate. However, while removing the influence of conflict and poverty, the national orphan prevalence rate due to AIDS is actually increasing as seen in the projected increase in the percentage of maternal and double AIDS orphans.

This trend, the increasing percentage of maternal and double AIDS orphans, is the same for South Africa; however, the increase is profoundly greater. In 1990, the percentage of maternal and double orphans due to AIDS was 6.4%. This was one fifth of Uganda's value for that same year. Nonetheless, by 2000, South Africa had surpassed Uganda as the percentage of maternal and double orphans due to AIDS increased to 62.1% compared to 55.3% for Uganda. The projection for 2010 indicates that South Africa will have close to twice the percentage of maternal and double AIDS orphans as Uganda (92.3% compared to 59.1%). Two critical trends emerge here regarding South Africa. First, the difference between the percentage of maternal and double AIDS orphans for 1990 and the projected percentage for 2010 is near 86 percentage points. This demonstrates a substantially rapid growth of maternal and double AIDS orphans most likely due to the simultaneously growing and destructive effect of the HIV/AIDS crisis. While Uganda's percentage of maternal and double AIDS orphans is growing, South Africa's is growing at an incomprehensi-

Table 14.2.   National Orphan and AIDS Orphan Trends for Uganda and South Africa, 1990-2010

Attributes	Uganda	South Africa
Orphans as % of all children 1990	10.0	10.0
Orphans as % of all children 1995	13.0	9.0
Orphans as % of all children 2000	15.0	10.0
Orphans as % of all children 2003	14.0	13.0
Orphans as % of all children 2010	11.0	19.0
% of maternal & double AIDS orphans 1990	29.1	6.4
% of maternal & double AIDS orphans 1995	45.5	17.3
% of maternal & double AIDS orphans 2000	55.3	62.1
% of maternal & double AIDS orphans 2005	58.0	85.0
% of maternal & double AIDS orphans 2010	59.1	92.3

Sources: Adapted from Hunter and Williams (2000) and UNAIDS/UNICEF/USAID (2004).

ble pace. Second, South Africa's 2010 projection of the percentage of maternal and double orphans due to AIDS (92.3%) indicates that the source of orphanhood will have close to completely shifted from traditional causes of orphanhood to HIV/AIDS. From 2000 to 2010, this shift is nearly twice as fast as Uganda's. To explain such a phenomenon, it is important to remember that South Africa is one of Africa's wealthiest and most developed countries. Because of this, much has been invested in the last 20 years to combat traditional causes of orphanhood such as poverty as a result of apartheid. But with the disregard for HIV/AIDS and its devastating effects due to governmental unresponsiveness and poor leadership, it appears that HIV/AIDS will soon be the leading cause of orphanhood in South Africa.

Comparing Regional Trends

Table 14.3 illustrates the regional orphan prevalence rate trends for the years 1999–2003 in Uganda's four geographic regions (Central, Eastern, Northern, and Western). These trends are divided into four cate-

Table 14.3.   Nonorphan and Orphan Prevalence Rates by Region for Uganda

Regions	Nonorphan	Maternal	Paternal	Double
1999/2000				
Uganda	84.0	3.0	9.0	3.0
Central	83.0	3.0	9.0	4.0
Eastern	90.0	2.0	6.0	2.0
Northern	86.0	4.0	10.0	2.0
Western	87.0	3.0	7.0	3.0
2002/2003				
Uganda	85.8	2.2	8.4	3.2
Central	83.7	2.9	8.8	4.1
Eastern	88.5	1.9	7.4	2.0
Northern	86.0	2.2	8.4	3.6
Western	84.8	2.2	10.0	3.3
Change (2002/2003–1999/2000)				
Uganda	+1.8	-0.8	-0.6	+0.2
Central	+0.7	-0.1	-0.2	+0.1
Eastern	-1.5	-0.1	+1.4	0.0
Northern	0.0	-1.8	-1.6	+1.6
Western	-2.2	-0.8	+3.0	+0.3

Sources: Adapted from Uganda Bureau of Statistics (2001, 2003).

gories: nonorphan, maternal orphan, paternal orphan, and double orphan. The category of double orphan signifies that the mother and father of a child are either deceased or absent. As of 1999–2000, Uganda had a nonorphan prevalence rate of 84%. The region with the highest nonorphan prevalence rate was Eastern Uganda with 90%; the region with the lowest was the Central with 83%.

In 1999–2000, Uganda had a 3% maternal, 9% paternal, and a 3% double orphan prevalence rate. Northern Uganda had the highest maternal and paternal orphan prevalence rates with 4% and 10% respectively. Again, the combination of HIV/AIDS and the devastating influence of rebel groups likely explain the Northern Region's high maternal and paternal orphan prevalence rates while the Central and Western Regions have benefited from political stability since Museveni overthrew the Milton Obote government. Central Uganda has the second largest paternal orphan prevalence rate behind Northern Uganda with 9%. The Northern Region would be expected to have the highest double orphan prevalence rates among the four regions; however, it is among the lowest with only 2%. Central Uganda has the highest double orphan prevalence rate with 4%. This figure patterns the high adult HIV prevalence rate in the region during the late 1980s and throughout much of the 1990s.

Regional orphan prevalence trends for 2002–2003 present a distinct picture from those portrayed from 1999–2000. Table 14.3 indicates that the nonorphan prevalence rate for Uganda increased 1.8 percentage points to 85.8% in 2002-2003. On the other hand, it appears that the nonorphan prevalence rate decreased for half of Uganda's regions. Both Eastern and Western Uganda decreased from 90% and 87% to 88.5% and 84.8%. The cause for these declining nonorphan prevalence rates is likely a result of HIV/AIDS and the spill-over conflict from neighboring Hutu extremist groups from Rwanda and the Democratic Republic of Congo and internal insecurity from indigenous rebel groups like the Lord's Resistance Army.

Additionally, Uganda encountered maternal and paternal orphan prevalence rates that decreased to 2.2% and 8.4% respectively. However, the double orphan prevalence rate increased to 3.2% in 2002-2003 from 3% in 1999-2000. Northern Uganda's maternal and paternal orphan prevalence rates decreased substantially from 4% and 10% to 2.2% and 8.4%. On the other hand, the double orphan prevalence rate increased from to 2.0% to 3.6%. Western Uganda experienced the largest increase of orphan prevalence rates with a paternal orphan prevalence rate of 10%. Finally, the Central Region topped all regions with maternal and double orphan prevalence rates of 2.9% and 4.1%. These orphan prevalence rates for the Central Region remained the same as 1999–2000.

South Africa, on the other hand, presents a picture of maternal orphans by province quite divergent than that of Uganda's. For Uganda, each of the four regions and Uganda itself experienced a decrease in their respective maternal orphan prevalence rate between 1999/2000 and 2002/2003. Table 14.4 displays the percent changes for the years 2000 to 2003 and 2000 to 2010 for the total number of maternal orphans, the number of maternal AIDS orphans, and the number of maternal non-AIDS orphans in each of South Africa's nine provinces and for South Africa respectively. From 2000 to 2003, the total number of maternal orphans increased by 50% for South Africa. Each of the nine provinces experienced a percent increase also during the same time period. The province with the largest percent increase was KwaZulu-Natal with 62%, and the province with the smallest percent increase was the Western Cape with 21%. Four additional provinces experienced an increase in the total number of maternal orphans of greater than 40%.

Table Percent 14.4.   Change in Maternal Orphans by Province for South Africa

Province	Percent Change 2000-2003			Percent Change 2000-2010		
	Total Maternal Orphans	Maternal AIDS Orphans	Maternal Non-AIDS Orphans	Total Maternal Orphans	Maternal AIDS Orphans	Maternal Non-AIDS Orphans
Eastern Cape	28	263	-8	237	1962	-33
Free State	42	227	-9	260	1337	-36
Gauteng	56	248	0	296	1398	-22
KwaZulu Natal	62	209	-10	325	1061	-35
Limpopo	27	248	-8	208	1686	-30
Mpumalanga	52	194	-9	260	945	-35
Northern Cape	29	298	0	214	2326	-13
North West	42	242	-6	260	1477	-28
Western Cape	21	290	+3	139	2264	-7
South Africa	50	213	-6	259	1102	-27

Source: Adapted from Dorrington et al. (2002).

With respect to the number of maternal AIDS orphans, this value has skyrocketed within each province and South Africa in general between 2000 and 2003. According to Table 14.4, the number of maternal AIDS orphans in South Africa increased by 213%. Additionally, eight out of the nine provinces experienced an increase greater than 200%. However, the only province below 200% was Mpumalanga with an increase of 194%. Essentially, because of how close 194 is to 200, it could be said that all nine provinces had maternal AIDS orphan populations that increased by a percent equal to or greater than 200%. The province with the largest percent increase between 2000 and 2003 was the Northern Cape with 298%.

As for the number of maternal non-AIDS orphans between 2000 and 2003, South Africa and six of the nine provinces experienced a decrease. South Africa experienced a decrease of 6%, and the province with the largest percent decline was KwaZulu-Natal with a 10% decline. The other five provinces with percent decreases in the number of maternal non-AIDS orphans experienced a percent decrease of 6% or greater. The province with the largest percent increase was the Western Cape with 3%. Two provinces did not have a percent increase or decrease concerning the total number of maternal non-AIDS orphans between 2000 and 2003.

Between the years 2000 and 2010, the total number of maternal orphans is projected to increase at a rate greater than the increase between 2000 and 2003. South Africa is projected to have an increase of 259%. This is 5 times greater than the value for 2000–2003. Eight of the nine provinces are projected to increase by more than 200%. The smallest projected increase in the total number of maternal orphans is the Western Cape with an increase of 139%. As it experienced the smallest decrease between 2000 and 2003, the Western Cape is projected to do so again between 2000 and 2010. While the largest increase was 62% among the provinces during 2000–2003, the largest projected increase between 2000 and 2010 is 325% from KwaZulu-Natal.

Following the projected and substantial increases of the total number of maternal orphans, between 2000 and 2010, the number of maternal AIDS orphans is projected to increase by percentages in the thousands. South Africa's total number of maternal AIDS orphans is projected to increase by 1102%. Again, this is 5 times greater than the value for 2000–2003. Among the nine provinces, Mpumalanga is projected to have the only increase less than 1,000% with 945%. Six provinces will have increases greater than 1,000%, and two provinces will have increases greater than 2,000% between 2000 and 2010. The largest projected increase in the number of maternal AIDS orphans for this time period is the Northern Cape with 2,326%.

While both the total number of maternal orphans and maternal AIDS orphans are projected to increase significantly between 2000 and 2010, the number of maternal non-AIDS orphans is projected to decrease. Between 2000 and 2010, South Africa will experience a 27% decrease in the number of maternal non-AIDS orphans, while at the provincial level, five of the nine South African provinces are projected to have decreases greater than 30%. The largest decrease will occur in the Free State with 36%. The projected provincial and national decrease in the number of maternal non-AIDS orphans signifies that the cause of orphanhood is shifting from traditional causes of orphanhood to others such as HIV/AIDS. This appears to be a logical conclusion as apartheid's influence has declined substantially allowing the former marginalized members of society access to health care, education, and employment.

Comparing Uganda and South Africa

After comparing Uganda and South Africa in terms of continental, national, and regional trends, several conclusions emerge that differentiate as well as provide evidence of strong similarities. First, according to continental, national, and regional trends, Uganda has experienced and is projected to experience a general decrease in the numbers of orphans. This cannot be said of South Africa. Evidence previously illustrated indicates that South Africa is moving in the opposite direction. As Uganda's orphan crisis is projected to improve, South Africa's orphan crisis is projected to degenerate to catastrophic levels. Second, continental, national, and regional trends provide no sign of improvement or assurance in the near future for South Africa. This is an indication of the gravity of the crisis. While Uganda is not out of the fire just yet, even with a present decline in HIV/AIDS and projections of a future decline in orphanhood, South Africa is 25 years away from considering such a state. For South Africa to reach where Uganda is projected to be, it might take 50 years and considerable changes in national policy concerning HIV/AIDS. If that does not happen, it could possibly take longer.

Third, continental, national, and regional trends indicate that a shift is occurring with respect to the cause of orphanhood. It appears that HIV/AIDS is replacing traditional causes of orphanhood in both countries. Nonetheless, this shift is occurring at distinct rates. In Uganda, HIV/AIDS has become the majority contributor to orphanhood. Conflict and poverty continue to be influential causes of orphanhood in Uganda; however, they are not as influential as HIV/AIDS. The shift from conflict and poverty to HIV/AIDS for the majority share has occurred gradually and over some time. In the case of South Africa, HIV/AIDS has rapidly and abruptly replaced nearly all competing causes of orphanhood in a short period of time. While other causes do exist, HIV/AIDS has procured a virual monopoly during a vacuum of causation. It appears that a contributing factor to this near monopoly is the unbridled and uncontrolled escalation of HIV/AIDS during the same period. Fourth, regional trends indicate that the orphan crisis and HIV/AIDS as the cause of orphanhood are distributed homogeneously within South Africa. Each South African province is experiencing similar orphan crises with projected increases in maternal AIDS orphans and decreases in non-AIDS orphans. In addition, HIV/AIDS has replaced apartheid as the central cause of orphanhood within South African provinces. On the other hand, the orphan crisis and HIV/AIDS as the cause of orphanhood are distributed heterogeneously within Uganda. Each region is experiencing a distinct orphan crisis with either decreasing nonorphan or maternal prevalence rates or increasing paternal or double orphan prevalence rates. Moreover, the cause of orphanhood for each region is distinct or is a combination of multiple causes. For example, Northern Uganda is also plagued by insecurity and poverty in addition to HIV/AIDS. All three are significant causes of orphanhood. This is not the case for Central Uganda.

OUTCOMES OF ORPHANHOOD IN UGANDA AND SOUTH AFRICA

Comparing Uganda and South Africa in terms of continental, national, and regional orphanhood trends has revealed that each country is headed in opposite directions with Uganda substantially improving and South Africa substantially deteriorating. While South Africa is currently and is projected to experienced a heightened orphan crisis, it should be noted that although declining numbers and positive projections present Uganda as a case of recovery, these numbers and projections mask the fact that orphanhood is still and will be continually problematic in Uganda whether it is 1.7 million orphans in 2001 or a decrease to 1.5 million orphans in 2010 (UNICEF, 2003a). Although each country is headed down distinct paths, one of recovery and the other of catastrophe, orphans in both countries will experience similar horrific outcomes. Therefore, the following section discusses the outcomes of orphanhood in Uganda and South Africa.

In general, orphanhood is caused by push factors such as HIV/AIDS, conflict, poverty, natural disaster, and abandonment, and pull factors including peer-influence and urbanization (Jacob et al., 2004). As previously stated, orphanhood in Uganda and South Africa is largely caused by HIV/AIDS. While the causes of orphanhood necessitate resolution for immediate and long term prevention, it is also imperative to address and alleviate the outcomes of orphanhood for immediate and short term recovery. Meier (2003) stated that, specifically referring to AIDS orphans, children who lose parents to AIDS are severely impacted medically, socially, and economically. Orphans in Uganda and South Africa experience one and possibly all four outcomes of orphanhood. These outcomes are the following: loss of parental care, extended family care, institutional care, and self-care.

Loss of Parental Care

According to Hutchinson (2001), more than likely orphans will have lost, due to various causes including HIV/AIDS, either a significant income producer such as the father or a significant caregiver such as the mother. Among a variety of outcomes and circumstances, losing the father signifies the likelihood of fewer financial resources for school fees and health care, while losing the mother represents the loss of the primary caregiver, child nurturer, and provider of social, psychological, physical, and cultural development.

The deficiency of basic education and health care are two tragic consequences of losing parental care. Ainsworth and Over (1994) and Hutchinson (2001) stated that double orphans in Sub-Saharan Africa, including countries like Uganda and South Africa, are significantly less likely to attend school and are almost twice as likely not to receive curative care as ill children with both parents alive. Additionally, Sengendo and Nambi (1997) asserted that the effect of losing one or both parents on a Ugandan children's education is brutal and disintegrating. Children that lose the income producer and the caregiver also lose the ability to pay school fees and purchase school materials and uniforms. This substantially perpetuates attendance disruption and drop out, and adversely impacts access, progression, and completion of primary and secondary education. Finally, as educational opportunities become out of reach for AIDS orphans in Uganda and South Africa, the lack of education increases the risk of infection by HIV. According to De Walque (2004), educated youth in Uganda have a greater likelihood of using condoms and visiting voluntary counseling and testing centers, and are less likely of being at risk for HIV infection.

Orphans emotionally and mentally suffer at great lengths as they watch parents die in severe pain without medical care (Bradshaw et al., 2002; Meier, 2003; Sengendo & Nambi, 1997). Considerable psychological effects, depression, and anxiety are due to losing parents, fearing of the future, experiencing HIV-related discrimination, and lacking the basic necessities for survival (Meier, 2003). A growing body of literature has discussed the major psychological effects experienced by AIDS orphans in Uganda, South Africa, and Sub-Saharan Africa (Bicego et al., 2003; Bradshaw et al., 2002; Garbus & Marseille, 2003; Hunter, 1990; Sengendo & Nambi, 1997; UNICEF, 1999, 2003a).

Extended Family Care

When both parents die or abandon their child, it is tradition in Uganda and South Africa, as well for many countries in Africa, for the extended family to assume responsibility for the orphan. This means that grandparents, aunts and uncles, and older siblings become the caregivers and income producers. Although the extended family has historically worked as an alternative to natural parents, according to Preble (1990), widespread orphanhood will cause the extended family, the traditional system of adoption, to be incapable and to have insufficient means to meet the escalating demands for child care. The HIV/AIDS epidemic in Uganda and South Africa profoundly affects how the traditional family structure is able to parent and provide for orphaned grandchildren, nieces and nephews, and brothers and sisters.

The Uganda AIDS Commission (UAC, 2002) stated that HIV/AIDS impedes the extended family from supplying children, their own or orphaned, with the basic essential needs such as education, health care, adequate food and water, shelter, and protection from abuse. This is the case for South Africa also. Ugandan and South African orphans cared for by their extended families will inevitably experience one or more of the following. First, orphans experience economic and social problems due to the lack of financial resources to cover their needs. It is probable that the orphan's extended family lives in the village under conditions insufficient to care and provide for the orphan (Ntozi, 1997). Second, orphans experience worse treatment from extended family caregivers. This could be in the form of domestic labor or the confiscation of inheritance such as land. Often orphans living with their extended family are forced to work as domestic labor to cover the costs of child care (Hunter, 1990). It is frequent that orphans lose their inheritance to uncles, aunts, or grandparents in order to compensate for childcare (UNICEF, 2003a). And third, orphans will experience the loss of another caregiver to old age and/or disease. Orphaned children in Uganda and South Africa are frequently cared for by older relatives such as grandparents that are too old and feeble to properly act as the caregiver. Additionally and tragically, the older caregivers are susceptible to death by old age, malaria, and HIV/AIDS leaving the orphan to experience the loss of another loved one (Ntozi, 1997; UNICEF, 2003a).

Institutional Care

The last line of defense other than the extended family is institutional care provided by government and nongovernment sponsored orphanages. While the intention and effort is sincere and amazing as to provide the necessary care for orphaned children, these institutions are rare and limited in reference to the ability to care for the magnitude of orphans, the isolated geographical locations, and the scarcity of resources needed to provide survival, educational, and medical care. In Uganda and South Africa, orphanages are very expensive to operate and require large amounts of resources to support education and health care facilities. The lack of financial resources restricts their power to properly be equipped and staffed. Many orphanage caregivers fear contamination by handling and caring for AIDS orphans, while many donors consider AIDS orphans a poor investment because of the inevitability of death (Preble, 1990). Because of the immense numbers, orphans lack individual care and treatment that is normally found in the home. The lack of individual care, discrimination and stigma, and the fact that many orphanages operate under poor conditions, leads many AIDS orphans to choose to leave the orphanage and live as street children. However, in areas where orphanages do not exist and the extended family is no longer capable of providing care, orphans have no choice to stay at the orphanage or not, they are forced to live on the streets to maintain survival.

Self Care

Uganda and South Africa have considerable quantities of street children. For Uganda, Jacob et al. (2004) stated that HIV/AIDS is the most influential determinant of street children. The majority of Ugandan and South African orphans on the streets are forced to the streets because, first, the child's parents have either deceased or are absent. Second, the extended family does not have the ability or the resources to care for the orphan. And third, government and nongovernment sponsored orphanages are not geographically available, no longer can provide sufficient care, or the orphan chooses to leave. While it is important to know why orphans have come to live on the streets, the conditions of Uganda's and South Africa's streets and the precarious atmosphere experienced by orphans there requires immediate consideration. Orphans living on the streets are vulnerable to some of the world's most merciless horrors including narcotic abuse, child labor, and child prostitution (Garbus & Marseille, 2003; Meier, 2003; UAC, 2002; UNICEF, 1999, 2003a).

The death of an orphan in Uganda and South Africa has the probability of occurring at each level of orphanhood. It occurs under the care of parents, extended family, and government and nongovernment care. Nevertheless, orphan mortality under the care of the streets of Kampala, Mbarara, Johannesburg, or East London is no longer a probability, it is a certainty especially when orphans experiment with harmful narcotics and are forced to labor in rock quarries, as domestic laborers, or as child prostitutes (UAC, 2002; UNICEF, 2003a). Many orphans abuse harmful narcotics as an escape from depression and the psychological scars of orphanhood, and doing so retards their decision making abilities and renders them defenseless against threats to their personal well-being. Orphans work often unpaid under brutal, harmful, and abusive conditions for food, clean water, and shelter (Garbus & Marseille, 2003; UNICEF, 2003a). More than likely the orphans working as child prostitutes will either become infected with a sexually transmitted disease such as HIV/AIDS, they will become prey to sexual predators, or possibly become sexual predators to prey on new cohorts of orphans (Garbus & Marseille, 2003; Meier, 2003; UNICEF, 1999).

Finally, orphans living on the streets are at risk of dying from illnesses considered preventable. Living conditions for orphans on the streets of Uganda and South Africa are appalling. There is no healthy food, clean water, sanitation, safe shelter, or health care. Many orphans survive by eating out of garbage cans, drinking filthy water, never bathing, defecating and urinating on the street, and sleeping in the same garbage cans where they gather food. These conditions breed dysentery and cholera, malaria, malnutrition, and ultimately orphan mortality unless treated. Tragically, while ill children with parents can be treated for malaria and dysentery or receive immunizations to fight off other illnesses, ill orphans on the street do not have the luxury of such health care and perish from what is considered preventable to nonorphans.

CONCLUSION

Considering the current state of the orphan crises, the positive and negative projections, and the horrific outcomes that orphans face, it is necessary that Uganda and South Africa design and implement policies at the national and local levels to address short term recovery and long term prevention. Both Uganda and South Africa are headed in distinct directions regarding orphanhood, and thus, it would be impossible and irrelevant to suggest universal policy recommendations that both countries could implement. In the case of Uganda and South Africa, it would be more effective to create individualized policies that recognize the current state, context, and direction of each orphan crisis. However, policy preconditions can be taken from the context of Uganda and implemented in the context of South Africa. The rationale behind the discussion of policy preconditions is the notion that the differentiating factor separating Uganda and South Africa is that presence and absence of policy preconditions. Therefore, it would be more rewarding to conclude by briefly presenting policy preconditions as a preliminary foundation to address, alleviate, and reverse the orphan crisis in South Africa based on the successes of Uganda.

Policies require specific preconditions to ensure that they can flourish and achieve their designed goals. Consistent with what occurred in Uganda, policy preconditions including open and progressive leaders, responsive and active governments, and collaboration between international, national, and nongovernmental organizations are crucial to overturning an orphan crisis. If one or more of these are absent, successful polices, no matter how perfect their design or funding, immediately become handicapped and vulnerable to failure.

Unfortunately, in the case of South Africa, the policy preconditions mentioned above were lacking during the principle stages of the orphan crisis and are vaguely present now. Changing the direction of South Africa's orphan crisis will require the full implementation of these policy preconditions. Moreover, implementation invariably will signify a change in the top level leadership's philosophy regarding the origin of AIDS, the transmission of the disease, the incessant rape and cultural stigma that occurs nationwide, the impact of HIV/AIDS on the affected and the unaffected, and the care for those affected and those left behind. When top level leadership, specifically referring to President Thabo Mbeki, begin to recognize and view HIV/AIDS and its consequences differently, not only will the national government become more active in the fight against HIV/AIDS and orphanhood, collaboration will materialize between international organizations, the national government, and nongovernmental organizations. Additionally, collaboration, especially in terms of philosophy, will allow for the effective allocation and utilization of resources in priority areas where before conflicting philosophies obstructed collaboration and the allocation and utilization of resources leaving priority areas neglected. Ultimately, the implementation of such policy preconditions will attract successful policies that will not only reduce and ameliorate the orphan crisis in South Africa, but will reduce and hopefully eliminate the predominant cause of South Africa's orphan crisis, HIV/AIDS.

REFERENCES

Africa Action. (2003). *South Africa: AIDS treatment action*. Washington, DC: Author.

AIDS Helpline. (2000). *HIV/AIDS/STD strategic plan for South Africa: 2000–2005*. Pretoria: Author.

Ainsworth, M., & Over, M. (1994). AIDS and African Development. *The World Bank Research Observer, 9*(2), 203-240.

Bennell, P., Hyde, K., & Swainson, N. (2002). *The impact of the HIV/AIDS epidemic on the education sector in Sub-Saharan Africa*. Brighton, England: Centre for International Education, University of Sussex.

Bicego, G., Rutstein, S., & Johnson, K. (2003). Dimensions of the emerging orphan crisis in Sub-Saharan Africa. *Social Science & Medicine, 56*(2003), 1235-1247.

Bradshaw, D., Johnson, L., Schneider, H., Bourne, D., & Dorrington, R. (2002). *Orphans of the HIV/AIDS epidemic: The time to act is now* (MRC policy brief). Tygerberg, South Africa: Burden of Disease Research Unit, Medical Research Council.

De Walque, D. (2004). *How does the impact of an HIV/AIDS information campaign vary with educational attainment? Evidence from rural Uganda* (WPS 3289). Washington DC: The World Bank.

Dorrington, R., Bradshaw, D., & Budlender, D. (2002). *HIV/AIDS profile for the provinces of South Africa: Indicators for 2002*. Cape Town, South Africa: Centre for Actuarial Research, University of Cape Town.

Fredriksson, J., & Kanabus, A. (2004). *HIV and AIDS in South Africa*. Horsham, England: Avert.

Garbus, L., & Marseille, E. (2003). *HIV/AIDS in Uganda*. San Francisco: University of California San Francisco.

Hunter, S. S. (1990). Orphans as a window on the AIDS epidemic in Sub-Saharan Africa: Initial results and implications of a study in Uganda. *Social Science & Medicine, 31*(6), 681-690.

Hunter, S. S., & Williamson, J. (2000). *Children on the brink: Updated estimates & recommendations for intervention (Executive summary)*. Washington DC: USAID.

Hutchinson, P. (2001). Combating illness. In Reinikka, R. & Collier, P. (Eds.), *Uganda's recovery: The role of farms, firms, and government* (pp. 407–449). Washington DC: The World Bank.

Jacob, W. J., Smith, T. D., Hite, S. J., & Cheng, S. Y. (2004). Helping Uganda's street children: An analysis of the Model for Orphan Resettlement and Education (MORE). *Journal of Children & Poverty, 10*(1), 3-22.

Johnson, L., & Dorrington, R. (2001). *The impact of AIDS on orphanhood in South Africa: A quantitative analysis*. Capetown, South Africa: Centre for Actuarial Research, University of Cape Town.

Meier, E. (2003). The growth of AIDS orphans and policy solutions. *Pediatric Nursing, 29*(1), 75-76.

Ntozi, J. P. M. (1997). Effect of AIDS on children: The problem of orphans in Uganda. *Health Transition Review, 7*(Suppl.), 23-40.

Preble, E. A. (1990). Impact of HIV/AIDS on African children. *Social Science & Medicine, 31*(6), 671-680.

Sengendo, J., & Nambi, J. (1997). The psychological effect of orphanhood: A study of orphans in Rakai District. *Health Transition Review, 7*(Suppl.), 105-124.

UAC. (2001). *Twenty years of HIV/AIDS in the world: Evolution of the epidemic and response in Uganda*. Kampala: Author.

UAC. (2002). *HIV/AIDS in Uganda: The epidemic and the response*. Kampala: Uganda Author.

UNAIDS/UNICEF/USAID. (2004). *Children on the brink 2004: A joint report of new orphan estimates and a framework for action*. Washington DC: USAID.

UNAIDS/WHO. (2004). *Epidemiological fact sheets on HIV/AIDS and sexually transmitted infections: 2004 update*. Geneva, Switzerland: Authors.

UNICEF. (1999). *Children orphaned by AIDS: Front-line responses from Eastern and Southern Africa*. New York: Author.

UNICEF. (2003a). *Africa's orphaned generation*. New York: Authors.

UNICEF. (2003b). *Children orphaned by AIDS in Sub-Saharan Africa*. New York: Authors.

Varga, C. A. (1997). Sexual decision-making and negotiation in the midst of AIDS: Youth in KwaZulu-Natal, South Africa. *Health Transition Review,* 7(3), 45–67.

ABOUT THE AUTHORS

Delius Asiimwe is a senior research fellow at the Makerere Institute of Social Research (MISR), Makerere University. He holds a master's degree in development studies and a postgraduate diploma in conflict resolution. For the past 14 years he has been at the MISR and has done considerable work and published in the area of public policy analysis and development mainly in health systems and financing. He has also been involved in a number of HIV/AIDS and sexual and reproductive health action-oriented research studies. These include a study titled, "Focus Group Discussions on Social Cultural Factors Impacting HIV/AIDS in Uganda, 2003" funded by UNDP and the "5th Country Program Baseline Survey Report, 2001," funded by the government of Uganda and UNFPA. His recent work focuses on the integration of family planning into voluntary counseling and testing (VCT), prevention of mother-to-child transmission (PMTCT), and antiretroviral therapy (ART) training services. Asiimwe is an editor of a forthcoming book titled *Decentralisation and Transformation of Governance in Uganda*.

Beatrice Bainomugisha is a counseling psychologist who specializes in child and adolescent counseling. She has been involved in HIV/AIDS mitigation activities as a counselor and program coordinator at the Family Planning Association of Uganda (FPAU) and School Environment Program Manager for the Straight Talk Foundation (STF). She has written and coordinated successful proposals, including a youth center in war-torn Gulu District in Uganda, a care and support project to cater for the HIV/AIDS-affected and infected youth involved in transient trades. As a member of the Uganda Reproductive Health Advocacy Network, Bainomugisha has trained adolescents, teachers, parents, religious leaders, service providers, and civil organization members on adolescent and social reproductive health, parenting, peer education, and counseling, adolescent friendly services, and life planning skills.

John M. Collins is a doctoral student in a joint degree program in Educational Theory and Policy and Comparative and International Education at Penn State University. Collins has a master of education from Brigham Young University (BYU) in Comparative and International Development Education. His current research includes the examination of education attainment inequality in Vietnam, Cambodia, and China and is particularly interested in education inequality and issues of equity. Collins is currently working on a two-country comparative study between Senegal and Uganda looking at HIV/AIDS-related education programs and issues of equitable participation, efficiency, and organizational effectiveness.

Alex Godwin Coutinho holds a MD degree, master of public health, master of science, and a diploma in tropical medicine and hygiene. He has had extensive experience working with HIV/AIDS in Uganda and Sub-Saharan Africa since 1983. Coutinho was previously the vice-chair of the Global Fund Technical Review from 2002-2004. He was also a member of the Interim Board of the Global Fund to Fight AIDS, Tuberculosis and Malaria representing TASO in the establishment of the fund in Uganda. He sits on the AIDS Information Centre Board and the International Partnership for Microbicides Board of Directors. Coutinho has also been a member of the strategic advisory group to the World Health Organization for the HIV/AIDS global strategy and member of the Scientific Committee of the Academic Alliance for HIV/AIDS.

Lynn R. Curtis is vice president of International Programs for ProLiteracy Worldwide (formally Laubach Literacy) where for 23 years he has advanced participatory education and community action in Latin America, Asia, Africa, the Middle East, and the United States. Having pioneered the development of ProLiteracy's *FAMA* and *Literacy Solutions* training systems, Curtis currently directs ProLiteracy's efforts to initiate, strengthen, or expand *literacy-for-social-change* partnership programs in 56 countries throughout the world. An internationally acknowledged authority on global literacy and development practice, Curtis is author of the books *Literacy for Social Change* and *Perceptions of Community-Oriented Literacy Facilitators* as well as the literacy and action manuals, *Picturing Change, How To Start and Grow Your Own Business, Good Health Begins at Home, Parents are Teachers* and *Overcoming AIDS* (coauthor).

Julie M. Hite is an assistant professor in the Department of Educational Leadership and Foundations in the McKay School of Education at BYU. Her research interests center on organizational and strategic leadership in the context of education, with a specific focus on organizational and social networks in public, private and international educational organizations. She has published articles in *Strategic Management Journal*, *Strategic Organization*, *Journal of International Business Studies*, *Entrepreneurship Theory and Practice*, *International Journal of Educational Leadership* and *Bilingual Research Journal*.

Steven J. Hite is professor of educational research theory and methodology at BYU. His current research and service endeavors include the application of geographical information systems with educational management information systems in the national and regional education sectors of Africa and South Asia, and the exploration of HIV/AIDS education efforts in secondary schools in Africa. Professor Hite's main professional and personal goal is to facilitate the real-life integration and use of the full range of quantitative and qualitative educational research and evaluation systems to improve the quality, efficiency, effectiveness, and equality of educational opportunities for disadvantaged individuals, families, and communities in developing countries.

W. James Jacob is assistant director at the Center for International and Development Education (CIDE) at the University of California, Los Angeles where he also received his PhD in education. His primary scholarly focus is on the planning, development, and evaluation of international organizations and programs with geographic emphases in Sub-Saharan Africa, China, and the Pacific Rim. He has worked as a policy analyst and evaluator of HIV/AIDS education programs in Uganda from 2001 to 2005, where he was simultaneously the principal investigator of a Sub-Saharan African HIV/AIDS literacy education research program. He is currently directing a Global Higher Education Trends Analysis (GHETA) study on the influences of the market economy on postsecondary education institutions.

Betty Kagoro is a Ugandan, working as an editor with the Straight Talk Foundation. She holds a diploma in journalism from the Uganda Institute of Business and Media Studies in Kampala. Currently she is pursuing an bachelor of arts degree in communication science at the University of South Africa (UNISA), which she will complete in 2005. She practiced journalism from 1996 to the year 2000 at Uganda's leading daily, *The New Vision*, before getting employed as an editor at the Straight Talk

Foundation. She is married to Julius Barungi and is blessed with two kids, Jerry and Joanita.

Linda L. Kavuma holds a master's of science degree from the University of London. She has worked at Makerere University's Institute of Public Health and the Uganda Ministry of Health. She currently coordinates the Uganda Infectious Disease Institute's research program for HIV-discordant couples, which was spearheaded by the University of Washington. In addition to working on HIV/AIDS projects in Uganda, Kavuma has extensive experience working in Botswana, India, Namibia, and South Africa. Much of her research and work involve disadvantaged people infected or affected by the AIDS epidemic, including discordant couples, single spouse families, orphaned children, and other vulnerable children.

Richard Kibombo is a professional statistician and a researcher with the Makerere Institute of Social Research (MISR), Makerere University. He has a master of science degree in statistics from the University of Wisconsin and a bachelor of science in statistics from Makerere University. He has been involved in a number of government- and NGO-supported research initiatives in the areas of HIV/AIDS and adolescent sexual and reproductive health. These include, among others: sociocultural factors impacting HIV/AIDS, integration of family planning into HIV/AIDS services, and primary students' perceptions on sexual maturation.

Jeremy Liebowitz lives in Kampala, Uganda, where he works as an independent consultant. His recent projects include a paper on "Faith-Based Organizations and HIV/AIDS in Uganda and KwaZulu-Natal" for the Health Economics and HIV/AIDS Research Division at the University of KwaZulu-Natal. He has done extensive research on the role of religion in society and politics at the community level in Uganda, including his doctoral research on the role of the Anglican Church of Uganda in shaping political culture. In addition, he also works on democracy and governance issues, and is currently the coordinator for the "Strengthening Political Pluralism" program of the International Republican Institute-Uganda. He holds a Ph. from the University of Wisconsin-Madison in political science with a minor in African Studies.

Albert James Lutalo-Bosa is the vice chancellor at Kyambogo University, the primary teacher education university in Uganda. He received degrees from the University of London (BSc) and McGill University (MSc and PhD). He has taught biochemistry at Makerere University to medical veterinary and science students; his primary research areas include enzymology and lipoproteins. Prior to becoming the vice chancellor at Kyambogo

University, Lutalo-Bosa served as deputy vice chancellor of Makerere University (1989–1993); Principal of the Institute of Teacher Education at Kyambogo University (ITEK) (1993–2001).

Christopher B. Meek completed a PhD in indudtrial and labor relations from Cornell University in 1993. He is an associate professor of organizational in the Marriott School of Management at BYU, where he also served as the coordinator of the International Development Studies and Asian Business Programs for 7 years. His research interests include stratgies for successfully facilitating economic and social development with noe-Western societies particularly among indigenous North Americans and in Southern Africa. Meek has also been involved in studying and writing about the impact of national culture and particularly systems of kinship structure, collective patterns of group subsistence maintenance, and practices of ancestor worship rites and rituals on organizational structures, management systems, and labor-management relations in non-Western societies. His primary geographic regions of focus include Japan, Korea, South Africa, Indonesia, Thailand, Western North American Indian tribes, and with most major trade unions in the United States.

Donald Morisky is currently professor and chair of the Department of Community Health Sciences at the UCLA School of Public Health, where he has been for the past 23 years. He also is director of the Pre-Doctoral Training Program in the Social and Behavioral Determinants of HIV/AIDS. Prior to that he was on the faculty of the Johns Hopkins School of Public Health where he received his doctorate of science in health education and health behavior. His research addresses the social and behavioral determinants of HIV/AIDS prevention both domestically and globally. He has received numerous National Institutes of Health-funded research grants directed to the conceptualization, implementation, and evaluation of community-based intervention programs for HIV/AIDS prevention as well as tuberculosis control. He has conducted research in the Philippines for over 30 years, addressing global health issues as maternal and child health, family planning, prevention, and control of infectious diseases such as tuberculosis and HIV/AIDS.

Alex Mugume has a master's degree in social sector planning and management and a bachelor's degree of social work from Makerere University. He currently works for UPHOLD as an HIV/AIDS specialist. Mugume worked as a project officer, monitoring and evaluation officer, and projects and planning coordinator for TASO from 1996 until 2004. He has also worked as the district deputy chief administrative officer. His primary research interests have related to social support initiatives that empower youth, orphans and other vulnerable children, and care and support activities for youth through educational and practical skills training for their economic survival.

Rosemary M. Nabadda is a medical doctor holding a master's degree in International Public Health of the University of Sydney. She also holds a master of arts in development studies from Uganda Martyr's University, Nkozi, Uganda. Nabadda is working as the senior medical officer for health services at Kyambogo University, Kampala, Uganda. As coordinator of the Peer Education Program at Kyambogo University, Nabadda has worked closely with the Ministry of Education and Sports. Since 2002, Dr. Nabadda has been actively involved initiating community activities. She is advocating for a more holistic approach in addressing HIV/AIDS issues including streamlining HIV/AIDS in all functions of the university such as welfare of faculty, staff, and students, and in the areas of teaching and research. Her current area of interest focuses on reducing vulnerability to HIV/AIDS among students and educators in higher educational institutions.

Sande P. Ndimwibo holds a bachelor of arts degree in social sciences, a diploma in education, and a diploma in project planning and management from Makerere University. He is the executive director of Uganda Youth Anti-AIDS Association (UYAAS) and has worked with youth in the area of HIV/AIDS for the past 13 years. He simultaneously holds a number of other positions related to HIV/AIDS and youth in Uganda including chairman of the Uganda Association for the Promotion for Adolescent Health (UAPAH), which is a network of Uganda-based NGOs that work with young people on adolescent and reproductive health issues; project manager for MOES research projects examining best practices of HIV/AIDS in Uganda schools; and national chairman of the Uganda Reproductive Health Bureau (URHB). Ndimwibo has received multiple certificates in HIV/AIDS, reproductive health and life planning skills from international and Ugandan institutions. His research focuses on planning, monitoring, and evaluation of HIV/AIDS programs in Uganda.

Stephen F. Noll is the current vice chancellor, Uganda Christian University. The Rev. Prof. Stephen Noll was appointed in October 1999 to be the first Vice Chancellor (President) of Uganda Christian University, the first chartered private university in Uganda (2004). The university was founded by the Anglican Church of Uganda in 1997 on the site of Bishop Tucker Theological College in Mukono (founded in 1913). In Uganda, Noll has served as chairman of the vice chancellors' forum and been active in the formulation of higher education policy. Noll received the Bachelor of Arts degree from Cornell University, the master of arts degree from the Graduate Theological Union in Berkeley, and a PhD from the University of Manchester, England. He has been ordained in the Episcopal Church since 1971. Before coming to Uganda, Noll served for 21 years as professor of biblical studies and academic dean at Trinity Episcopal School for Ministry, in Ambridge, Pennsylvania. He is author of four books and numerous articles.

Yusuf K. Nsubuga holds a master's degree in education (planning and management) from Makerere University, where he also obtained bachelor of arts degree in economics and rural economy. He has also had postgraduate training at the University of East Anglia, Norwich (England) in planning for social and economic impact of HIV/AIDS in developing countries. Prior to joining the Uganda AIDS Commission and the National AIDS Control Program in 1994, Nsubuga served as a school administrator for 11 years. Along with some colleagues, Nsubuga established the Uganda Network on Law Ethics and HIV/AIDS and later became coordinator of the African Network on Law Ethics and HIV/AIDS. Nsubuga was appointed commissioner for secondary education a position he holds to date. He is also the HIV/AIDS coordinator for the entire education sector. As vice chairperson of the Uganda Network on Law Ethics and HIV/AIDS, Nsubuga coordinates a national body that is spearheading the legal and ethical response to HIV/AIDS. He sits on several national committees, including the Partnership Forum and the National Coordination Committee of the Global Fund to Fight AIDS, Tuberculosis and Malaria.

Robert Ochai has a master's degree in social sector planning and management and a bachelor of arts in social work and social administration from Makerere University. He has had an extensive career at TASO. Robert started off as a manager of one of the TASO branches and is currently the deputy executive director in charge of program management. His roles include providing oversight in the implementation of all TASO programs. Prior to working with TASO, he served as a project coordinator in a youth center where he worked closely with children and youth. These experiences have increased his interest and engagement in the areas of children in the face of HIV/AIDS in Uganda.

Acou Sam Ogojoi was a senior probation and welfare officer working with the Ministry of Gender, Labour and Social Development in Uganda. The late Ogojoi served as the national coordinator for the Promotion of Children and Youth Project. He held a bachelor of arts in social sciences and a master of arts in youth and community studies. He had a long experience working with street children in Uganda. He was responsible for spearheading the Model for the Removal, Rehabilitation, and Reintegration of Street Children in Uganda, which has seen over 2,000 children reunited with their families in the last 3 years. He has attended and presented papers in international conferences on a wide range of issues related to vulnerable children in Uganda. He has also coauthorized publications and notable among these is "Practice Guidelines for Work with Street Children in Uganda" which has contributed to the better practice in towns, municipalities, and divisions in Uganda in addressing the challenges of street children. Acou Sam Ogojoi died in August of 2005.

Terrance D. Olson earned a PhD in marriage and family living from Florida State University in 1973. He is a professor in the school of family life at BYU. He taught at the University of New Mexico from 1971–1974. As the principal investigator on grants from the U.S. Department of Health and Human Services from 1981–1987, he addressed problems associated with adolescent pregnancy. From 2000–2003, he assisted with a grant to the National Council for Adoption. Olson focuses on how the philosophies of science inform intervention practices. His work on moral agency, drawing on the work of Levinas and Warner, is applied to issues of adolescent sexuality, AIDS, adoption, marital interaction, parenting, the moral dimension of short story and film writing, and family life education. He studies the intersection of social science and religion. He has served as a department chair and as an associate dean of the College of Family, Home, and Social Sciences.

W. Joshua Rew is pursuing a doctoral degree in international education in the Department of Educational Leadership and Policy Studies at Florida State University. His current interests include the examination of education attainment inequality in Viet Nam and postapartheid South Africa, school effectiveness and student performance in Uganda, and the role of geographic information systems as tools for education policy analysis.

Troy D. Smith is a research associate for CRA International where he is involved in work on economic litigation. He has previously been affiliated with the Foundation for International Community Assistance (FINCA), where he evaluated the impact of FINCA's national microfinance programs in Uganda and Zambia. He has also conducted a comparative study of comprehensive higher education institutions in East Africa. His research interests are in the areas of economic development, microfinance, equity, program evaluation, policy, and the human rights of street children and AIDS orphans. His regional emphasis is on Africa and the African Diaspora.

Catharine Watson studied biology at Princeton University and then trained as a nurse in the England. She has lived in Uganda since 1986, working first as a foreign correspondent. In 1993 she started *Straight Talk* newspaper. In 1997, she and Anne Akia Fiedler turned *Straight Talk* into an NGO, Straight Talk Foundation (STF). Since then STF has evolved into a fully fledged communications not-for-profit organization with a staff of 60 of which Watson is joint director. Watson has managed the development of many more social change newspapers, including *Young Talk*, *Parent Talk*, *Teacher Talk*, *Tree Talk*, *Farm Talk* as well as radio shows and newspapers in nine languages.

Richard G. Wilkins is the managing director and founder of the World Family Policy Center at BYU. He is a professor of law at the J. Reuben Clark Law School in Provo, Utah, and has written numerous articles on constitutional law, international law, family policy, federal jurisdiction, and legal advocacy. Wilkins conducts an annual survey of U.S. Supreme Court voting trends published in the *Hastings Constitutional Law Quarterly*. He is a former assistant to the solicitor general, U.S. Department of Justice. Recently, he was invited to work with an advisory committee analyzing the newly adopted constitution for the European Union. He has participated in numerous international negotiations dealing with emerging issues in international human rights. He has testified before legislative bodies in the United States, Australia, Sweden, and the European Union.

INDEX